Mechanisms and Machine Science 133

This book series establishes a well-defined forum for monographs, edited Books, and proceedings on mechanical engineering with particular emphasis on MMS (Mechanism and Machine Science). The final goal is the publication of research that shows the development of mechanical engineering and particularly MMS in all technical aspects, even in very recent assessments. Published works share an approach by which technical details and formulation are discussed, and discuss modern formalisms with the aim to circulate research and technical achievements for use in professional, research, academic, and teaching activities.

This technical approach is an essential characteristic of the series. By discussing technical details and formulations in terms of modern formalisms, the possibility is created not only to show technical developments but also to explain achievements for technical teaching and research activity today and for the future.

The book series is intended to collect technical views on developments of the broad field of MMS in a unique frame that can be seen in its totality as an Encyclopaedia of MMS but with the additional purpose of archiving and teaching MMS achievements. Therefore, the book series will be of use not only for researchers and teachers in Mechanical Engineering but also for professionals and students for their formation and future work.

The series is promoted under the auspices of International Federation for the Promotion of Mechanism and Machine Science (IFToMM).

Prospective authors and editors can contact Mr. Pierpaolo Riva (publishing editor, Springer) at: pierpaolo.riva@springer.com

Indexed by SCOPUS and Google Scholar.

Daniela Tarnita · Nicolae Dumitru · Doina Pisla ·
Giuseppe Carbone · Ionut Geonea
Editors

New Trends in Medical and Service Robotics

MESROB 2023

Springer

Editors
Daniela Tarnita
University of Craiova, Applied Mechanics
Craiova, Romania

Nicolae Dumitru
University of Craiova, Applied Mechanics
Craiova, Romania

Doina Pisla
Technical University of Cluj-Napoca, CESTER
Cluj-Napoca, Romania

Giuseppe Carbone
University of Calabria, DIMEG
Rende, Italy

Ionut Geonea
University of Craiova, Applied Mechanics
Craiova, Romania

ISSN 2211-0984 ISSN 2211-0992 (electronic)
Mechanisms and Machine Science
ISBN 978-3-031-32445-1 ISBN 978-3-031-32446-8 (eBook)
https://doi.org/10.1007/978-3-031-32446-8

This Springer imprint is published by the registered company Springer Nature Switzerland AG
The registered company address is: Gewerbestrasse 11, 6330 Cham, Switzerland

Preface

From the point of view of research and applications, medical and service robotics are enjoying a growing interest, at the same time as the obvious growth of the market.

The eighth edition of the International Workshop on New Trends in Medical and Service Robots (MESROB 2023) was organized by the University of Craiova, Romania, from June 7 to 10, 2023, under the patronage of IFToMM - International Federation for the Promotion of Mechanism and Machine Science. MESROB is one of the main conferences for the IFToMM Technical Committees on Biomechanical.

The aim of the MESROB Workshop is to provide an international platform for researchers, engineers and PhD students involved in the general field of medical and service robotics, to exchange the latest research results and exchange views on future research directions in these areas.

Since the first symposium, in 2012 in Cluj-Napoca, Romania, MESROB has attracted eminent experts and provided a forum for researchers working in the field of medical and service robots. Continuing with the editions: MESROB 2013 in Belgrade, Serbia, MESROB 2014 in Lausanne, Switzerland, MESROB 2015 in Nantes, France, MESROB 2016 in Innsbruck and Graz, Austria, MESROB 2018 in Cassino, Italy, and MESROB 2020 and 2021 in Basel, Switzerland, the Workshop continued to grow in terms of number of participants and scientific impact.

A collection of 42 papers that were selected based on a peer-review process, with authors from Europe, North America, Asia, covers a wide range of highly modern interdisciplinary research topics such as: 1) Surgical robotics, 2) Design of medical devices, 3) Exoskeletons and prostheses, 4) Biomechanics, 5) Kinematics and dynamics of medical robotics, 6) Anthropomorphic hands.

We wish to express our gratitude to the authors, the reviewers, and Scientific Committee for their valuable contribution to ensure the scientific quality of MESROB 2023.

Finally, we would like to thank Ministry of Education and Dolj County Council for the financial support of this important scientific event.

Daniela Tarnita
Nicolae Dumitru
Doina Pisla
Giuseppe Carbone
Ionut Geonea

Organization

General Chair

Daniela Tarnita	University of Craiova, Craiova, Romania

Co-chairs

Doina Pisla	Technical University of Cluj-Napoca, Cluj-Napoca, Romania
Nicolae Dumitru	University of Craiova, Craiova, Romania
Giuseppe Carbone	University of Calabria, DIMEG, Rende, CS, Italy
Georg Rauter	University of Basel, Switzerland

International Scientific Committee

Bernard Bayle	University of Strasbourg, France
Hannes Bleuler	EPFL, Switzerland
Branislav Borovac	University of Novi Sad, Serbia
Mohamed Bouri	EPFL, Switzerland
Giuseppe Carbone	University of Calabria, Italy
Philippe Cattin	University of Basel, Switzerland
Marco Ceccarelli	University of Rome Tor Vergata, Italy
Christine Chevallereau	CNRS, France
Gery Colombo	IISART, Switzerland
Carlo Ferraresi	Technical University of Turin, Italy
Paolo Fiorini	University of Verona, Italy
Niklaus Friederich	University of Basel, Switzerland
Nicolas Gerig	University of Basel, Switzerland
Irini Giannopulu	UNSW-RCIT, France
Michael Hofbaur	Joanneum Research, Austria
Manfred Husty	University Innsbruck, Austria
Yeongmi Kim	Management Center Innsbruck, Austria
Med Amine Laribi	University of Poitiers, France
Juana Mayo	University of Seville, Spain
Jean-Pierre Merlet	Inria, France
Vesna Novak	University of Wyoming, USA

Doina Pisla	TU of Cluj-Napoca, Romania
Annika Raatz	Leibniz University, Hannover, Germany
Georg Rauter	University of Basel, Switzerland
Aleksandar Rodić	Mihajlo Pupin Institute, University of Belgrade, Serbia
Daniela Tarnita	University of Craiova, Romania
Philippe Wenger	CNRS, France
Akio Yamamoto	University of Tokyo, Japan
Azhar Zam	University of Basel, Switzerland
Teresa Zielinska	Warsaw University, Poland

Awards Committee

Giuseppe Carbone
Med Amine Laribi
Daniela Tarnita

Local Organizing Committee

Daniela Tarnita
Nicolae Dumitru
Ilie Dumitru
Ionuț Geonea
Cristian Copiluși
Lucian Gruionu
Adrian Roșca
Călin Vaida
Gabriela Marinache

Contents

Anthropomorphic Hands

Surgical Robotics

Soft Robot Assistance for Tumor Biopsy and Ablation in Magnetic Resonance Imaging

Kira Schlockermann[1], Jan Peters[1(✉)], Bennet Hensen[2], J. Joaquin Löning C.[2], Frank Wacker[2], and Annika Raatz[1]

[1] Institute of Assembly Technology, University of Hannover, Hannover, Germany
peters@match.uni-hannover.de

[2] Institute of Diagnostic and Interventional Radiology, Hannover Medical School, Hannover, Germany
https://www.match.uni-hannover.de

Abstract. This work presents a soft robotic system that supports interventionalists in tumor diagnostics through biopsy and ablation in the magnetic resonance imaging (MRI) environment. The system is designed to indicate the location of the puncture, assist in holding the biopsy and ablation needles, and support the fine adjustment of the puncture angle. The robot consists of a six-chamber soft actuator that can be extended with additional actuators or end effectors using a connector system. Two end effector designs are presented, a needle holder, and a system for indicating and, if necessary, marking the puncture site. The soft robot components are prototyped and characterized in an experimental set-up regarding the bending capabilities and evaluated with the help of an experienced interventionalist. A minimum bending angle of 23.51° was achieved, which satisfies the predefined requirements.

Keywords: soft robotics · interventional radiology · tumor ablation

1 Introduction

Percutaneous tumor ablation is a promising option for treatment of malignant tumors of the liver in patients unable to undergo transplantation or surgical resection. For the treatment, an antenna is inserted directly into the tumor, which is then locally heated and destroyed by using microwaves. The procedure takes place with the help of imaging systems such as computer tomography or magnetic resonance imaging [1–3]. The lower ionizing radiation level, good spatial and temporal resolution, but above all, the ability to construct in-vivo temperature mapping make MRI-guidance an ideal tool for minimal invasive interventions [4]. Additionally, MRI provides dynamic procedural guidance through real-time imaging. However, in close bore magnets a relevant drawback for performing interventions in MRI is the limited range of motion for the interventionalist and the resulting difficulty in performing the procedure inside the MRI bore. As a result, there is continued research interest in robotic solutions

D. Tarnita et al. (Eds.): MESROB 2023, MMS 133, pp. 3–12, 2023.
https://doi.org/10.1007/978-3-031-32446-8_1

to assist or automate the medical procedure. Most of the following concepts use computed tomography (CT) scans rather than the MRI. This includes the Needle Positioning System (NPS) from DEMCON Advanced Mechatronics as well as the robotic surgical assistance Guidoo [5,6]. DEMCON's NPS is a system for image-guided percutaneous needle placement using CT. The system is used for thoracic and abdominal applications and consists of a robotic arm with two degrees of freedom (DOF) and a reusable end effector with a ball joint (3 DOF) [5,6]. Guidoo is a robotic assistance system designed to increase the speed as well as the reliability of percutaneous biopsy. The system uses of a robotic arm that can guide a biopsy needle to the puncture site after prior planning. The robot holds the position and the medical staff can insert the needle into the target site [7]. However, these systems are designed for CT imaging and are not MRI compatible. One example for a MRI-compatible system is the INNOMOTION Robot by Melzer et al. This system is designed to support percutaneous needle placement [8]. The main drawback are the large dimensions of the system in the limited space of the MRI-bore. In contrast, two alternative systems have established themselves on the market: The Micromate from ISYS Medizintechnik GmbH with seven DOF is universally applicable for different ablations as well as the Remote Controlled Manipulator (RCM) from Soteria Medical BV (5 DOF) for the use on the prostate [9,10]. The main drawback of the Micromate system is the electric motor, which makes this system unsuitable for real time MRI interventions. The RCM from Soteria Medical BV can be used in MRI but is limited to the use for prostate biopsies.

Further examples are the Sunram 5 a MRI robot for breast biopsy, and the Interreg Project SPIRITS (Smart Printed Interactive Robots for Interventional Therapy and Surgery). Both robots are mostly made from 3D printed MRI compatible materials. The robot of the SPIRITS project can be controlled with the help of a hydraulic control system. The ablation applicator can perform rotational as well as translatory movements autonomously [11–13]. The Sunram 5 can also move the needle autonomously using a stepper motor system. An interesting feature of this approach is the integrated safety ejection mechanism that can pull the needle out of the body within 0.31 s [12]. Another advanced research project that is focusing on breast cancer diagnosis is the MURAB project (MRI and Ultrasound Robotic Assisted Biopsy). The robotic approach combines MRI and ultrasound imaging to leverage the advantages of the two imaging processes. A commercial available Kuka MED robot is used to autonomously approach the target area after planning the path with the MRI. An end effector (3 DOF) with an ultrasound probe and needle holder assists the treating interventionalist [14].

While each of the mentioned MRI compatible robots represent an innovative solution for their respective use case, there is room and the need for further development and optimizations. On the one hand, the working space is limited in many systems, due to the non-variable length of the robot as well as the missing flexibility in the mounting system. On the other hand, the respiratory motion of the patient remains an unsolved problem, which is why these systems cannot be used in areas of large respiratory motion [15].

The proposed system developed here addresses the mentioned challenges of existing systems and offers both a variable robot length and secure positioning even during respiratory motions. In addition, this new concept should also reduce the workload for the treating interventionalist and increase the safety while reducing the intervention time. Our proposed system leverages multiple core advantages that are inherent for soft robots. This includes the material (silicone) that enables MRI compatibility as well as the softness of the robotic systems. This is not only safe with respect to the patient but also for the interventionalist. In addition, actuators of different sizes can be easily and inexpensively manufactured and combined. Our soft robotic approach is developed for indicating and, if necessary, marking the puncture site as well as securely holding the medical puncture needle in place.

Section 2 explains the concept and methods that were used for manufacturing the soft robot, the supporting structures and applicators. The experimental protocol describes the experiments that were carried out to characterize and validate the proposed soft robotic assistance system (Sect. 3). The results of the respecting experiments are summarized in Sect. 4 followed by the discussion in Sect. 5.

2 Concept and Methods

The soft robotic assistance system must meet task-specific requirements that are defined in Sect. 2.1. Section 2.2 describes the procedure of the intervention using the proposed system. The individual parts are developed and prototypically implemented in this work (Sect. 2.3). The overall concept is shown in Fig. 1.

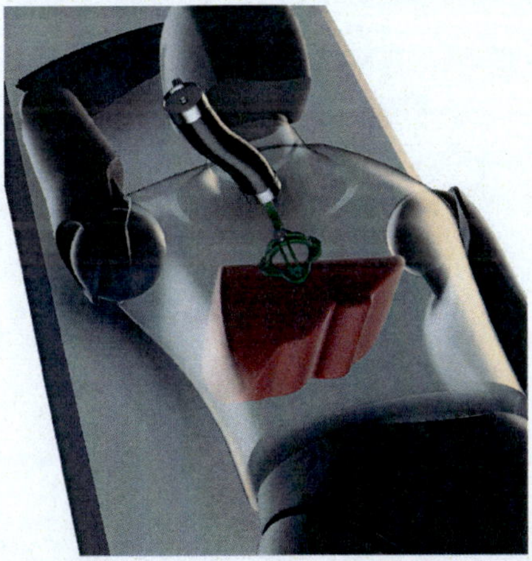

Fig. 1. Soft robot assistance system for percutaneous tumor biopsy and ablation. The robot is mounted directly in the MRI bore with an easy-to-use connector system which allows for flexible positioning. The variable robot length helps to adapt for body dimensions.

2.1 Requirements for Percutaneous Interventions Using the Assistance System in MRI

A robot for MRI ablation applications must meet the ASTM F2503-13 (renewed to ASTM F2503-20) compatibility standard as well as not cause electromagnetic interference in the MRI [16]. Therefore, during the characterization phase, measurements were taken in the MRI with the prototypes through a gradient echo and a spectrum measurement. Since there are different MRI sizes, the requirement for an MRI bore with a 70 cm radius was adapted for the time being. However, one of the main advantages of our proposed system is in contrast to the previous mentioned examples, that the soft robot has a modular design so that it can be lengthened or shortened. Thus, the robot can be flexibly adapted to different MRI sizes and areas of application.

2.2 Procedure of the Medical Intervention with the Assistance System

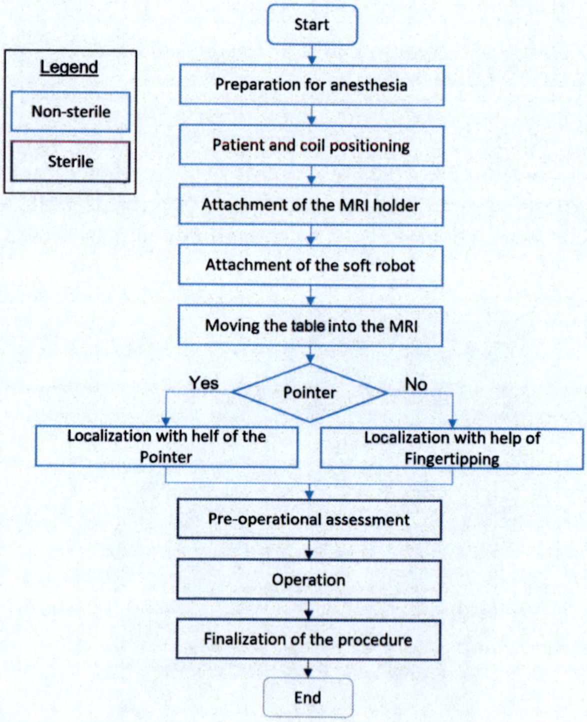

Fig. 2. Procedure of the medical intervention with the developed soft robotic system.

The procedure of the intervention with the assistance of the developed robotic system is shown in a simplified way in the flow chart (see Fig. 2). After the patient is prepared for anaesthesia and placed on the MRI patient table, the soft robot is mounted, at this point without the end effector. Before the procedure begins, the puncture is planned using real-time imaging of the MRI. Instead of the usual finger tipping, a manual process to find the puncturing location, the pointer system is used. The entire process takes place in a non-sterile room. The patient is then sterilely prepared for the tumor removal procedure. After the pre-operational assessment is done, the operation itself is performed by the interventionalist and the procedure is finalized afterwards.

2.3 Conceptual Design of the Robotic System

The development process was designed in accordance with the VDI guideline 2221 [18], and requirements that were set regarding the feedback of the interventionalists who are performing the medical process in their work. The overall system consists of the actuator, the connector as well as two end effector applicators. This includes the needle holder and the pointer system. The individual concepts are described below.

Concept of the Soft Actuator. The soft actuator used for the approach is inspired by Azadeh Shariati et al. [17] and was adapted for this project, due to the actuator dimensions and the good bending characteristics. The soft actuator manufactured from Ecoflex 00-50 consists of six fiber-reinforced pressure chambers. An additional channel is located in the centre. The tubes for the pneumatic connection are located on the side of the actuator to ensure the connection of the connector system. The dimensions and arrangements of the actuator used are illustrated in Fig. 3.

Concept of the Connector System. In order to connect the soft actuator reversibly to an end effector or further actuators, a modular connector concept was designed (see Fig. 4a). The two sides can be connected to each other using a rotary motion of male to female counterparts. Prototypically, these adapters are fixed with a polymer screw. In the further development, this is to be replaced by a quick-action clamping system. The actuators are glued onto the outer connector surfaces, whereby the walls have been designed for a better adhesion by an increased bonding surface area.

Concept of the Pointer (End Effector 1). Two end effectors were designed to support the procedure in the operating room (OR). The system for indicating the puncture location marks the position or indicates it with a laser system (Fig. 4b). This allows the interventionalist to visually inspect the subsequent puncture site. For this purpose, a system has been designed in which a marker or a laser pointer can be attached to the robot. The end effector connects to the soft actuator through the described connector system. In this way, the two concepts for marking the puncture site can easily be chosen within the procedure. If the puncture site is to be marked with a surgical skin pen, the system

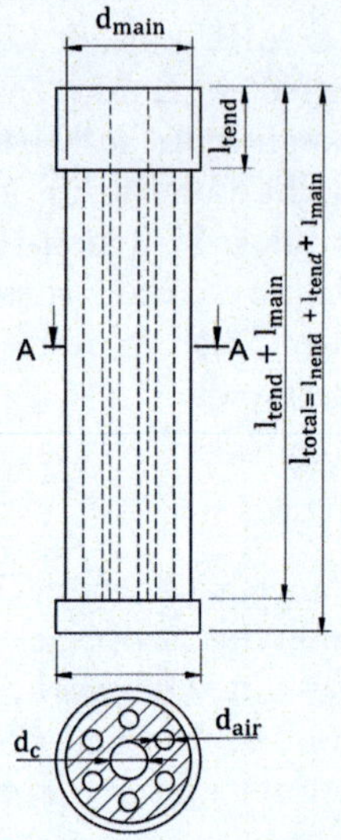

Geometry	Size	Unit
l_{total}	133	mm
l_{main}	105	mm
l_{tend}	20	mm
l_{nend}	8	mm
d_{end}	35	mm
d_{main}	30.4	mm
d_{air}	4.5	mm
d_c	9	mm
m	0.11	kg

Fig. 3. Actuator based on the model of Azadeh Shariati et al. [17]. The cap including the tubes (l_{tend}) is thicker than the other end (l_{nend}).

could also be replaced by a more advanced and automated solution by using a pneumatic marking end effector. In this case, a medical marker head located in a cylinder is pushed forward with the help of compressed air and the contracted by a spring. The advantage of this system compared with the manual holding system where the marker head always sticks out is that it prevents any possible accidental marking. The pneumatic system is only activated when the pointer reaches the target position. These proposed systems are meant for a future automation of the whole intervention process and would not be needed as long as the interventionalist is present during the planning process.

Concept of the Needle Holder (End Effector 2). The needle holder system is intended to support the interventionalist during diagnostics or ablation. The soft robot should be able to hold the needle in position and ensure simple needle alignment. The physician inserts the needle manually. The following system is inspired by the SeeStar (Apriomed). Two orthogonal axes each with a rail system, allow the needle to rotate freely around the injection site (Fig. 4c)). The axis system together with the needle holder can be fixed with a screw. The needle is inserted into the end effector via the holder system. This end effector is also attached to the actuator using the above described connector system. The needle should be aligned according to the orientation predicted on the basis of previous planning. The soft manipulator moves to the target site and is attached to the patient's skin with a medical adhesive (applied to the flat bottom side of the end effector). In this way, accidental movement of the end effector is prevented. In addition, the patient's breathing movement is taken into account, by

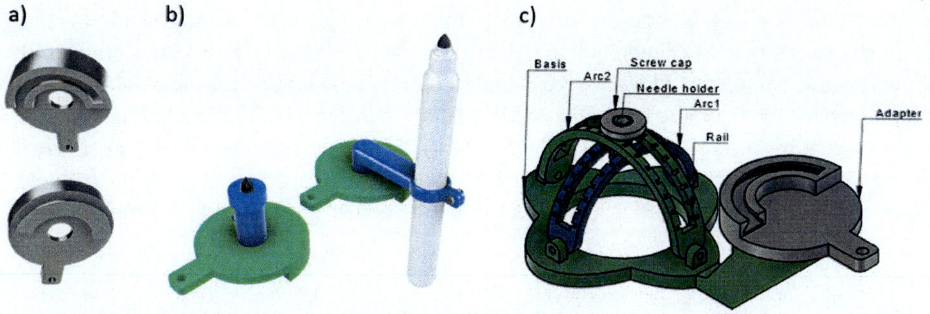

Fig. 4. a) Connector system including a male and female part. b) Hydraulic pointer system and manual pen or laser holding system with adapter connection. b) Designed needle holder system which allows the needle to rotate freely around the injection site.

attaching the end effector to the skin. The soft robot passively follows the movement, because of the robot's inherent compliance. By that, forces exterted to the patient are minimised. Attaching the end effector to the patient also has the advantage of compensating for the weight of the needle. After the attachment, the needle is inserted. As a future development, the system will calculate the needed angle based on the MRI data and the interventionalist can arrange the system accordingly, which would be a major advantage over the completely manual insertion of the needle. For easier handling, the axes are colored differently.

2.4 Sterility Concept

The soft robot must meet certain sterility standards to be used during surgery. The concept provides for the following: The actuator is covered with a sterile foil attached to the connector and the foil is fixed at the upper end. The needle holder end effector as well as the adapters, which are not covered by the foil, are supplied separately in sterile packaging and are initially to be seen as a single-use product. In the future, the end effector will be further developed so that it can be sterilized and used multiple times.

2.5 Fabrication of the Soft Robot

The actuator is manufactured with Ecoflex 00-50 silicone. For this purpose, the molds are printed using the fused deposition modeling (FDM) 3D printing process. First, the fiber reinforcement is prepared with sewing yarn. For this purpose, the yarn is tied around a three-part rod. Six of these rods for the air channels are fixed with another larger rod in a main mold and poured in with the silicone. After the silicone has cured and the outer rods have been removed, thinner rods are inserted to cast the inside of the fiber reinforcement as described in [17]. Once the silicone has cured and the thinner air duct rods are removed, the openings on one actuator side are covered with silicone. After that, tubes are glued at the other side 10 mm deep into each chamber. Once the glue has dried, the actuator is placed with the tube side in a mold. The tubes hang out sideways and the end is closed with silicone. Finally, the adapters are attached to the respective ends of the actuator with a silicone adhesive. The end effectors and adapters are manufactured using the FDM 3D printing process. The pointer and the adapters are printed from PLA (polylactide). The stereolithography process is used for the needle holder in order to achieve a higher precision and surface finish.

3 Characterization and Validation of the Soft Robotic Assistance System

3.1 Bending Characteristics of the Soft Robot

The characterization of the bending properties takes place in a test rig with six OptiTrack cameras. A Simulink interface is used to control the compressed air supply for the actuator system. Two air chambers of the actuator are actuated. The position and orientation of the end effector is tracked using infrared markers and the camera system. To characterize the soft actuator in terms of bending capabilities, the soft robot is attached to a fixture in the experimental setup (Fig. 5) so that the robot is oriented along the z-direction. A base with infrared markers is attached to the lower end of the actuator using the connector system. These markers are tracked with OptiTrack cameras and processed in Motive [19]. Two air chambers are then pressurized which leads to a bending motion in the x-z plane. The end effector moves in positive x-direction. To calculate the bending angle, the direction vector in z is calculated at the beginning (z_1) and at the end (z_{end}) using:

$$\alpha = arccos(\frac{z_1 \cdot z_{end}}{|z_1| \cdot |z_{end}|}) \tag{1}$$

The angle between the direction vectors is used as the bending angle.

4 Results of the Bending Characterization

Each measurement was performed three times with one actuator, two actuators attached to each other, and with one actuator and a rigid needle holder including a coaxial needle. The pressure ranged up to 60 kPA. An average angle of 24.75° (SD = 0.04°) was measured with one actuator. With a coaxial and diagnostic needle, the average bend decreased to 23.51° (SD = 0.18°). The two actuator system achieved 26.44° (SD = 0.94°).

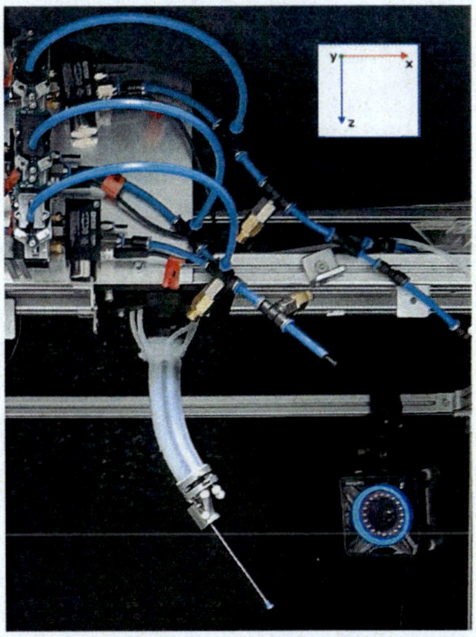

Fig. 5. Experimental setup with a soft robot with six integrated air channels and a rigid end effector to easily hold a medical needle (In this case a coaxial needle) for experimental purposes. Two pneumatic channels are actuated and allow bending in the x-z plane.

5 Discussion

The presented assistance system is a new approach to the field of MRI guided intervention. By attaching the end effector to the patient and using a soft robot, the system should not restrict the natural body movement due to its low stiffness but moves with the breathing movement. With our proposed system, the respiratory motion can be taken into account while maintaining the correct positioning of the needle. These advantages will be tested in the further course of the project. The assisting system is also characterized by the adaptability of the actuator due to a high DOF and the possibility of combining different actuators and thus varying the length. However, the overall bending for two actuators did not increase significantly. This is because of the additional weight of the second actuator. To mitigate this, future designs will incorporate a stiffening mechanism to help increasing the payload. In addition, the robot can be used to locate the puncture site. The system simplifies the procedure of the entire process for the interventionalist by eliminating the need for manual finger tipping and holding the needle in an unergonomic pose. The concepts presented here will be manufactured, optimized and tested under conditions that are similar to the real medical setup. In an ongoing effort to improve the system, the safety of the system must be tested extensively. Finally, while the system was developed in collaboration with the systems' end users, the entire soft robotic system must be tested in a medical environment by the medical staff. In a first step, the parts that are used in sterile environment must be adapted according to sterility standards.

References

1. Simon, C., Dupuy, D., Mayo-Smith, W.: Microwave ablation: principles and applications. Radiographics **25**, S69–S83 (2005)
2. Boss, A., Dupuy, D., Pereira, P.: Microwave ablation. In: Percutaneous Tumor Ablation in Medical Radiology, pp. 21–28 (2008)
3. Vogl, T.: Basic principles in oncology. In: Percutaneous Tumor Ablation in Medical Radiology, pp. 3–5 (2008)
4. Yang, N., et al.: Magnetic resonance imaging-guided microwave ablation of hepatic malignancies: feasibility, efficacy, safety, and follow-up. J. Cancer Res. Ther. **16**, 1151–1156 (2020)
5. Arnolli, M., Buijze, M., Franken, M., Jong, K., Brouwer, D., Broeders, I.: System for CT-guided needle placement in the thorax and abdomen: a design for clinical acceptability, applicability and usability. Int. J. Med. Robot. Comput. Assist. Surg. MRCAS (2018)
6. Heerink, W., et al.: Robotic versus freehand needle positioning in CT-guided ablation of liver tumors: a randomized controlled trial. Radiology **290**, 826–832 (2019)
7. Fraunhofer-Institut für Produktionstechnik, Guidoo (2022)
8. Melzer, A., et al.: Innomotion for percutaneous image-guided interventions: principles and evaluation of this MR- and CT-compatible robotic system. IEEE Eng. Med. Biol. Mag. **27**, 66–73 (2008)
9. Interventionals Systems GmbH Micromate: Tomorrow's medical robot today (2021)
10. Schouten, M., et al.: Evaluation of a robotic technique for transrectal MRI-guided prostate biopsies. Eur. Radiol. **22**, 476–483 (2012)
11. Fraunhofer-Institut für Produktionstechnik und Automatisierung IPA Medizinroboter aus dem Drucker - Fraunhofer IPA (2022)
12. Groenhuis, V., Siepel, F., Welleweerd, M., Veltman, J., Stramigioli, S.: Sunram 5: an MR safe robotic system for breast biopsy. In: The Hamlyn Symposium on Medical Robotics, pp. 85–86 (2018)
13. Fraunhofer-Institut für Produktionstechnik SPIRITS (2022)
14. Welleweerd, M.K., Siepel, F.J., Groenhuis, V., Veltman, J., Stramigioli, S.: Design of an end-effector for robot-assisted ultrasound-guided breast biopsies. Int. J. Comput. Assist. Radiol. Surg. **15**(4), 681–690 (2020). https://doi.org/10.1007/s11548-020-02122-1
15. Kägebein, U.: MRT-geführte Ablation mit Hilfe des optischen Moiré Phase Trackingsystems. (Universitäts- und Landesbibliothek Sachsen-Anhalt) (2018)
16. Naefe, P., Luderich, J.: Einführung. Konstruktionsmethodik Für Die Praxis, pp. 1–13 (2020)
17. Shariati, A., Shi, J., Spurgeon, S., Wurdemann, H.: Dynamic modelling and viscoelastic parameter identification of a fibre-reinforced soft fluidic elastomer manipulator. In: Proceedings of the 2021 IEEE/RSJ International Conference on Intelligent Robots and Systems (IROS 2021) (2021)
18. Design of technical products and systems Model of product design. (VDI 2221) Verein deutscher Ingenieure VDI Guidelines, pp. 1–4 (2019)
19. Wiese, M., Runge-Borchert, G., Cao, B.-H., Raatz, A.: Transfer learning for accurate modeling and control of soft actuators. In: 2021 IEEE 4th International Conference On Soft Robotics (RoboSoft), pp. 51–57 (2021)

Workspace-aware Planning of a Surgical Robot Mounting in Virtual Reality

Murali Karnam[1(✉)], Marek Zelechowski[2], Philippe C. Cattin[2], Georg Rauter[1], and Nicolas Gerig[1]

[1] BIROMED -Lab, Department of Biomedical Engineering, University of Basel, Allschwil 4123, Switzerland
murali.karnam@unibas.ch
[2] CIAN, Department of Biomedical Engineering, University of Basel, Allschwil 4123, Switzerland
https://biromed.dbe.unibas.ch

Abstract. When placing a redundant surgical robot in an operating room, the robot should be able to reach all desired trocar locations. At the same time, robots have a limited position and orientation reach that is not intuitive to take into account for a user while verifying the desired reachability. Therefore, identifying feasible mounting locations for a surgical robot in an operating room depends on required trocar locations, reachable workspace, and operating room constraints. In this work, we aimed to find feasible locations to fix a redundant surgical robot in an operating room. As an alternative to formulating this as a mathematical optimization problem, we provided an interactive planning tool in VR to visualize the robot and its workspace, and to allow identification of a suitable placement for the robot. As a proof-of-concept, we used our interactive VR planning tool to find a suitable placement for the robot, and design a fixture to mount the robot in the room.

Keywords: medical robots · robotics · design · VR

1 Introduction

Typically, surgical robots are moved into operating rooms on push carts. Subsequently, the personnel check if robots can reach the desired trocar locations on the patient. Although this provides flexibility, robots usually come in the way of medical personnel and other equipment in a crowded operating room. Furthermore, positioning and setting the robot takes considerable time depending on the surgery and has an opportunity for reduction [1]. In our project, we plan to fix the robot to an operating room ceiling, clearing up space for the medical personnel and easing the surgeon-robot interaction, and increasing the usable range of the robot workspace. We use a robot with large workspace to reach an operating table completely so that the robot can go to any pose on the patient. It would, for example, be useful in Maxillofacial surgeries where bone from the patient's tibia (an autograft) is harvested and placed in the same patient's jaw.

D. Tarnita et al. (Eds.): MESROB 2023, MMS 133, pp. 13–19, 2023.
https://doi.org/10.1007/978-3-031-32446-8_2

Planning the exact location of the robot's fixed structure in the room needs to consider the robot's workspace and the reach through the trocars on a patient with respect to an operating table. The requirements can be posed as constraints to an optimization problem to maximize the robot's reach on a patient and solve for a feasible or optimal robot placement. However, encoding some constraints and formulating their cost into a mathematical framework is not trivial. For example, a design with the robot structure parallel to a wall is easier and cheaper to manufacture and assemble compared to a rotated robot structure. Weighing such soft constraints as a cost during optimization is difficult, while these constraints are intuitive to understand or test by a user. As an alternative, we propose to use virtual reality (VR) to plan the robot fixture (Fig. 1).

Recently, many applications have used VR and augmented reality (AR) [2] solutions, including robot-assisted surgery (RAS) [3]. For example, AR was used to show optimal port positions on a patient [4] and aid the first assistant to the surgeon during a surgery [5]. For industrial applications, the robot workspace was visualized, and a user could add safety zones for path planning [6]. In this work, we visualized the robot's workspace to the user in different ways. The user could freely move the robot and inspect whether the robot's reach is satisfactory. The desired location of the {robot_root} would then be used as an input to design a mounting structure to fix the robot e.g. to the ceiling.

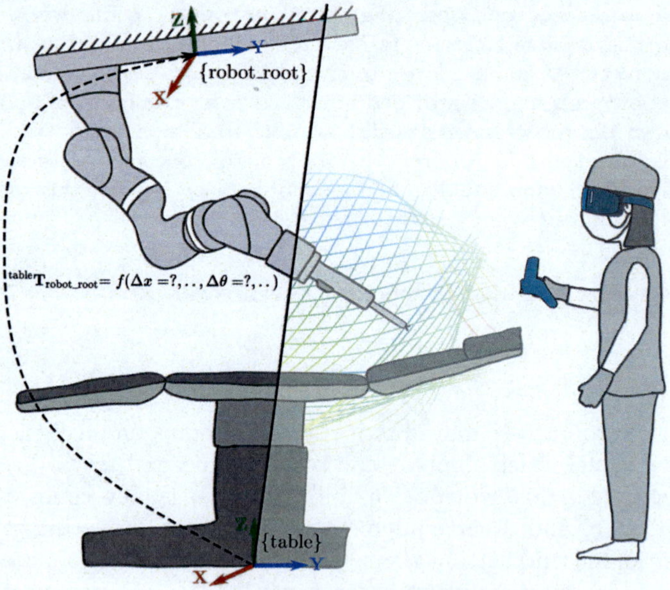

Fig. 1. Overview of the planning problem (left): The 6 degrees of freedom (DoF) transform between a fixed pose of the {robot_root} with respect to a fixed {table} must be found, such that the robot can reach most desired locations on a patient. The proposed solution (right): Equip the user with a VR headset that allows moving a virtual {robot_root} freely and inspecting the workspace (a representative mesh with a color map) to find suitable position and orientation parameters. The function f maps the translation and rotation (Euler angles) to a transformation matrix.

2 Materials and Methods

2.1 Apparatus

A virtual operating room was visualized with a Meta Quest 2 VR headset (Meta Platforms, USA). This virtual room included a surgical table and an 8-DoF redundant robot [7], consisting of a KUKA LBR iiwa (KUKA AG, Ausburg, Germany) extended with a linear axis with a motion range of 1.5 m at the base and a generic endoscopic tool at the tip. The ceiling in the room where we plan to mount the robot was at a height 3.5 m from the floor. Interaction with the virtual objects was realized with a handheld VR controller (Fig. 2). The operating table was height adjustable, but was fixed to 0.9 m (motion range center).

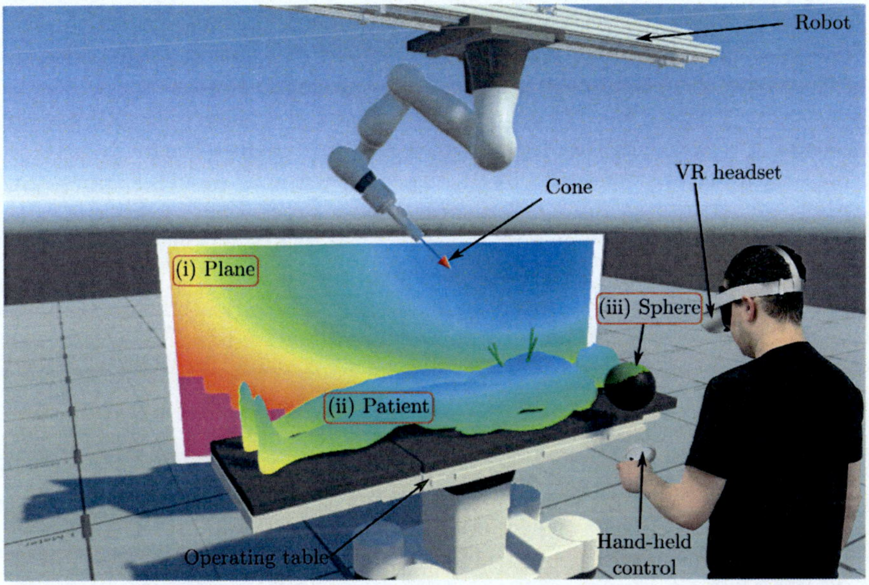

Fig. 2. Virtual operating room and user wearing a Meta Quest 2 VR headset while holding the hand-held controller to plan the {robot_root} location. The 5-DoF reachable workspace (position and pitch-yaw) of the robot was represented using simplified rotation heat-map textures on a movable plane (i) and patient (ii) with a texture representing heat-map of the simplified 1D rotation workspace, and a sphere (iii) that shows a green-colored surface for all possible orientations for which the endoscope tip can reach the center of the sphere. (Color figure online)

2.2 Workspace Calculation, Visualization, and Interaction

A discretized workspace of the 8-DoF robot was calculated by extending the forward kinematics approach for the 7-DoF robot that we presented in a previous work [8]. The workspace region of interest was divided into 5D voxels at a resolution of 0.1 m in position and 4° in orientation. Through an iterative process, the 5D reachability map of the robot with respect to the {robot_root} consisting of all the possible yaw and pitch angles at each position was recorded. This calculated workspace included the 3D position and 2D orientation (pitch and yaw of the tool) but is specific to the robot and tool design. This calculation of the workspace took approximately 6 h on a computer with Intel Xeon E5-2620 @ 2.4 GHz CPU and 64 GB RAM running 16 threads in parallel. It has to be noted that this a one time calculation for the robot and the same workspace can be calculated with a higher voxel resolution if necessary.

For a simplified workspace visualization, the 2D rotational workspace at each position was reduced to a single value between 0 and 1. This value represented the fraction of the achievable rotation over the maximum possible rotational workspace, calculated by covering a total surface area of a hemisphere. The workspace was visualized to the user in three different options similar to previous work [8] (Fig. 2): movable plane (i) and patient (ii). Unreachable endoscope tip positions were represented in magenta, while reachable rotational workspace was represented from red (little angular freedom to reach position) to blue (large angular freedom to reach position) along the rainbow color map. Complete 2D rotational workspace could be inspected with the movable sphere (iii). The sphere's surface was rendered in green for all directions, from which the endoscope could reach the center of the sphere, and in black for the remaining directions.

Virtual objects could be moved in 6 degrees of freedom by pointing the hand-held control at the virtual object and pressing a button to grasp them. The workspace could be inspected by grasping the moving plane, patient or sphere. Furthermore, the robot could be grasped to move the {robot_root}, and all the workspace visualizations were updated accordingly. In addition to the workspace, robot motion could also be inspected by moving the red cone to a desired pose. The inverse kinematics solution of the displayed robot to the desired cone pose was calculated on the same real-time computer that controls an equivalent, actual, physical robot [9] and communicated back to the VR in a work that was previously presented.

2.3 Evaluation

We evaluated our VR planning using the system ourselves as a qualitative proof-of-concept. The {robot_root} was moved to different poses to inspect the feasible workspace of the robot while keeping these additional design constraints and preferences in mind:

- The patient model should be entirely within the workspace limits.
- Fixed elements of the robot should be as far as possible from the patient.
- Having the linear axis parallel or at a right angle to the ceiling is preferable due to mounting cost and complexity.
- The physical room's ceiling space constraints must be respected. The mountings cannot interfere with the electrical, ventilation, and fire safety installations of the building.

For a selected {robot_root}, two metrics were calculated: {robot_root} pose with respect to {table}, and minimum safety distance between the lowest fixed structure of the robot and the highest point of the patient model. The minimum safety distance indicated the free space above the patient that would allow the surgeon to use other tools Based on the identified location of the robot root, a first draft for the ceiling mount was designed.

3 Results

We calculated the robot workspace and realized the planner as an interactive work tool. We successfully demonstrated usage by finding a feasible pose for the {robot_root}. A final robot root location with only a positional shift ($\Delta z = 2.0$ m) with respect to the {table} was found to be sufficient to cover the required workspace completely (Fig. 3 (top)). Based on a chosen operating table height of 0.9 m, the minimum safety distance between the robot structure and the patient for the given pose was 0.6 m (shown in Fig. 3). Based on the planned location, a representative mounting structure was designed to support the robot from the ceiling located at 3.5 m from the floor (Fig. 3 (bottom)).

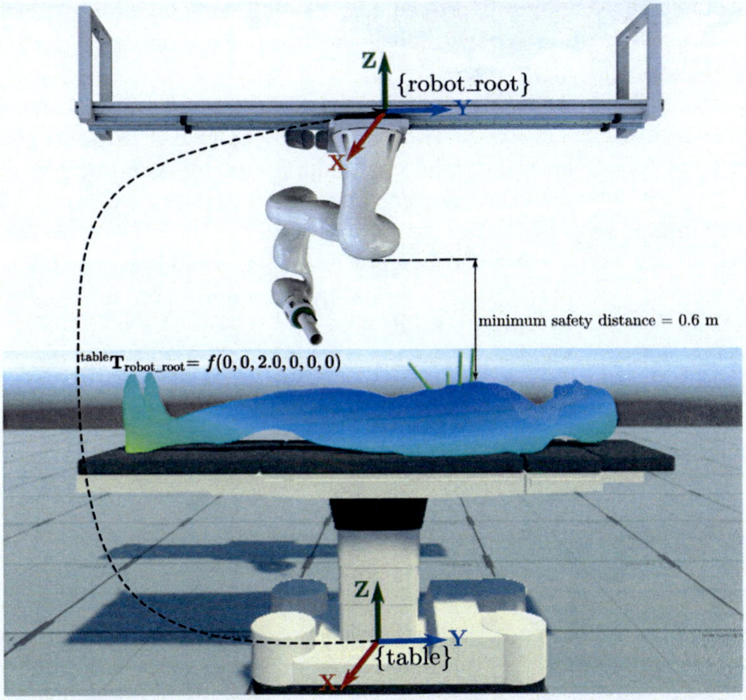

Fig. 3. CAD rendering of the robot mounted to the ceiling at the planned location (top) with respect to the operating table. Simplified 1D rotation workspace of the robot as a heat map on the patient (bottom).

4 Discussion

We observed that in our case, a feasible solution did not need {robot_root} to be rotated with respect to the ceiling (Fig. 3). It was also the initial and default rotation that was provided to the user. We found that the rotational workspace of the robot was higher in regions below the robot's center compared to the outer edges of the operating table. It implied that the robot can reach positions below the robot center with many different orientations. It was also the region with the minimum safety distance to the robot structure. The final resulting solution is to have the robot base exactly above the operating table, at a height displacement of 2.0 m, with an approximate safe distance from the patient of 0.6 m.

Once the robot is fixed, patient positioning can further be optimized to ensure that the robot can reach the desired poses, as suggested in our previous work [8]. Our method also has the potential to solve the equivalent problem of positioning a robot on a cart near the operating table, which seems more prevalent in certified surgical robot setups.

The workspace was visualized only for one generic tool. Therefore, the reachable workspace would differ based on the exact tool dimensions. We plan to include multiple tools and calculate the workspaces for each of them in the future. In this first approach, we are yet to consider the capabilities or limits of an adjustable OR table. However, the current implementation already allows the user to inspect the OR table range by moving the plan or patient model accordingly.

For the single fixed mounting that was realized as a proof-of-concept, an optimization-based approach could have also been realized. Positioning a cart-mounted surgical robot is a non-trivial challenge for many different procedures. However, OR lamps or any other device would not limit our approach. In the contrary, the simple usage of our system would indicate its advantages over any other approach that we have seen so far. For example, we did not consider other equipment in the operating room, such as the lamps, monitoring devices that are also attached to the ceiling through multi-segmented passive arms. We consider the effort of the mathematical formulation of optimization goals and constraints for each specific procedure and operating room as not feasible. Often, only the clinicians know their preferences and constraints, so an intuitive interactive tool for them is needed.

5 Conclusion

We used VR to intuitively visualize a robot's workspace and assist a user to plan robot placement in an operating room. In future, we want to allow surgeons to interact with a virtual operating room and test if the tool can reach all required poses during surgery.

Acknowledgements. We gratefully acknowledge funding by the Werner Siemens Foundation through the MIRACLE project, and we thank Prof. Dr. med. Niklaus F. Friederich and Prof. Dr. med Michael Hirschmann for their continuous support to medical questions. We also thank Balázs Faludi and Norbert Zentai for their support with VR software development.

References

1. Kozminski, D.J., Cerf, M.J., Feustel, P.J., Kogan, B.A.: Robot set-up time in urologic surgery: an opportunity for quality improvement. J. Robot. Surg. **14**(5), 745–752 (2020). https://doi.org/10.1007/s11701-020-01049-8
2. Suzuki, R., Karim, A., Xia, T., Hedayati, H., Marquardt, N.: Augmented reality and robotics: a survey and taxonomy for AR-enhanced human-robot interaction and robotic interfaces. In: Proceedings of the 2022 CHI Conference on Human Factors in Computing Systems, CHI 2022. Association for Computing Machinery, New York, NY, USA (2022). https://doi.org/10.1145/3491102.3517719
3. Qian, L., Wu, J.Y., DiMaio, S.P., Navab, N., Kazanzides, P.: A review of augmented reality in robotic-assisted surgery. IEEE Trans. Med. Robot. Bionics **2**(1), 1–16 (2020). https://doi.org/10.1109/TMRB.2019.2957061
4. Weede, O., Wünscher, J., Kenngott, H., Müller-Stich, B.P., Wörn, H.: Knowledge-based planning of port positions for minimally invasive surgery. In: 2013 IEEE Conference on Cybernetics and Intelligent Systems (CIS), pp. 12–17 (2013). https://doi.org/10.1109/ICCIS.2013.6751571
5. Qian, L., Deguet, A., Wang, Z., Liu, Y.H., Kazanzides, P.: Augmented reality assisted instrument insertion and tool manipulation for the first assistant in robotic surgery. In: 2019 International Conference on Robotics and Automation (ICRA), pp. 5173–5179 (2019). https://doi.org/10.1109/ICRA.2019.8794263
6. Puljiz, D., Krebs, F., Bosing, F., Hein, B.: What the hololens maps is your workspace: fast mapping and set-up of robot cells via head mounted displays and augmented reality. In: 2020 IEEE/RSJ International Conference on Intelligent Robots and Systems (IROS), pp. 11445–11451 (2020). https://doi.org/10.1109/IROS45743.2020.9340879
7. Karnam, M., Cattin, P., Rauter, G., Gerig, N.: Comparing cascaded real-time controllers for an extended KUKA LBR iiwa robot during physical human-robot interaction. In: Siebte IFToMM D-A-CH Konferenz. Technische Universität Ilmenau (2021). https://doi.org/10.17185/duepublico/74060
8. Żelechowski, M., Karnam, M., Faludi, B., Gerig, N., Rauter, G., Cattin, P.C.: Patient positioning by visualising surgical robot rotational workspace in augmented reality. Computer Methods in Biomechanics and Biomedical Engineering: Imaging & Visualization, pp. 1–7 (2021). https://doi.org/10.1080/21681163.2021.2002192
9. Karnam, M., Zelechowski, M., Cattin, P.C., Rauter, G., Gerig, N.: Augmented reality for 6-DOF motion recording, preview, and execution to enable intuitive surgical robot control. Curr. Dir. Biomed. Eng. **8**(2), 225–228 (2022). https://doi.org/10.1515/cdbme-2022-1058

Structural Study of a Robotic System for Sils Surgery

Doina Pisla[1], Nicolae Crisan[2], Ionut Ulinici[1], Bogdan Gherman[1], Corina Radu[2], Paul Tucan[1], and Calin Vaida[1](✉)

[1] CESTER, Technical University of Cluj-Napoca, 400114 Cluj-Napoca, Romania
calin.vaida@mep.utcluj.ro
[2] "Iuliu Hatieganu" University of Medicine and Pharmacy, 400347 Cluj-Napoca, Romania

Abstract. The use of smart robot technologies is slowly eliminating the limitations of manual single incision laparoscopic surgery (SILS). In this paper, the authors present a parallel robotic structure designed for use in SILS surgery, the mechanical structure of the robotic device is presented and its motion capabilities relative to the surgical task. Furthermore, a FEM analysis of the components of the robotic structure that are most subjected to strain during operation was carried out, as to study the components capability of maintaining the structural integrity of the robotic system without being subjected to deformations that could impede the functioning of the robotic device.

Keywords: Robotic SILS · Parallel Robot · FEM

1 Introduction

Single incision laparoscopic surgery (SILS) is a further evolution of minimally invasive surgery (MIS) and differs from it by requiring a single incision into the patient's body through which the instrumentation for the surgical procedure is inserted. Though the procedure presents clear advantages [1] there are several complexities entailed by the procedure's characteristics, mainly difficulty in instrument manipulation and increased chance of collision between instruments and between instruments and the laparoscope/laparoscopic camera, considering the increased proximity of the instruments as all together with the camera are introduced and manipulated within the limitations of a singular incision. For this purpose, specialized instrumentation such as curved and flexible instruments have been developed for use in manual surgery. Furthermore, to increase the ease of the procedure and taking into account its risk, robotic systems have been implemented. These have been shown to reduce risks associated with SILS and the capacity to bypass instrument manipulation difficulties.

1.1 State of the Art in Robotic SILS

Robotic systems dedicated for use in single incision laparoscopic surgery can be classified based on end-effector configuration, in that regard there are:

D. Tarnita et al. (Eds.): MESROB 2023, MMS 133, pp. 20–31, 2023.
https://doi.org/10.1007/978-3-031-32446-8_3

1. **Systems with a single hyper-flexible end-effector for the instruments and camera**: Of these there is the da Vinci SP robotic system [2, 3].The instruments and cameras are contained within a tubular structure that is inserted through the incision, and such a construction removes the need for a conventional SILS port. The flexible instruments and laparoscopic camera of the SP system offer increased visibility and high dexterity when compared to classical SILS instruments though this comes at the cost of a reduced manipulation force for tissue handling, due to the structure of the instruments that presents multiple bends.
2. **Multi-arm independent robotic structures each arm guiding a single instrument:** Of these there is the Senhance robotic system [4, 5] which has three independent serial robotic arms, one for each instrument and another for the laparoscopic camera. This robotic device maintains the need for a conventional SILS port for the procedure, and while the triple-arm structure implies greater motion outside the surgical space, its configuration allows for increased forces and stability at the level of the end effector.
3. **Multi-arm robotic structures positioned on a single central platform/column:** Of these there is the SPORT robotic system [6, 7] which contains two articulated arms and two lighted cameras placed on a platform attached to an actuated column Other devices are also being developed for minimally invasive procedures and are the subject of research dedicated towards ensuring efficient surgical procedures with patient safety and ease of use in mind [8-13].

Following the introduction, Sect. 2 describes the inclusion of a robotic system into a SILS surgical procedure and details how the proposed robotic device can mechanically achieve the tasks pertaining to each step of the surgical procedure. Section 3 presents the robot assembly, and its mechanical subassemblies are studied detailing the role of each component in executing the motions at the level of the end-effector followed by Sect. 4 where FEM analyses of the more strained components in scenarios of interest are presented. In Sect. 5 the final ideas about the paper are presented.

2 Parallel Robotic System for SILS

2.1 Robotic Integration in Medical Procedure

The SILS robotic system proposed in this paper [13, 14] must be assimilated in the medical protocol pertaining to the respective procedure. In (Fig. 1.), where the steps of the medical procedure encompassing the medical (non-robotic tasks) and technical (robot related tasks) for each step are presented [15]. The medical procedure is divided into 6 separate steps. The first step "preplanning" has the purpose of ensuring that the parameters for the medical procedure and the integration of the robotic system are well defined. The second step "preparation" deals with preparing the patient and operative space for the procedure and readying the robotic device for the surgical task. This is followed by the "insertion" step in which the robotic device is used to introduce the instruments and camera within the operative space. The fourth step "positioning & orientation" ensures that the robotic system is prepared for safe and efficient instrument manipulation. The fifth step "Surgical task" refers to instrument manipulation while finalization aims to lead to the patient's safe removal from the surgery room and returning the robotic system to its initial state.

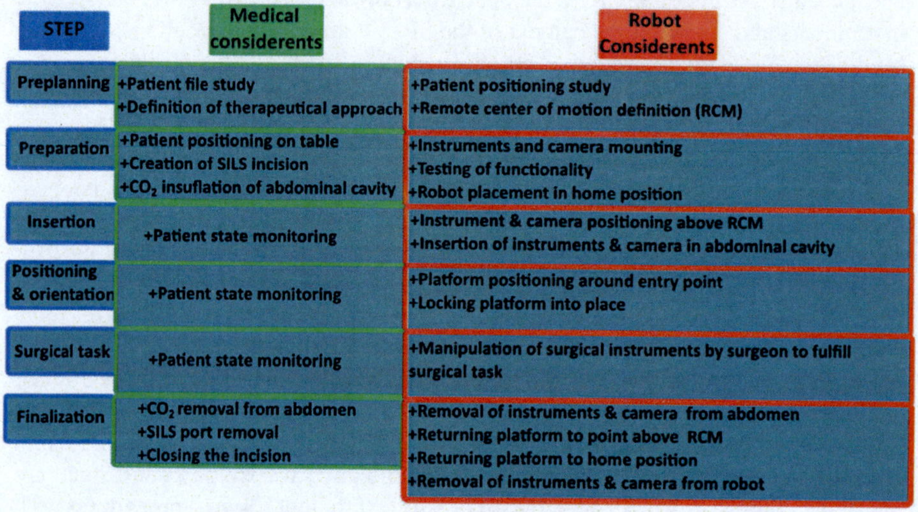

Fig. 1. Medical procedure with robot integration

2.2 The SILS Robot Platform Motions

In Fig. 2. The kinematic scheme used in the mechanism definition is overlayed on the robotic platform. With respect to the medical procedure steps illustrated in Sect. 2.1, the first robot action is represented by the definition of the remote center of motion. This is done taking into account the patients position on the table, the configuration of the SILS port inserted into the incision and the position of the point on the instrument platform (which in this stage represents the end-effector) that is used to define the tool center point of the end effector, taking into account the current construction of the platform and the configuration of the instruments and camera on the platform, is represented by the point at the tip of the laparoscopic camera mounted on the platform. That point is aligned with the entry into the incision, and it represents the remote center of motion for the camera and instrument assembly in Fig. 2 it is marked as the entry point and represents the RCM for the procedure. It is to be noted that the instruments themselves have independent RCM-s, which are defined relative to this point.

For the **preparation stage**, the instruments and camera are mounted and their functionality is tested after which the robot is brought into its homing position.The homing position represents a configuration in which the end-effector is placed as far away from the insertion point while also maintaining a orientation of the instrument platform perpendicular to the patient bed.To ensure homing, joints q5, q4, q3, q1, and q2 are actuated along their respective vertical axes in tandem, to maintain the laparoscope's tip colinear with the entry direction into the abdominal cavity (not moving the joints in tandem and maintaining set distances between them, in the vertical plane can result in the tilting of the instrument platform).

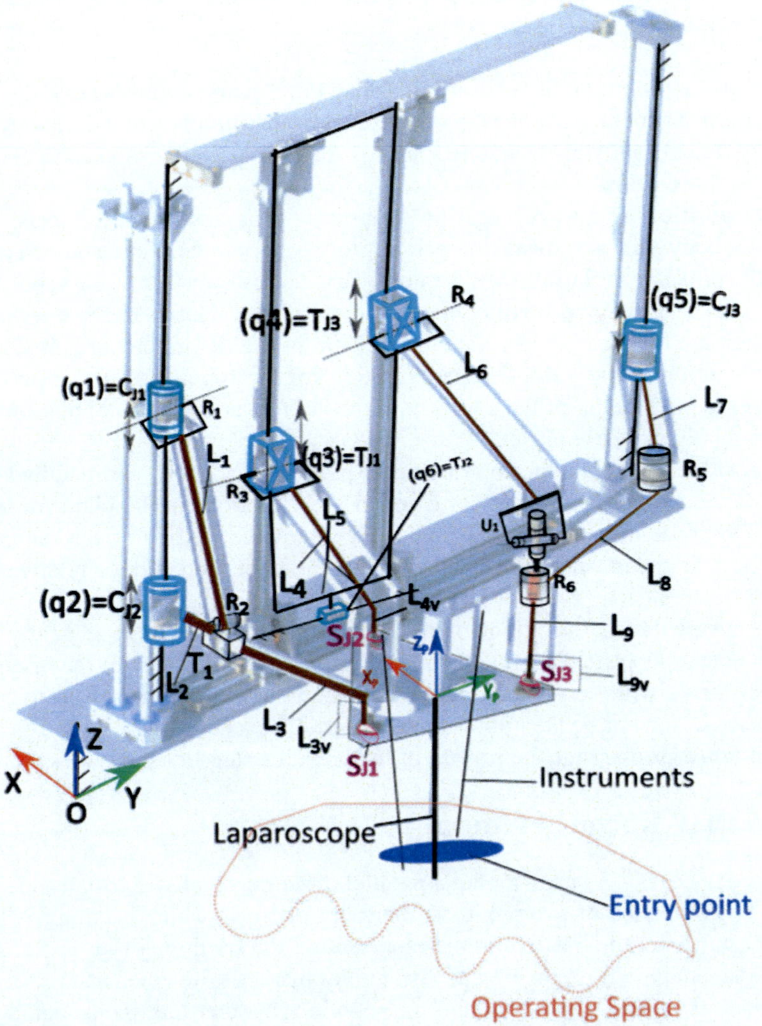

Fig. 2. Kinematic scheme overlaid on robotic platform

For homing it must be ensured that:

- the distance between q1 and q2 on the vertical axis is at 393 mm;
- the distance between q3 and q2 on the vertical axis is set at 158 mm in the positive direction of the Z axis;
- the distance between q4 and q3 is set at 218 mm in the positive direction of the Z axis;

- the distance between q5 and q4 is set at 277 mm in the negative direction of the Z axis.

The q6 joint assembly does not have a set distance at which it must be placed during operation, as it moves though, the previous distances between the other joints must be ensured.

For the **insertion stage** the platform is carried in a point slightly above the RCM. After this, the instrument platform is moved in the negative direction of the Z axis (down), into the abdominal cavity, by actuating joints q1 through q5 in tandem and maintaining q6 at its current position.

For the **positioning and orientation stage** it is to be noted that the incision into the patient's body will not always be parallel to the horizontal plane and as such the tilting of the instrument platform will be necessary. In this eventuality, the set distances between joints q1 through q5 will contain different values relative to the ones defined above (which are for the case in which the incision is parallel to the horizontal plane). It is for this purpose that a 6 DOF configuration for the robot platform is necessary, as it allows the positioning of the platform in the vertical and horizontal planes and its orientation relative to these planes.

After positioning around the entry point the platform's motion is limited by locking q6, while at this point the necessity of compensatory motions of the platform relative to the motion of the instruments in the next stage, requires the q1 through q5 joints to no longer be actuated in tandem, only allowing their independent motion relative to one another.

For the **surgical task**, the motion of the instruments is induced independently by the instrument actuation systems, while the platform only compensates for the orientation of the instruments with very small and precise motions in the order of up to 50 mm displacements of the non-locked joints on their vertical axes.

For the **finalization stage** the reverse of the previous steps must be carried out.

3 The 6 DOF Robotic Platform

The robotic device (Fig. 3.) has a modular parallel structure which was adopted in similar devices [15], comprised of two modules, the robot platform which is comprised from the fixed base/frame, the 6 active joints representing the q1 through q6 in Sect. 2.2, marked in magenta in Fig. 3, their respective guides marked with green and red, a series of passive joints marked with cyan and the robotic arms that link the actuated joints to the mockup instrument platform through three passive spherical joints mounted on the platform (cyan). The robotic device is actuated by 6 motors, each of them actuating one of the joints. The second module is represented by the instrument platform, which contains the mechanisms necessary to actuate the instruments after insertion in the patient's abdomen.

When referring to the robot platform, the instrument platform is the end-effector of the device. The end-effector is actuated through three kinematic chains from here on referred to as motion chains, all of which are connected to the platform through three spherical joints. The motion chains are highlighted with a dotted line in Fig. 3 from left to right in yellow, orange and black.

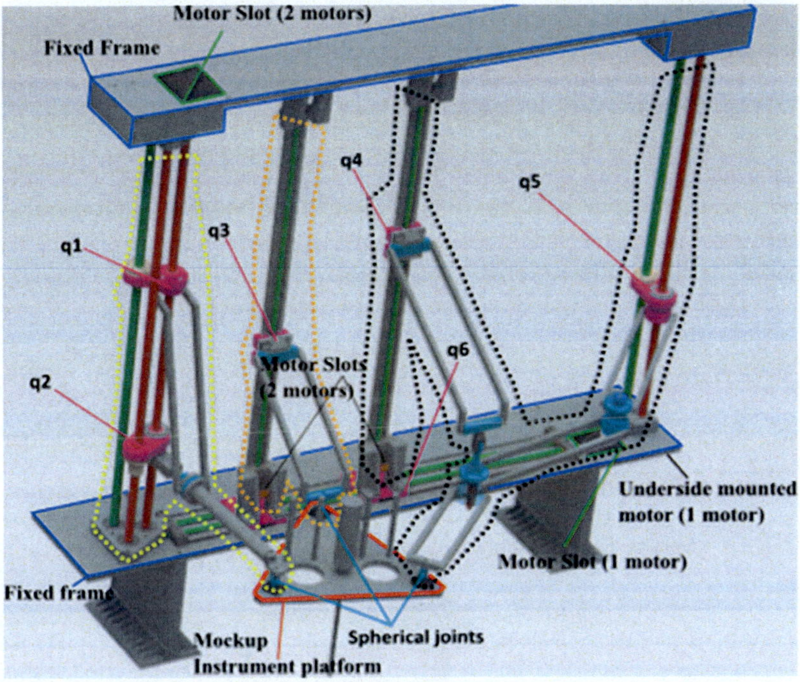

Fig. 3. The parallel SILS robotic system

3.1 The First Motion Chain

The first motion chain (Fig. 4) is comprised of two motors (1) actuating the translation joints with free rotation (7), (9).

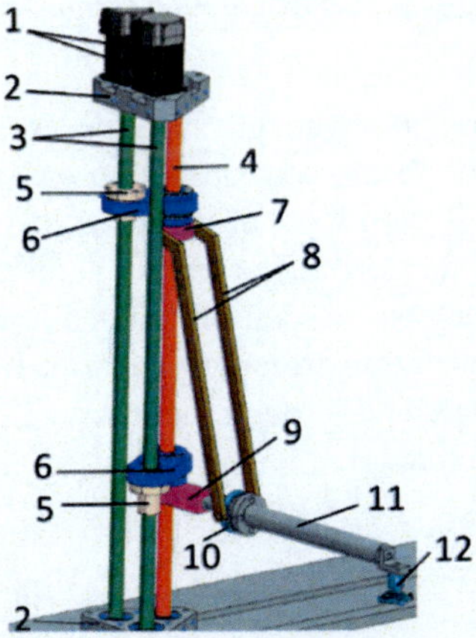

Fig. 4. The first motion chain

The transmission of the motion from the motors is done through a screw(3)-nut(5) mechanism connected to the linear bearing assemblies forming the active joints (7),(9) through a connector comprised of two parallel axial bearings mounted in a aluminum case (6) connecting the nut to the linear bearings. As the linear bearings move along their axis (4), the distance between them can remain either constant, in which case the end of the kinematic chain represented by the passive spherical joint assembly (12) executes a motion in the vertical plane. If the joints move relative to one another, the arms (8) actuate a passive translation joint (10) which is constrained by a piston assembly (11). This motion allows the tilting of the spherical joint, and can induce tilting in the instrument platform, as constrained by the other two motion chains.

3.2 The Second Motion Chain

The second motion chain (Fig. 5.), uses one motor (8') to actuate a linear slider (3') through a screw-nut mechanism (2'), along its vertical axis (1').

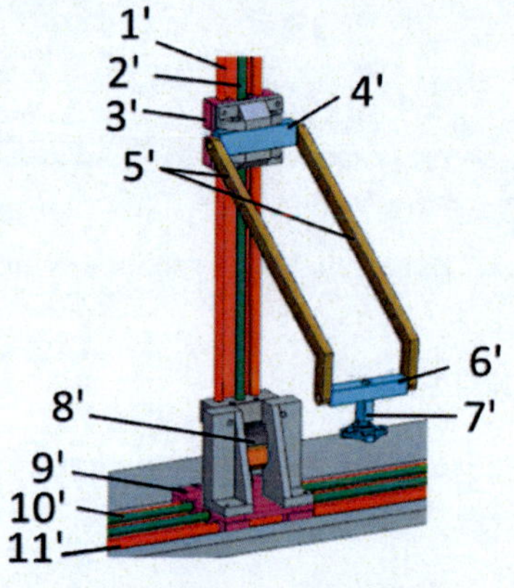

Fig. 5. Second motion chain

This moves the arms (5') along the vertical axis of the assembly, which is constrained to the instrument platform through the spherical joint assembly (7'). In order for the motion to be without stutters, at both ends of the arms, there are two passive rotation joints (4') and (6'). If the other motion chains are not actuated in tandem with this one, the spherical joint assembly and passive rotation joints allow for the forward/backward tilting of the spherical joint and the instrument platform, for sideways tilting, the rail (11') – slider (9') assembly is actuated through the screw (10'), which is a part of the q6 translation joint as presented in Sect. 3.

3.3 The Third Motion Chain

The third motion chain (Fig. 6.), is the amplest of the three, containing two motors for actuation (9") and (15"), being also connected to the q6 joint and directly linked through it to the second motion chain. The motion of the first part of the motion chain represented by the assembly containing elements (1") through (7") and (9") through (13") is an exact copy of the second motion chain with the difference being that the spherical joint at the end is replaced by an universal joint (7"). This in turn is connected to a passive rotation joint (8"). For the second part of the motion chain, in a similar manner to the first motion chain, the motor 15" transmits motion through the screw (17")-nut (8") mechanism to the linear bearing assembly that comprises the active joint q5 (20") through an aluminum casing (19") with parallel axial bearing connecting the nut to the joint assembly. This motion in turn is transmitted to a passive rotation joint assembly (22") through the arms (21") which also have a free passive rotation at both edges. Through arms (23") rotation joint (22") is connected to rotation joint (8") which represents the common connection between the first part of the motion chain, the second part and the spherical joint (14") connected to the instrument platform, which as in the case of the second motion chain also contains two passive rotation joints at both ends. If motor (9") is actuated in tandem with motor (15") and the other motors from the other motion chains the spherical joint assembly achieves a motion along the vertical axis. If (9") and (15") are actuated separately, tilting motions in both directions can be achieved, provided that the other motion chains are also actuated in order to compensate. Elements (11") through (13") represent the q6 joint.

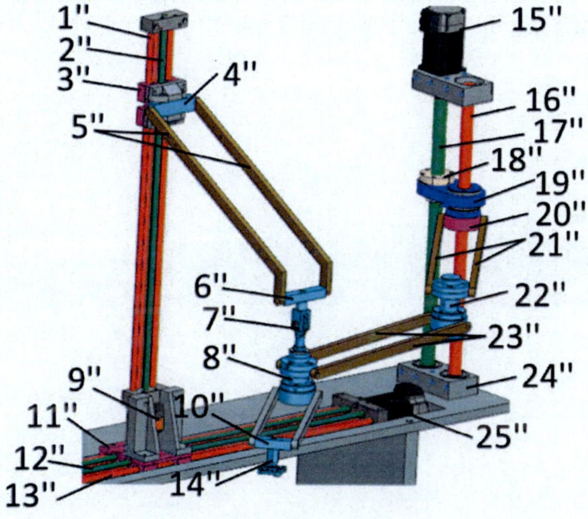

Fig. 6. The third motion chain

It should be noted that due to the particular configuration of the entire robotic system, and all three motion chains being connected through the instrument platform, actuating only a single motion chain while the others are not will only result in needless exertion of the motors, and possible strain on the mechanical structure of the actuated chain, as such the robot cannot work without full actuation of all three motion chains at all times.

4 FEM Analysis of System Components

While the construction of the robotic system ensures negligibly small forces being exerted upon the robot's components, a FEM analysis of what would be the most strained components has been done, to minimize any risks during its interaction with patients [16, 17]. The elements that were studied are represented by the connecting arms between the actuated joints and the instrument platform (highlighted with brown in Sects. 3.1 to 3.3). As these arms take on the total weight of the instrument platform, instruments and laparoscope it was deduced that the arms are the elements that would be most susceptible to mechanical deformations during operation, which could lead to errors during the surgical procedure, as such a FEA was performed to assess their stiffness.

Figure 7. Represents one of the arms connecting q1 to the piston assembly that is in turn connected to the instrument platform through the spherical joint (all part of the first motion chain at 3.1). The conditions considered were that the minimum distance between the q1 and q2 joints has been set, and the second and third kinematic joints are inactive and only hold the platform via mechanical blocking owing to the structure of each chain (no motor breaking included), as such it was calculated that the studied arm would have to undergo pressure equivalent to slightly under $\mathbf{F_1} = \mathbf{10N}$ perpendicular to the arm's length, at the point of contact between it and the piston assembly. It can be observed that in this case the arm made from aluminum would be subjected to a 0.0836 mm deformation at the tip (a negligible value).

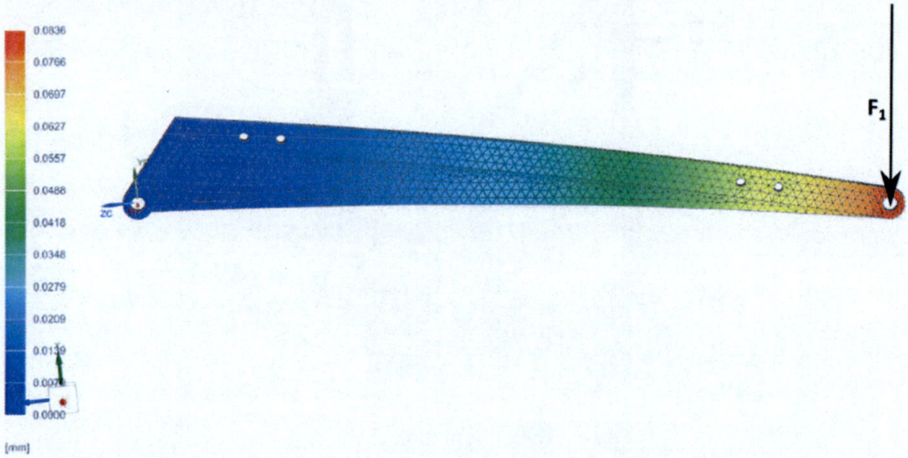

Fig. 7. The deformations of the q1 arm under the effect of a vertical force

In Figs. 8 and 9 the same situation in which the other kinematic chains were disabled, was studied. This results in a similar force parallel to the arm lengths at the point of contact with the spherical joints. In the case of Fig. 8. The arm is the one connecting the q3 joint to the passive spherical joint on the platform, and it was considered that the weight of the platform dragged the arm and placed it in a as near to vertical position as possible given mechanical limitations, under these conditions the aluminum arm would suffer a

0.0812 mm deformation at the connecting point between it and the spherical joint under the action of a force of $\mathbf{F_i = 10N}$.

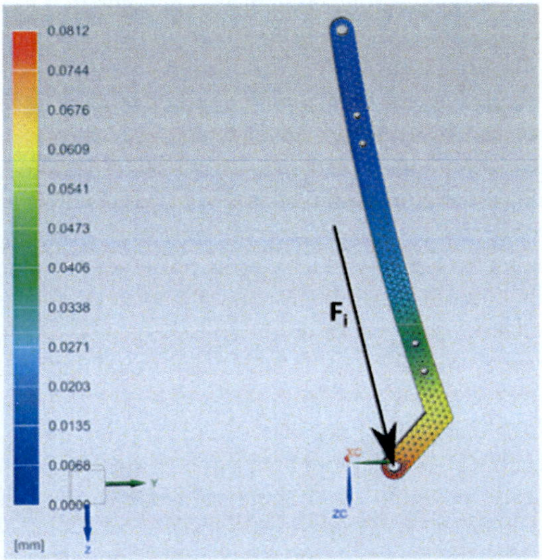

Fig. 8. The deformations of the q2 arm under the effect of a 10N force

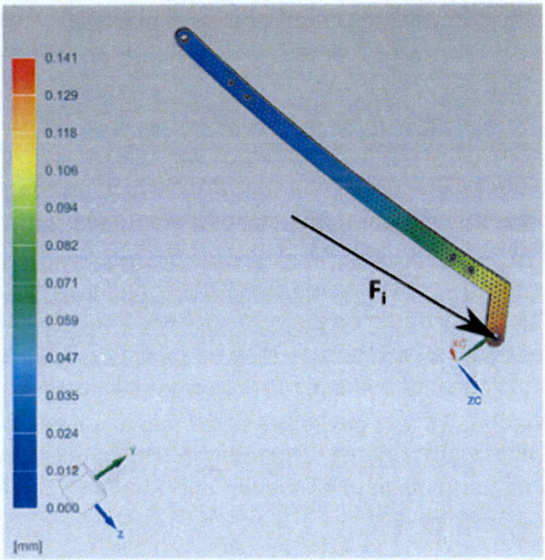

Fig. 9. The deformations of the q4 arm under the effect of a 15N force

In Fig. 9. The arm connecting the q4 joint to the platform was studied, under the same conditions. This arm is connected to a universal joint which links it to an assembly containing 4 passive rotation joints, the passive spherical joint the connecting arms between these two and the instrument platform, as such, in this case a $\mathbf{F_i = 15N}$ force was considered to exert pressure upon the arm which has been brought in the same position as the arm in 8a. The result is a 0.141 mm deformation at the point of contact. This represents a near twice as large of a deformation compared to the previous arms, though only in a scenario where the rest of the robot joints are completely inactive, and the assembly held by the arm is basically a deadweight.

While the forces studied here are rather small, they are slightly above the estimated weight of the platform and instruments, when divided between each arm. A doubled force would result in deformations over 1mm, which could potentially pose a threat as precision during surgical operation should be under 1mm [18]. Fortunately the platform is expected to remain still once instrument insertion inside the patient's body is done, and as such any additional forces acting upon the arms of the robot cannot occur, therefore it was determined from these FEM simulation that the most strained components of the robotic arm, would not suffer any major deformations under the set conditions, and as such during normal systems operation the robotic arms would most definitely be capable of without any danger.

Additionally, during singular positions when the platform is rotated around its vertical axis most of the concentrated forces would act directly upon the spherical connectors, fortunately to reach those positions all 6 actuators would have to be set for a set of specific values which cannot be reached accidentally.

5 Conclusions

This paper focuses on the mechanical design of a parallel modular robot with 6 degrees of freedom developed for use in SILS surgery. The design of the robotic structure and its subassemblies have proven to be capable of fulfilling the necessary tasks implied by the medical protocol pertaining to a SILS procedure. Each of the three motion chains that make up the robotic structure have shown a rigid structure capable of ensuring the precision and stability of the instrument platform, which are imperative in the safe execution of the robotic surgical tasks. The robotic arms that support the full weight of the instrument platform, instruments and laparoscope have been subjected to a FEM analysis studying the deformations that would occur during an erroneous functioning of the device when these elements would be forced to independently maintain the platform's position and orientation. The deformations observed were negligible enough to support the capacity of the device to maintain the platform stable. The results shown in this paper present the robotic structure as a viable solution for a SILS robotic system and have shown the device's mechanical structure's capability of safely operating the instruments and instrument platform and withstand its weight and forces implied during operation without having any risk to the patient.

Acknowledgement. This work was supported by a grant of the Ministry of Research, Innovation and Digitization, CNCS/CCCDI – UEFISCDI, project number PCE171/2021 – Challenge within PNCDI III and by the project POCU/380/6/13/123927-ANTREDOC, "Entrepreneurial competencies and excellence research in doctoral and postdoctoral studies programs", co-funded from the European Social Fund through the Human Capital Operational Program 2014–2020.

References

1. Far, S.S., Miraj, S.: Single-incision laparoscopy surgery: a systematic review. Electron Physician, pp. 3088–3095 (2016)
2. Peters, B.S., Armijo, P.R., Krause, C., Choudhury, S.A., Oleynikov, D.: Review of emerging surgical robotic technology. Surg. Endosc. **32**(4), 1636–1655 (2018)
3. Harky, A., et al.: The future of open heart surgery in the era of robotic and minimal surgical interventions. Hear. Lung Circ. **29**, 49–61 (2019)
4. McCarus, S.D.: Senhance robotic platform system for gynecological surgery. JSLS J. Soc. Laparoendosc. Surg. **25** (2021)
5. Rumolo, V., Rosati, A., Tropea, A., et al. : Senhance robotic platform for gynecologic surgery: a review of literature. Updates Surg. **71**, 419–427 (2019)
6. Gosrisirikul, C., Don Chang, K., Raheem, A.A., Rha, K.H.: New era of robotic surgical systems. Asian J. Endosc Surg. **11**, 291–299 (2018)
7. Seeliger, B., Diana, M., Ruurda, J.P., Konstantinidis, K.M., Marescaux, J., Swanström, L.L.: Enabling single-site laparoscopy: the SPORT platform. Surg. Endosc. **33**(11), 3696–3703 (2019)
8. Rassweiler, J.J., et al.: Future of robotic surgery in urology. BJU Int. **120**, 822–841 (2017)
9. Pusca, A., et al.: Workspace analysis of two innovative parallel robots for single incision laparoscopic surgery. Acta Tehnica Napocensis, **65**(II), 407–414 (2022)
10. Pisla, D., et al.: Singularity analysis and geometric optimization of a 6-DOF parallel robot for SILS. Machines **10**(9), 764 (2022)
11. Gherman, B., et al.: Singularities and workspace analysis for a parallel robot for minimally invasive surgery, 2010 IEEE (AQTR), pp. 1–6 (2010)
12. Plitea, N., et al.: Innovative development of surgical parallel robots. Acta Electronica, Mediamira Science, Cluj-Napoca, pp. 201–206 (2007)
13. Ulinici, I., Crisan, N., Vaida, C., Andras, I., Pisla, D.: Analysis and preliminary design of a new parallel robot for SILS. 2022 2022 IEEE Int. Conf. on Automation, Quality and Testing, Robotics (AQTR) (2022)
14. Ulinici, I., Vaida, C., Antal, T., Pisla, D.: Kinematics and workspace simulation of a new parallel robot for SILS. Acta Tehnica Napocensis, Series: App. Math. Mech. And Eng. **65**(II), 505–514 (2022)
15. Pisla, D., et.al.: Kinematics and workspace analysis of an innovative 6-DOF parallel robot for SILS. Proceedings of the Romanian Academy, Series A, **23**(3), 279–288 (2022)
16. Tucan, P., Vaida, C., Plitea, N., Pisla, A., Carbone, G., Pisla, D.: Risk-based assessment engineering of a parallel robot used in post-stroke upper limb rehabilitation. Sustainability **11**, 2893 (2019)
17. Papadakis, M., et al.: The WHO safer surgery checklist time out procedure revisited: Strategies to optimise compliance and safety. Int. J of Survery **69**(19), 22 (2019)
18. Vaida, C., Pisla, D., Schadlbauer, J., Husty, M., Plitea, N.: Kinematic analysis of an innovative medical parallel robot using study parameters. In: New Trends in Medical and Service Robots, Springer, Cham, Mechanism and Machine Science **39**, 85-99 (2016). https://doi.org/10.1007/978-3-319-30674-2_7

Design and Functional Analysis of a New Parallel Modular Robotic System for Single Incision Laparoscopic Surgery

Doina Pisla[1], Iulia Andras[2], Alexandru Pusca[1](✉), Corina Radu[2], Bogdan Gherman[1], Paul Tucan[1], Nicolae Crisan[1], Calin Vaida[1], and Nadim Al Hajjar[2]

[1] CESTER, Technical University of Cluj-Napoca, 400114 Cluj-Napoca, Romania
alexandru.pusca@mep.utcluj.ro
[2] "Iuliu Hatieganu" University of Medicine and Pharmacy, 400347 Cluj-Napoca, Romania

Abstract. This paper presents the design and functional analysis for a new parallel modular robotic system for Single Incision Laparoscopic Surgery (SILS). The development of this robotic structure was carried out based on the kinematic scheme, with respect to the surgical instruments required by the medical protocol of SILS, using both mechanically processed and commercially available elements was achieved based on a validated kinematic model and a medical protocol for SILS procedure. The simulation and workspace analysis for the robotic structure were performed and validated using the inverse kinematic model of the robot structure. The detailed design of the robotic system was completed and validated by applying the finite elements analysis for the elements that guide the mobile platform, which are prone to large deformations of the structure.

Keywords: Parallel modular robot · design · Robotic assisted SILS · kinematics · workspace · simulation · FEA

1 Introduction

Single incision laparoscopic surgery (SILS) was firstly introduced in 1922 in gynecology where good results were obtained using this technique in over 400 patients however, it started to be used on a large scale only in the last 10–15 years. SILS has become a standard procedure in gynecology, becoming one of the most used methods, due to its benefits such as short recovery time, less blood loss, good cosmesis, and postoperative scars reduced after the medical procedure [1]. This method involves the insertion of the medical instruments required for the medical act (a laparoscopic camera and 1 or 2 surgical instruments) through a single multi-lumen port that is inserted into the patient's body by making an incision of 15–25 mm made at the navel compared to classic surgery where the incision is between 10 and 15 cm and the patient's body is open. The SILS technique is described in general surgery in 1997 and presently, this technique is expanding in inguinal hernia repair, appendicectomy, adrenalectomy, gastric banding, sleeve

D. Tarnita et al. (Eds.): MESROB 2023, MMS 133, pp. 32–41, 2023.
https://doi.org/10.1007/978-3-031-32446-8_4

gastrectomy, cholecystectomies, and splenectomy. SILS offers two configurations (X and Y) regarding the insertion of instruments into the multi-lumen port, each configuration comes with a few specific advantages and disadvantages. The X configuration offers a large intraoperative workspace but comes with the disadvantage of triangulation, while the Y configuration comes with the elimination of triangulation but reduced intraoperative workspace, these configurations were extensively presented in [2]. Due to the successful results obtained following the use of SILS, robotics systems have been developed that have the role of improving these results and at the same time reducing the disadvantages of this method [3, 16], disadvantages such as the tremor of the surgeon's hand, ergonomics, precision, dexterity, and instrument triangulation are eliminated using the robotics systems [4, 17]. The first robotic assisted surgery using the SILS method was performed in 2008, with the help of the da Vinci S robot using two standard instruments and a laparoscopic camera inserted in the middle of the trocar, the operation representing a real success at the time, thus eliminating the main disadvantages of classical surgery, such as the tremor of the surgeon's hand, dexterity, patient safety, accuracy, and poor ergonomics [5, 6]. The procedure ergonomics and efficiency are increased due to the master-slave concept [7], configuration in which surgeon occupies a sitting position at the master console from where he controls the slave structure, master-slave concept is described in detail in [7]. The first robot dedicated to SILS with Food and Drug Administration (FDA) approval was developed in 2018 by Intuitive Surgical, namely da Vinci SP, this system having a dedicated port for SILS where all instruments for surgery are attached (active instruments and laparoscopic camera) [8]. Another commercial robotic system used in SILS is the Senhance system, a multi-arm robot developed by Asensus Surgical, this system is a competitor to Intuitive Surgical, and is extensively presented in [4] and a comparison between da Vinci SP and Senhance is presented in [9]. The robotic systems presented above have a serial structure and have disadvantages such as the low rigidity, and collisions between robotic arms.

This paper presents the functional design analysis of a new parallel modular robotic structure used for SILS. The SILS instruments are attached to the robotic structure via a mobile platform reducing some disadvantages encountered in the previous robotic systems for SILS (such as collisions between robotic arms, rigidity, and ergonomics). Following the Introduction section, the paper is structured as follows: Section II presents the kinematic scheme for the parallel modular robotic system for SILS, Section III illustrates its detailed design, Section IV presents the robot simulation and the workspace generation using Siemens NX software [10], Section V presents a stiffness analysis of the main components of the parallel modular robot structure using (FEA) finite element analysis followed by conclusions regarding the developed work.

2 Kinematic Scheme for a New Parallel Modular Robotic System

The parallel robot presented in this paper belongs to a family of 6-DOF parallel robots with active translational joints [11, 18], its detailed kinematics being presented in [12]. The kinematic scheme is presented in Fig. 1 where three identical kinematic chains of the robot can be observed (KC_1, KC_2, KC_3). The degree of freedom for the parallel robot structure was calculated based on the formula presented in [13], having the general form:

$$M = (6 - F) \cdot N - \sum_{i=1..5} (i - F) \cdot C_i \tag{1}$$

where: M represents the mobility degree of the mechanism; F represents the mechanism family; N the mobile elements within the mechanism; C_i the class i, joints. Each input kinematic chain represents a class 3 joint, $F = 0$ (mobile platform has no constraints), $N = 4$, and $C_3 = 6$. The results of the Ec. (1) are presented in Ec. (2).

$$M = 6 \cdot N - 3 \cdot C_3 = 6 \tag{2}$$

The parallel modular robotic system has 6 - DOF and the robot structure has all the active joints in the same plane.

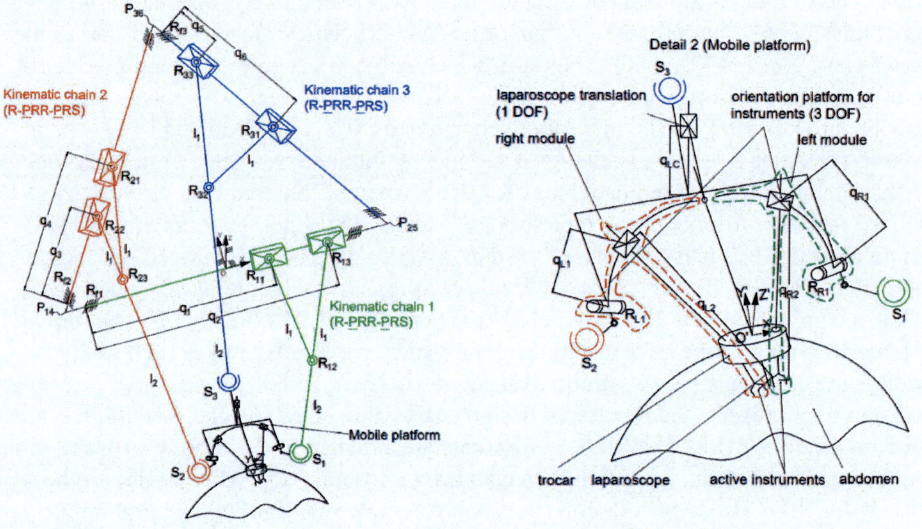

Fig. 1. Kinematic scheme for the parallel modular robotic system and mobile platform details

The 3-R-PRR-PRS robotic system has its base connected to the mobile platform through three identical kinematic chains, with each kinematic chain containing the following components: two active prismatic joints (q_1, q_2 for kinematic chain 1; q_3, q_4 for kinematic chain 2; q_4, q_5 for kinematic chain 3), one cylindrical joint for each kinematic chain (R_{f1} for kinematic chain 1, R_{f2} for kinematic chain 2 and R_{f3} for kinematic chain 3), three passive revolute joints (R_{11}, R_{12}, and R_{13} for kinematic chain 1, R_{f2}, R_{21}, R_{22}, and R_{23} for kinematic chain 2 and R_{f3}, R_{31}, R_{32}, and R_{33} for kinematic chain 3), and one spherical joint (S_1 for kinematic chain 1, S_2 for kinematic chain 2, S_3 for kinematic chain 3). An extensive analysis of this structure and the kinematic scheme is presented in [12] and [14]. The kinematic chains of the parallel modular robotic system are connected with the mobile platform using the three spherical joints (S1, S2, S3), as illustrated in detail in Fig. 1. The mobile platform is also composed of three modules, two modules with 3-DOF used for orientation and insertion of active instruments and one module with 1-DOF used for inserting the laparoscopic camera, these modules are attached to the aluminum frame of the mobile platform. The orientation modules used for the active instruments attached to the mobile platform (right and left modules) are composed of two active revolute joints (R_{L1} for the left active instrument and R_{R1} for the right active instrument), and four active translational joints (q_{L1} and q_{L2} for the left instrument and q_{R1} and q_{R2} for the right instrument). The laparoscopic camera has only one active translational joint which performs the camera insert/retraction (q_{LC}).

3 Constructive Design of a New Parallel Modular Robot for SILS

The design of the parallel modular robot used in SILS was carried out based on the kinematic scheme (Fig. 1). For the design of the robot, commercially available parts are used, as well as elements that will be processed using CNC machines (computer numerical control) or using 3D printing techniques. The 3D printing will be used for parts that have a complex shape. Figure 2 shows the constructive design of the parallel robot, highlighting the three identical kinematic chains that have the following 3-R-PRR-PRS configuration.

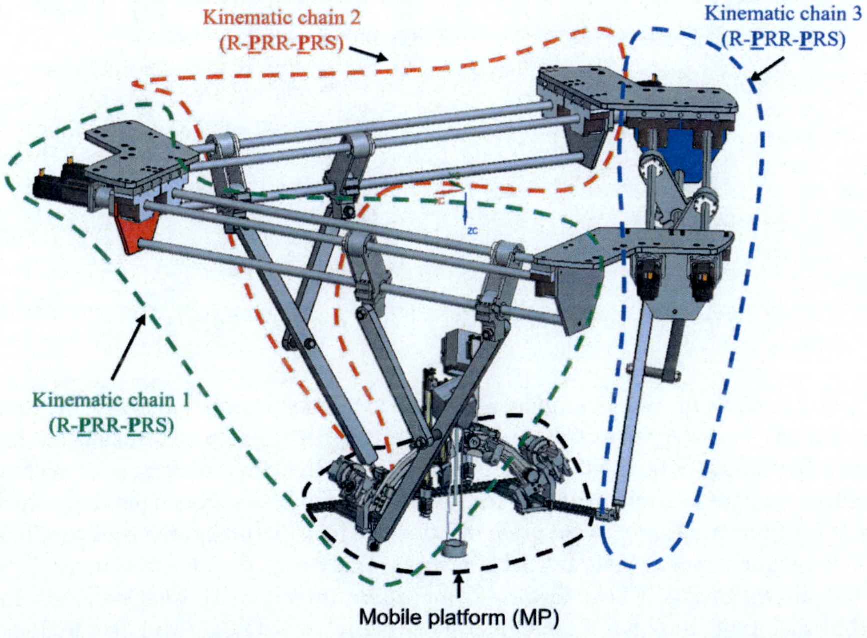

Fig. 2. Modeling and design of a new parallel modular robotic system for SILS

All three kinematic chains of the robot structure shown in Fig. 2 are connected using the spherical joints that attach to the mobile platform (MP), which have the role of orienting and inserting the instruments necessary for the medical act. Each kinematic chain is actuated by two motors connected with flexible couplings at the kinematic chain of the robot. Since the kinematic chains of the robot are identical, only one kinematic chain will be presented below according to Fig. 3.

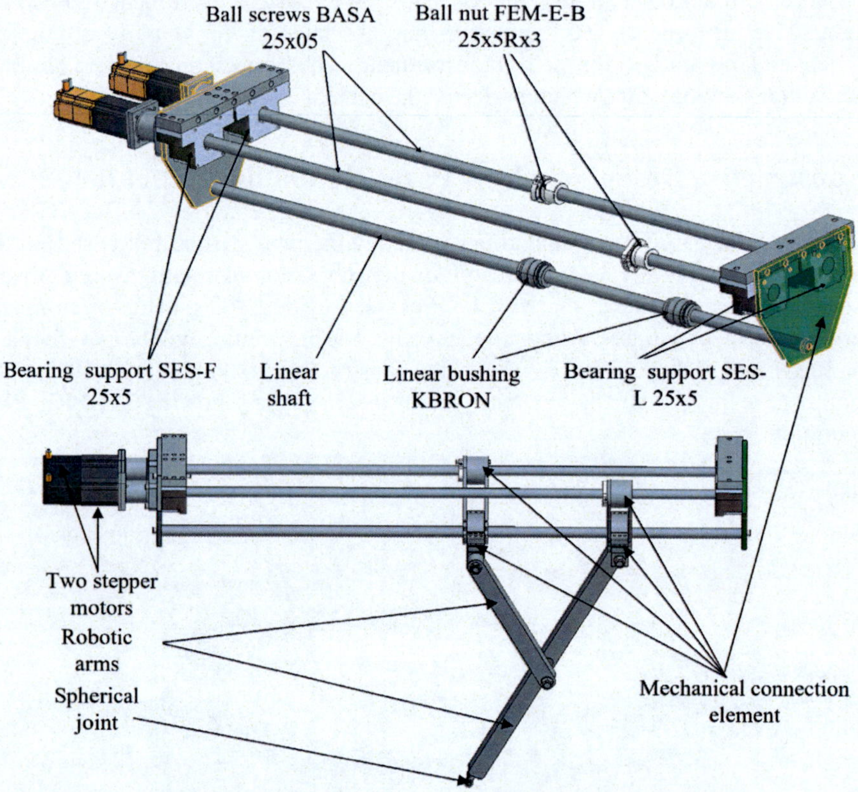

Fig. 3. Robot kinematic chain for main components details

Figure 3 shows the main components of the kinematic chain, the kinematic chain is actuated by two stepper motors connected to two ball-screw-nut mechanisms that transmit the sliding motion to the joined linear shaft of the kinematic chain. In order to perform the passive rotation of the two arms of the robot structure around the linear shaft, two KBRON linear bushings were used, this type of linear bushings create a cylindrical joint (translation along the axis and rotation around the axis). The two arms in the robot structure shown in Fig. 3 have in their composition three passive rotation joints and one spherical joint. To connect the two arms of the robot with the two KBRON linear bushings, two bushing housings were used attached to the body of the rotation of the bushings, these housings have a reaming in the lower part on which the two arms of the robot will be fixed with two threaded pins, sleeve bearings were used to reduce the friction between the linear shafts and the flanges. The third passive rotation joint has the role of connecting the two arms.

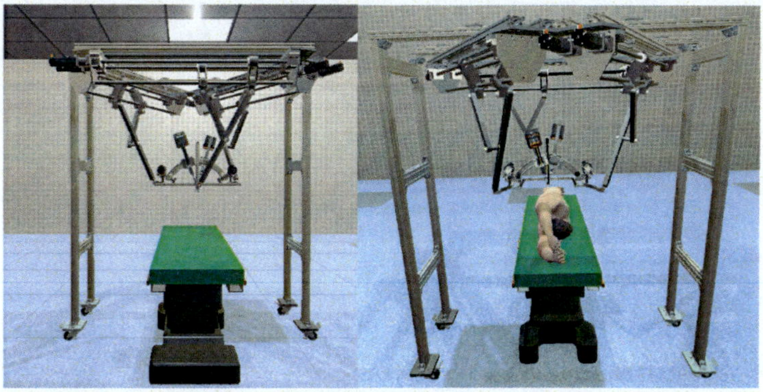

Fig. 4. The parallel robot for SILS integrated in operating room

Figure 4 shows the virtual design of the parallel robot used for SILS and the integration of this structure in the operating room without the patient and with the patient.

4 Robot Simulation and Workspace Generation in Siemens NX

The simulation of the robotic structure presented in this paper was carried out based on the inverse kinematic model presented in [12], using as input data values of the coordinates tip of the laparoscopic camera (X_E, Y_E, Z_E, ψ, θ, φ) located in an arbitrary position. The motion will reposition the tip of the laparoscopic camera (TCP) at the coordinates of the insertion point (X_B, Y_B, Z_B, $\psi = 0$, $\theta = 0$, $\varphi =$ -60°), inside the patient, namely the RCM (Remote Center of Motion). The value of $\varphi =$ -60° was selected based on the previous study [12] which demonstrated a workspace increase of the mobile platform with respect to the surgical procedure. In Fig. 5, the geometric parameters used in the simulation are presented, as the motion parameters, and the initial and final pose for the robot TCP. In Fig. 6, all linear dimensions are expressed in millimeters and the angular ones in degrees.

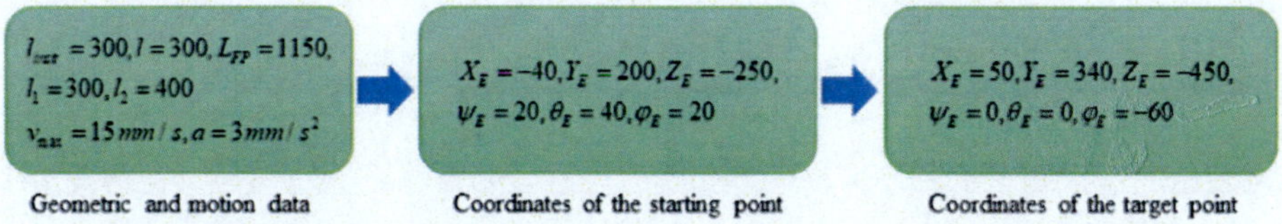

Fig. 5. Numerical data for the simulation trajectory of the parallel robot for SILS

For this trajectory, the graphs shown in Fig. 6 represent the displacement (green), velocity (blue) and acceleration (red) variation of the end-effector coordinates from the starting to the target point of the defined motion.

The validation of the robot functionality was done by computing the variation of the active joints in MATLAB [15] (Fig. 6) based on the inverse kinematic model, the same

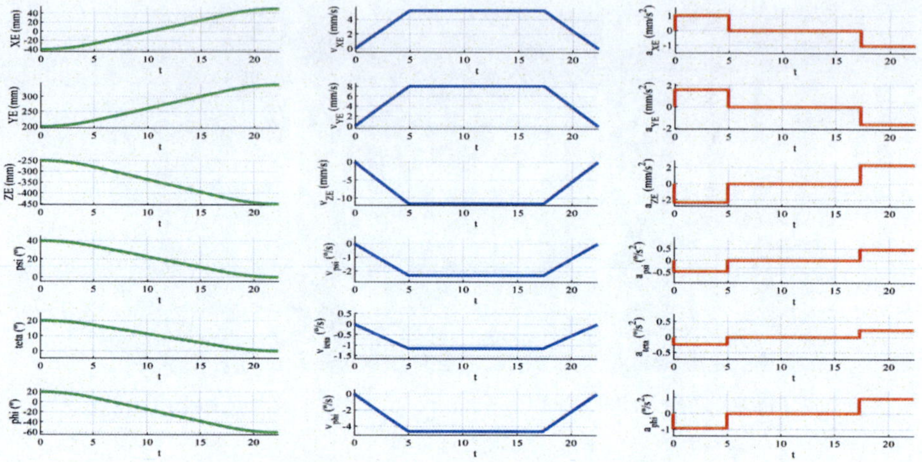

Fig. 6. Motion trajectory of the parallel robot for SILS

input data being used in the Siemens NX [10] program in the simulation module, where the MATLAB [15] generated trajectory (Fig. 6) is used as input for the robot TCP. Both sets of data have as outputs the displacements, velocities, and accelerations at the level of the active joints. Being a kinematic simulation, friction is not considered, and the mechanism has an ideal behavior in the 3D model. The results are illustrated in Fig. 7 where it can be observed that the active joints have similar behaviors in both applications validating both the mathematical model and the 3D model of the robot.

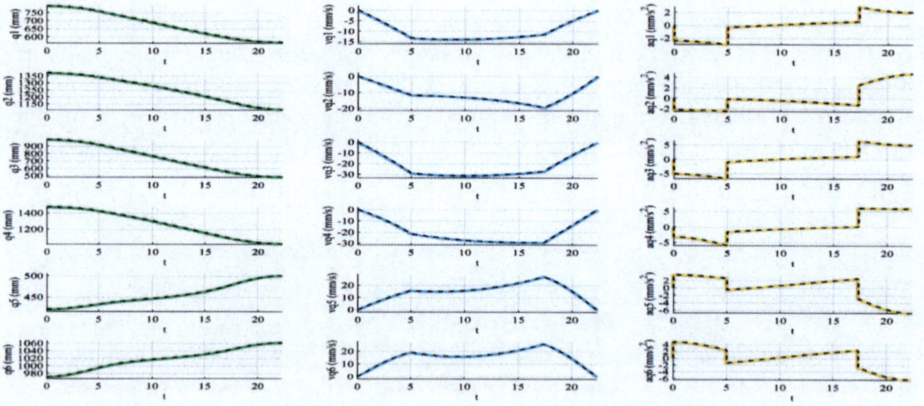

Fig. 7. Active joints displacements, velocities, and accelerations (MATLAB – coloured, NX – black dashed lines)

The robot workspace is generated using a virtual hemisphere attached to the RCM of the mobile platform (Fig. 8), on this hemisphere the trace function from the Siemens NX [10] simulation was applied, after which a simulation of the robot structure based on the inverse kinematic model was performed and the results are shown in Fig. 7.

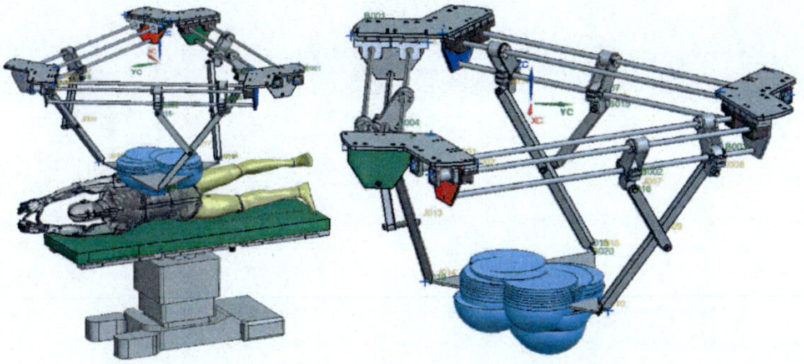

Fig. 8. Robot workspace generated with the trace function in Siemens NX

5 Finite Element Analysis for Main Components of the Robot

The last step in validating the design of the robot structure is to perform the finite element analysis (FEA), to simulate the mechanical deformation level of the moving parts which can influence the functional parameters of the robot (e.g., accuracy, stiffness). These analyzes were carried out by assigning material to all the component elements of the robot structure, thus accurately calculating the mass of both the robot structure and the mobile platform handled by the robot, this mass of the mobile platform will be used as a first input for the finite element analysis. The main elements subjected to FEA are the linear shaft, the mechanical elements connecting the active joints to the mobile platform, the robot arms, and the spherical joint (Fig. 3), as they are most prone to deformations. Finite element analysis is generated by following the next steps: applying the materials to each previously described component element (the robot arms, as well as the mechanical connecting elements, will be made of aluminum, and the precision axis and the spherical joints of steel), 3D tetrahedral mesh defines, defining fixed elements, applying different forces to stress areas, generating analysis, and extracting data. The most significant results generated from the FEA are presented in the figures below (Figs. 9, 10, 11 and 12), where we can see the maximum displacements and von Mises stresses suffered by the component elements of the robot structure following the application of a force between 60 and 300 N, depending on the load of each component. This force was applied on all three axes (*OX*, *OY*, and *OZ*) of these components, the most important results being: 0.07 mm displacement and 6.07 MPa von Mises stress for the linear shaft (*OX* axis loading); $4.7*10^{-4}$ mm displacement and 0.6 MPa von Mises stress for the mechanical connection element (*OY* axis loading); 0.09 mm displacement and 4.7 MPa von Mises stress for the main robot arm (*OY* axis loading); 0.18 mm displacement and 8.1 MPa von Mises stress for the secondary robot arm (*OZ* axis loading). The results of the FEA show that the designed elements are resistant from a mechanical point of view, so during the use of the system there will be no deformations that can create elasticity in the mechanism, reduce accuracy or create any safety issues during the procedure.

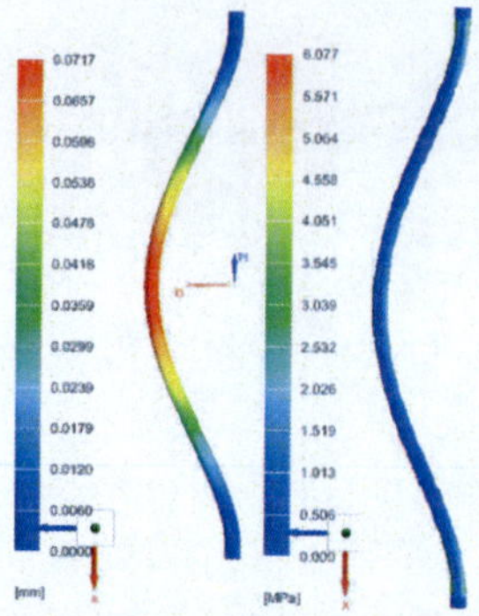

Fig. 9. Displacement and von Mises stress of the linear shaft

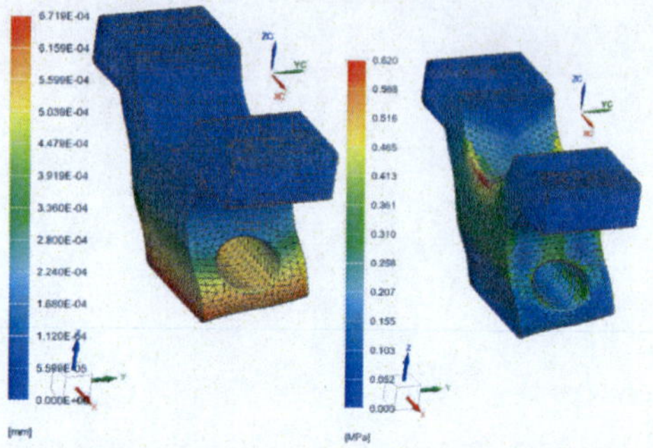

Fig. 10. Displacement and von Mises stress of the mechanical connection element

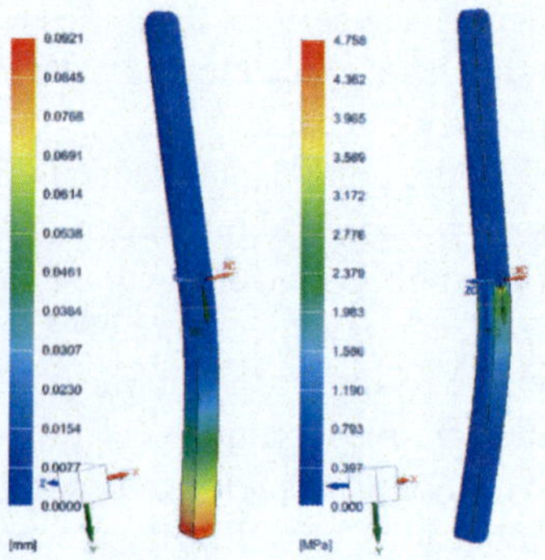

Fig. 11. Displacement and von Mises stress of the main robot arm

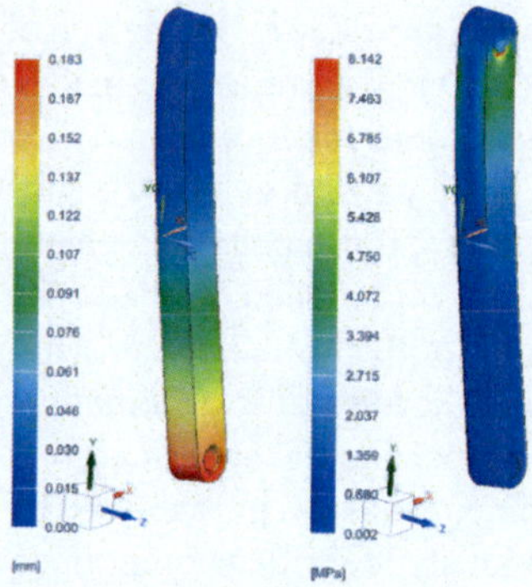

Fig. 12. Displacement and von Mises stress of the secondary robot arm

6 Conclusions

This paper presents the functional design validation of a parallel modular robot for SILS with 6-DOF, having three identical kinematic chains mounted on a triangular frame (the mobile platform). The kinematic scheme of the robot was used as a starting point for the constructive design of the robot. The design and assembly of the robot are validated based on the inverse kinematic model and simulations presented in this paper, to which is added the FEA for the components that guide the mobile platform, which are prone to large deformations of the structure. By validating the design of the proposed robotic structure, the development of the robot may proceed to the following stage: achievement of the experimental model and the implementation of the control system.

Acknowledgments. This work was supported by a grant of the Ministry of Research, Innovation and Digitization, CNCS/CCCDI – UEFISCDI, project number PCE171/2021 - Challenge within PNCDI III.

References

1. Chamberlain, R.S., Sakpal, S.V.: A comprehensive review of single-incision laparoscopic surgery (SILS) and natural orifice transluminal endoscopic surgery (NOTES) techniques for cholecystectomy. J. Gastrointest Surg. **13**(9), 1733–1740 (2009)
2. Vaida, C., Andras, I., Birlescu, I., Crisan, N., Plitea, N., Pisla, D.: Preliminary control design of a single-incision laparoscopic surgery robotic system. In: 2021 25th International Conference on System Theory, Control and Computing (ICSTCC), pp. 384–389 (2021)
3. Dreifuss, N.H., Chang, B., Schlottmann, F., et al.: Robotic inguinal hernia repair: is the new Da Vinci single port platform providing any benefit?, Surg. Endosc. (2022)
4. Hirano, Y., et al.: Robot-assisted surgery with Senhance robotic system for colon cancer: our original single-incision plus 2-port procedure. Tech. Coloproctol **25**, 467–471 (2021)
5. Harky, A., et al.: The future of open heart surgery in the era of robotic and minimal surgical interventions. Heart Lung Circ. **29**(1), 49–61 (2022)
6. Wang, W., Sun, X., Wei, F.: Laparoscopic surgery, and robotic surgery for single-incision cholecystectomy: an updated systematic review. Updates Surg. **73**(6), 2039–2046 (2021)
7. Pisla, D., et al.: New approach to hybrid robotic system application in single incision laparoscopic surgery. Acta Tehnica Napocensis **64**(3), 369–378 (2021)
8. Kwak, Y., et al.: Da Vinci SP Single-port robotic surgery in gynecologic tumors: single surgeon's initial experience with 100 cases. Yonsei Med J. **63**(2), 179–186 (2022)
9. Rao, P.P.: Robotic surgery: new robots and finally some real competition. World J Urol. **36**, 537–541 (2018)
10. plm.automation.siemens.com/global/en/products/nx.html. Accessed 19 Dec 2022
11. Koukourikis, P., Rha, K.H.: Robotic surgical systems in urology: what is currently available? Investig Clin Urol. (2021)
12. Pisla, D., et al.: Family of modular parallel robots with active translational joints for single incision laparoscopic surgery. OSIM A00733/03.12.2021
13. Pisla, D., et al.: Application oriented modelling and simulation of an innovative parallel robot for single incision laparoscopic surgery. ASME 2022, IDETC/ CIE 2022, St. Louis, Missouri, **7**, DETC2022–89968, V007T07A032, 10 (2022)
14. Pisla, D., Plitea, N., Vidrean, A., Prodan, B., Gherman, B., Lese, D.: Kinematics and design of two variants of a reconfigurable parallel robot. ASME/IFTOMM International Conference on Reconfigurable Mechanisms and Robots **2009**, 624–631 (2009)
15. mathworks.com/products/matlab.html Accessed 19 Dec 2022
16. Gherman, B., et al.: Singularities and workspace analysis for a parallel robot for minimally invasive surgery. In: 2010 IEEE International Conference on Automation, Quality and Testing, Robotics (AQTR), pp. 1-6 (2010)
17. Plitea, N., et al.: Innovative development of surgical parallel robots. Acta Electronica, Mediamira Science, Cluj-Napoca **4**, 201–206 (2007)
18. Tucan, P., Vaida, C., Plitea, N., Pisla, A., Carbone, G., Pisla, D.: Risk-based assessment engineering of a parallel robot used in post-stroke upper limb rehabilitation. Sustainability **11**, 2893 (2019)

Design and Development of a 6-Degree-Of-Freedom Robotic Device for Cochlear Implantation Surgery

Xiangyu An and Mingfeng Wang(✉)

Department of Mechanical and Aerospace Engineering, Brunel University London, London UB8 3PH, UK
Mingfeng.Wang@Brunel.ac.uk

Abstract. In this paper, we proposed a conceptual design of a robotic device that uses the 6-degree-of-freedom (DoF) 3-PRRS parallel manipulator for Cochlear Implant (CI) surgery. The kinematic analysis of this robotic platform has been studied and the constant and variable parameters describing the geometry and inverse kinematics of the analyzed parallel manipulator are determined. A 3D CAD model of the proposed 6-DoF 3-PRRS robotic device is built in SolidWorks®, which was subsequently converted into a prototype for practical testing. Finally, the prototype of the platform has been developed by using rapid prototyping technology. A series of preliminary experiments have been carried out in which the motion ranges, manoeuvrability and stability of the parallel manipulator platform have been tested.

Keywords: Parallel Manipulators · Cochlear Implant · Medical Robots · Kinematics

1 Introduction

The cochlear implant is used to treat or restore children and adults with severe or profound bilateral sensory nerve hearing impairment [1]. An electrode array with a microphone, transmitter-receiver pair and speech processor will be implanted and stimulates the neurosensory auditory nerves directly to achieve the goal of recovery. There are more than 600,000 patients have undertaken CI treatment in the last 30 years [2]. However, the post-operative hearing outcomes of the patients are variable and partly limited after recovery. It is widely believed that the residual hearing loss is caused by the trauma induced during the surgery.

To prevent implantation trauma induced by cochlear implant surgery and preserve residual hearing, the research focus on the improvements in the outcome of the surgical procedures and some developments have been carried out by studying the surgical approach, the materials used and the technical design. In the surgical approaches, the concept of "soft surgery" was introduced in 1993 by Lehnhardt [3], in which the primary goal was to minimize the amount of mechanical stress transmitted to the cochlea by using

D. Tarnita et al. (Eds.): MESROB 2023, MMS 133, pp. 42–49, 2023.
https://doi.org/10.1007/978-3-031-32446-8_5

drills and to limit the trauma caused by electrode advancement [4]. The round window (RW) approach has also been proven to be more beneficial during surgery and more helpful for the patient's recovery after surgery [5, 6]. It's worth noting that the key operation of CI surgery is to insert the electrode array (EA) into the inner ear, which requires high precision and stability [7]. Despite the advantages of these approaches, the manual process for cochlear implants still faces many challenges and technical limitations (e.g., human tremors and jitters). Therefore, robotic/robot-assisted CI surgery has been researched and developed to further reduce trauma in internal structures of the ear and improve the accuracy of the surgery [3], as well as provide standard and independent surgical processes via different EA characteristics. Vittoria et al. built a remote-controlled robotic system, RobOtol, as an endoscope or a micro instrument holder for middle ear surgery and CI surgery [8]. Specifically, the robot arm in RobOtol consists of a serial kinematic chain of three perpendicular linear links at the base and three rotatory links at the distal arm with a total of 6 DoFs [9]. In the work of [10], a conceptual method of EA insertion and guidance in the ear was proposed by developing an actuation system with a sensing and data-driven control strategy. The actuator system was equipped with 3 DoFs, and different trajectories of the insertion can be generated by three different insertions. Henslee et al. [11].proposed a robot-assisted CI surgery concept by using the ECochG. The proposed system demonstrates the real-time signals monitor and adaption during the EA insertion process. Once the system detects the change in the ECochG signal, a notification will be presented immediately.

Although the above robotic devices could improve the CI surgery with certain assistance, the performance may be limited either by the unitized serial mechanisms or reduced DoFs (i.e., DOF < 6). On the other hand, thanks to the inherent high dynamic advantages, parallel manipulators become more and more popular in applications for manufacturing [12], space [13], humanoids [14], as well as medical usage [15–18]. Among medical applications, Jose et al. propose an asymmetrical spherical parallel manipulator as a prosthetic wrist, which is inspired by the range of motion of the human wrist [15]. Yangmin et al. proposed to perform cardio-pulmonary resuscitation using a 3-PUU parallel manipulator with a frequency of 100 times per minute [16]. In the work [17], Dalvand et al. introduced a novel robot-assisted system for invasive surgery/microsurgery by using the 6-RRCRR parallel robot (PRAMiSS). The robot can perform micro manipulations with the control algorithm of this robotics system. Because of the excellent kinematic and dynamic characteristics of the parallel manipulator, PMs are also employed in the surgery application such as haptic minimally invasive surgery [18] and rehabilitation of shoulder and elbow [19] However, to the authors' knowledge, few studies can be found in the literature by applying parallel manipulators in CI surgery.

Taking the initiative of applying parallel manipulators for CI surgery, in this paper, a novel design of a 6-DoF parallel manipulator is proposed as a robotic device for CI surgery. The CI insertion with an assistant of the proposed 6-DoF robotic device is illustrated in Sect. 2. The inverse kinematic analysis of the proposed design is carried out in Sect. 3. In Sect. 4, a prototype of the proposed design is built and presented with test results of a series of preliminary experiments. Conclusions and discussion are in Sect. 5.

2 Design

2.1 System Overview

In Fig. 1(a), a conceptual CI surgery approach is illustrated that employs a 6-DoF parallel manipulator to assist the insertion of EA. To achieve this approach, the design objectives can be divided into three stages: firstly, the dimensions, functions, and rest of the requirements are specified for the model development. The concepts of the platform with cochlear implant insertion setup were proposed. Moreover, the design of the platform prototype, analysis, and optimization is conducted in the final stage of the design process.

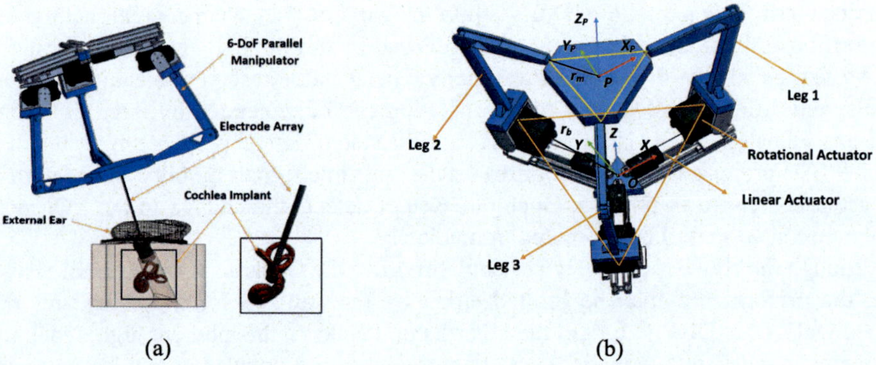

Fig. 1. Illustration of cochlear implant insertion by the proposed 6-DoF parallel manipulator

2.2 Design of 3-PRRS Parallel Manipulator

In this paper, a novel design of a 3-$\underline{\text{PR}}$RS parallel manipulator is proposed, where P, R and S, respectively, denote prismatic, revolute and spherical joints in which the underline ($\underline{\ }$) represents the actuated ones. As shown in Fig. 1(b), the moving platform is connected to the fixed base through three identical legs and in each leg, there are two actuators (linear and rotatory) to perform actuated joints. Moreover, at the initial configuration (see Fig. 1(b)), these three legs are symmetrically distributed, namely, the connection points on both moving and fixed platforms can form an equilateral triangle, where the linear actuators are at their shortest length and rotational actuators are at the neutral position.

According to Chebychev-Grübler-Kutzbach's formula, the DoF of the proposed mechanism can be obtained as:

$$DoF = m(N_l - 1 - N_j) + \sum_{k=1}^{N_j} f_k = 6(11 - 1 - 12) + 18 = 6 \tag{1}$$

where m represents the DoF of the space in which a mechanism is intended to function and for the spatial case, $m = 6$, N_l and N_j represent the numbers of the links and joints in the mechanism, respectively, and f_k represents the degrees of relative motion permitted by joint i. Therefore, the proposed 6-DoF 3-PRRS parallel manipulator can be fully actuated by 3 linear and 3 rotatory actuators. Furthermore, according to the study in [20, 21], the maximum value for the Jacobian determinant, $|J|$, of the 3–3 6-DoF parallel manipulators would occur when the base size is two times of the moving platform. Taking this into account, the dimension relation between moving and base platforms in this design is determined and we can obtain as $r_b = 2r_m$ at the initial configuration.

3 Analysis

To evaluate the mobility of the proposed design, a kinematic analysis is conducted in this section. In Fig. 2, the schematic diagram of the parallel manipulator is illustrated with only one leg demonstrated to reduce the complexity. Two Cartesian coordinate systems *{O}:O-UVW* and *{P}:P-XYZ* are fixed on the centres (i.e. points O and P) of the base and the moving platform, respectively. In the i-th leg, the joint points are denoted by O_{1i}, O_{2i}, O_{3i}, and O_{4i}, , (i = 1, 2, 3), respectively. The length of linear actuator i is denoted by $OO_{1i} = a_i = a + l_i$. The rotatory actuator i is attached at the point O_{1i} and its rotation axis is perpendicular to OO_{1i} with an offset of h. It can be noted that OO_{1i} is the translating along X-axis, forming the prismatic kinematic pair. Linkage $O_{2i}O_{3i}$, with the length of b, is connected with rotatory actuator i which rotates about Z_{2i}-axis at point O_{2i}. Then linkage $O_{3i}O_{4i}$, with the length of f, is connected to the linkage $O_{2i}O_{3i}$ and rotates about Z_{3i}-axis at point O_{3i} and another side was connected to the moving platform at the point O_{4i} through a spherical kinematic pair.

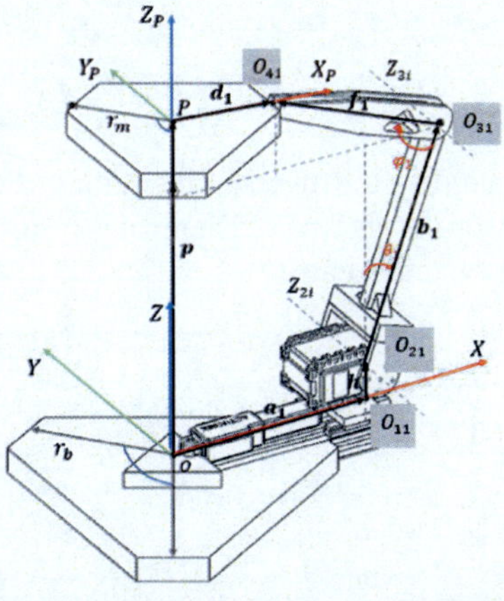

Fig. 2. Kinematic scheme of the proposed 3-PRRS parallel manipulator

3.1 Inverse Kinematic Analysis

In this subsection, inverse kinematic analysis is conducted, namely, to obtain input translation of $L = \left[l_1, l_2, l_3\right]^T$ and rotation of $\Theta = \left[\theta_1, \theta_2, \theta_3\right]^T$ with the known desired pose of moving platform $P = [X_P, Y_P, Z_P, \alpha, \beta.\gamma]$.

The homogeneous transformation matrix between the two coordinate systems $\{O\}$ and $\{P\}$ can be expressed as:

$$ {}^{O}T_P = \begin{bmatrix} {}^{O}R_P & P \\ 0 & 1 \end{bmatrix} = \begin{bmatrix} t_{11} & t_{12} & t_{13} & X_P \\ t_{21} & t_{22} & t_{23} & Y_P \\ t_{31} & t_{32} & t_{33} & Z_P \\ 0 & 0 & 0 & 1 \end{bmatrix} \tag{2} $$

where rotation matrix ${}^{O}R_P = R_z(\gamma)R_y(\beta)\,R_x(\alpha)$ and we can obtain that

$$ \begin{aligned} &t_{11} = c\gamma c\beta,\ t_{12} = c\gamma s\beta s\alpha - s\gamma c\alpha,\ t_{13} = c\gamma s\beta c\alpha + s\gamma s\alpha \\ &t_{21} = s\gamma s\beta,\ t_{22} = s\gamma s\beta s\alpha + c\gamma c\alpha,\ t_{23} = s\gamma s\beta c\alpha - c\gamma s\alpha \\ &t_{31} = -s\beta,\ t_{32} = c\beta s\alpha,\ t_{33} = c\beta c\alpha \end{aligned} $$

where s and c represent the *sin* and *cos* respectively.

In the i-th leg, the close-chain vector expression can be obtained as:

$$ \boldsymbol{p} = \boldsymbol{a}_i + \boldsymbol{h} + \boldsymbol{b}_i + \boldsymbol{f}_i - \boldsymbol{d}_i \tag{4} $$

where
$\boldsymbol{a}_1 = (r_b + l_1)[1, 0, 0]^T$, $\boldsymbol{a}_2 = (r_b + l_2)[-\frac{1}{2}, \frac{\sqrt{3}}{2}, 0]^T$,$\boldsymbol{a}_3 = (r_b + l_3)[-\frac{1}{2}, -\frac{\sqrt{3}}{2}, 0]^T$
$\boldsymbol{b}_1 = b[s\theta_1, 0, c\theta_1]^T$, $\boldsymbol{b}_2 = b[-\frac{1}{2}s\theta_2, \frac{\sqrt{3}}{2}s\theta_2, c\theta_2]^T$, $\boldsymbol{b}_3 = b[-\frac{1}{2}s\theta_3, -\frac{\sqrt{3}}{2}s\theta_3, c\theta_3]^T$,
$\boldsymbol{d}_1 = r_m{}^{O}T_P[1, 0, 0]^T$, $\boldsymbol{d}_2 = r_m{}^{O}T_P\,[-\frac{1}{2}, \frac{\sqrt{3}}{2}, 0]^T$, $\boldsymbol{d}_3 = r_m{}^{O}T_P\,[-\frac{1}{2}, -\frac{\sqrt{3}}{2}, 0]^T$,
$\boldsymbol{f}_1 = f[-c\delta_1, 0, s\delta_1]^T$, $\boldsymbol{f}_2 = f[\frac{1}{2}c\delta_2, -\frac{\sqrt{3}}{2}c\delta_2, s\delta_2]^T$, $\boldsymbol{f}_3 = f[\frac{1}{2}c\delta_3, \frac{\sqrt{3}}{2}c\delta_3, s\delta_3]^T$,
$\delta_i = \theta_i + \varphi_i - \frac{\pi}{2}$, and $\boldsymbol{h} = [0, 0, h]^T$, $\boldsymbol{p} = [X_P, Y_P, Z_P]^T$

It is worth noting that to simplify the inverse kinematics, the angle of φ_i are obtained by the additional rotation sensor in this work. Therefore, bring all of known parameters into Eq. (4), we can obtain the L and Θ are

$$ L = \begin{bmatrix} \frac{r_m}{2}t_{31} + Z_P \pm \sqrt{f^2 - \left(\frac{r_m}{2}t_{11} + X_P - \frac{r_b}{2}\right)^2 - \left(\frac{r_m}{2}t_{21} + Y_p\right)^2} \\ -\frac{r_m}{4}d_{31} + \frac{\sqrt{3}r_m}{4}t_{32} + Z_p \pm \sqrt{f^2 - \left(-\frac{r_m}{4}t_{11} + \frac{\sqrt{3}b}{4}t_{12} + X_p + \frac{r_b}{4}\right)^2 - \left(-\frac{r_m}{4}t_{21} + \frac{\sqrt{3}b}{4}t_{22} + Y_p - \frac{\sqrt{3}r_b}{4}\right)^2} \\ -\frac{r_m}{4}d_{31} - \frac{\sqrt{3}r_m}{4}t_{32} + Z_p \pm \sqrt{f^2 - \left(-\frac{r_m}{4}t_{11} - \frac{\sqrt{3}b}{4}t_{12} + X_p + \frac{r_b}{4}\right)^2 - \left(-\frac{r_m}{4}t_{21} - \frac{\sqrt{3}b}{4}t_{22} + Y_p + \frac{\sqrt{3}r_b}{4}\right)^2} \end{bmatrix} \tag{5} $$

$$ \Theta = \begin{bmatrix} \tan^{-1}\frac{\frac{r_m}{2}t_{21} + Y_p}{L_1 - \frac{r_m}{2}T_{31} - Z_p} \\ \tan^{-1}\frac{\frac{\sqrt{3}r_m}{4}t_{11} - \frac{3r_m}{4}t_{12} - \sqrt{3}X_p + \frac{r_m}{4}t_{21} - \frac{\sqrt{3}r_m}{4}t_{22} - Y_p}{2L_2 + \frac{r_m}{2}t_{31} - \frac{\sqrt{3}r_m}{2}t_{32} - 2Z_p} \\ \tan^{-1}\frac{-\frac{\sqrt{3}r_m}{4}t_{11} - \frac{3r_m}{4}t_{12} + \sqrt{3}X_p + \frac{r_m}{4}t_{21} + \frac{\sqrt{3}r_m}{4}t_{22} - Y_p}{2L_3 + \frac{r_m}{2}t_{31} + \frac{\sqrt{3}r_m}{2}t_{32} - 2Z_p} \end{bmatrix} \tag{6} $$

Based on the mathematical model and analyses performed in this kinematic analysis, the cochlear implant robot has good manufacturability and function-ability, as well as a relatively simple control algorithm when compared with other manipulators with six degrees of freedom. As a result of these features, the 3-PRRS parallel manipulator is well suited for use in medical applications, in this case cochlear implants, hence its application in this project.

4 Experiment

4.1 Experimental Setup

In Fig. 3, a prototype of the proposed 6-DoF 3-PRRS parallel manipulator is built up by utilizing rapid prototyping technology. The fixed base consists of three flexible bars with a linear actuator mounted on each of them. The linkages and moving platform are built by 3D printing with PLA materials. It is noted that the inserted electrode array for the CI surgery [9] (not included in Fig. 3) can be mounted on the moving platform by three fasten holes.

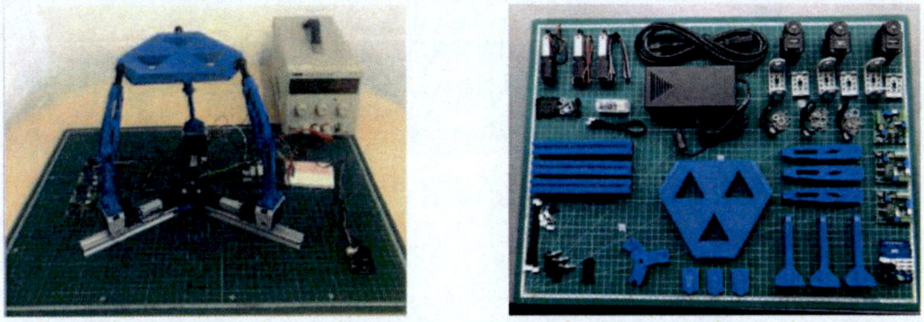

(a) (b)

Fig. 3. (a)The prototype of the proposed 6-DoF 3-PRPS PM (b) layout of elements

In this prototype, the selected rotatory motor is Dynamixel AX-12A which is driven by a Dynamixel motor shield. This combination not only has satisfied dimensions but also provides the potentiality to apply advanced control by reading various sensing data (e.g., position, velocity, and temperature). The Actuonix L12 with its default driver LAC board is selected for the linear actuator due to its compact size and position feedback.

A PID controller is built on an Arduino UNO board by sending a controlling signal to corresponding motor drivers. There are a couple of advantages that combine the Arduino board with LAC and Dynamixel motor shield boards. The boards provide the position feedback signal and researchers can monitor the position of the actuator in real-time. In the meantime, the boards offer direct control of the speed, sensitivity, extended end-of-stroke limits, and retracted end-of-stroke limits.

4.2 Insertion Test

The difficulty during the current cochlear implant surgery is the visibility in the inner ear structure and damage caused by the insertion device. Therefore, the test aimed to examine the stability and maneuverability of the parallel manipulator platform during the operation.

In Figs. 4 and 5, sequential movements are performed by the built prototype to preliminarily evaluate the mobilities required by cochlear implant insertion, in terms of linear insertion range and rotation range. The input movement commented for each motor is obtained from the kinematics analysis in Sect. 3.

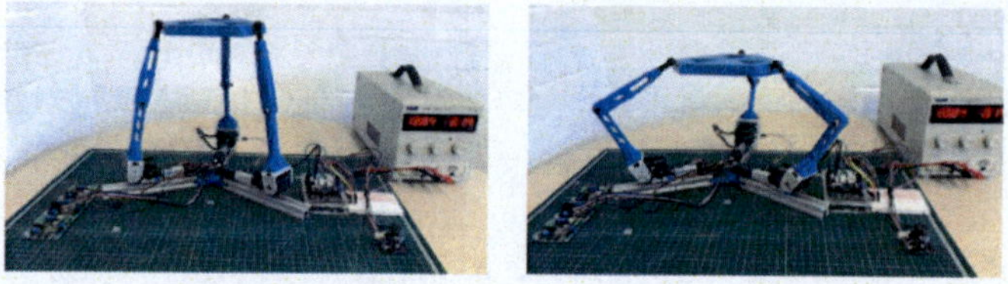

Fig. 4. Linear movements of the platform,

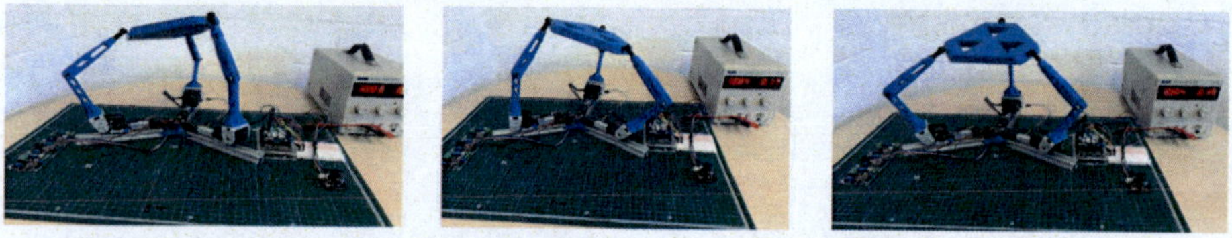

Fig. 5. Rotation movements of the platform.

5 Conclusion

In this paper, a novel design of a 6-DoF 3-PRRS parallel manipulator is proposed to perform robot-assisted cochlear implant insertion. Inverse kinematic analysis is carried out based on the close-loop vector chain method and only one set of solutions is chosen for moving the actuators due to the physical setup. A preliminary prototype is built to test the motion range of the proposed design and to evaluate its functionality for further performing cochlear implant insertion surgery in future work.

Acknowledgments. This work was supported by Brunel University London BRIEF funding.

References

1. Eshraghi, A.A., Nazarian, R., Telischi, F.F., Rajguru, S.M., Truy, E., Gupta, C.: The cochlear implant: historical aspects and future prospects. I Wiley Periodicals Inc. THE ANATOMICAL RECORD **295**, 1967–1980 (1967)
2. Wilson, B.S., Dorman, M.F.: Cochlear Implants: Current Designs and Future Possibilities. **45**(5), 695–730 (2008)

3. Auinger, A.B., Dahm, V., Liepins, R., Riss, D., Baumgartner, W.D., Arnoldner, C.: Robotic cochlear implant surgery: imaging-based evaluation of feasibility in clinical routine. Front Surg **8**, 423 (2021)
4. [Intracochlear placement of cochlear implant electrodes in soft surgery technique] - PubMed'. https://pubmed.ncbi.nlm.nih.gov/8376183/. Accessed 29 Jan 2023
5. Friedland, D.R., Runge-Samuelson, C.: Soft cochlear implantation: rationale for the surgical approach. Trends Amplif. **13**(2), 124 (2009)
6. Wanna, G.B., et al.: Impact of electrode design and surgical approach on scalar location and cochlear implant outcomes. Laryngoscope **124**(S6), S1–S7 (2014)
7. Bhavana, K., Bharti, B., Vishwakarma, R.: Round window insertion in veria technique of cochlear implantation: an essential modification. Indian J Otolaryngol Head Neck Surg. **71**(Suppl 2), 1586–1591 (2019)
8. Vittoria, S., et al.: Robot-based assistance in middle ear surgery and cochlear implantation: first clinical report. Eur. Arch. Otorhinolaryngol. **278**(1), 77–85 (2020)
9. Miroir, M., Nguyen, Y., Szewczyk, J., et al.: Design, kinematic optimization, and evaluation of a teleoperated system for middle ear microsurgery. Sci. World J. (2012)
10. Hafeez, N., et al.: Real-time data-driven approach for prediction and correction of electrode array trajectory in cochlear implantation. Applied Sciences **12**, 6343 (2022)
11. Henslee, A.M., Kaufmann, C.R., Andrick, M.D., Reineke, P.T., Tejani, V.D., Hansen, M.R.: Development and characterization of an electrocochleography-guided robotics-assisted cochlear implant array insertion system. Otolaryngology-Head and Neck Surgery **2**, 334–340 (2022)
12. Camacho-Arreguin, J.I., Wang, M., Russo, M., Dong, X., Axinte, D.: Novel reconfigurable walking machine tool enables symmetric and nonsymmetric walking configurations. IEEE/ASME Transactions on Mechatronics (2022)
13. Olazagoitia, J.L., Wyatt, S.: New PKM tricept T9000 and its application to flexible manufacturing at aerospace industry. SAE Technical Paper Series (2007)
14. Wang, M.F., Ceccarelli, M., Carbone, G.: Experimental tests on operation performance of a LARM leg mechanism with 3-DOF parallel architecture. Mechanical Sci. **6**(1), 1–8 (2015)
15. Leal-Naranjo, J.-A., Wang, M., Paredes-Rojas, J.-C., Rostro-Gonzalez, H.: Design and kinematic analysis of a new 3-DOF spherical parallel manipulator for a prosthetic wrist. J. Braz. Soc. Mech. Sci. Eng. **42**(1), 1–12 (2019)
16. Li, Y., Xu, Q.: Design and development of a medical parallel robot for cardiopulmonary resuscitation. IEEE/ASME Trans on Mechatronics **12**(3), 265–273 (2007)
17. Dalvand, M.M., Shirinzadeh, B.: Remote centre-of-motion control algorithms of 6-RRCRR parallel robot assisted surgery system (PRAMiSS). Proc IEEE Int Conf Robot Autom, pp. 3401–3406 (2012)
18. Chaker, A., Mlika, A., Laribi, M.A., Romdhane, L., Zeghloul, S.: Synthesis of spherical parallel manipulator for dexterous medical task. Front. Mech. Eng. **7**(2), 150–162 (2012)
19. Nunes, W.M., Rodrigues, L.A.O., Oliveira, L.P., Ribeiro, J.F., Carvalho, J.C.M., Gonçalves, R.S.: Cable-based parallel manipulator for rehabilitation of shoulder and elbow movements. In: IEEE International Conference on Rehabilitation Robotics (2011)
20. Lee, J.: Investigation of quality indices of in-parallel platform manipulators and development of web based analysis tools. PhD Dissertation, University of Florida, Gainesville, FL (2000)
21. Baigunchekov, Z.Z., Kaiyrov, R.A.: Direct kinematics of a 3-PRRS type parallel manipulator. Int. J. Mechanical Eng. Robotics Res. **9**(7), 967–972 (2020)

Fuzzy Logic Systems: From WisdomofAge Mentoring Platform to Medical Robots

Rus Gabriela[1], Bogdan Gherman[1](✉), Laurentiu Nae[2], Calin Vaida[1], Adrian Pisla[1], Eduard Oprea[2], Claudiu Schonstein[1], Tiberiu Antal[1], and Doina Pisla[1]

[1] CESTER, Technical University of Cluj-Napoca, Memorandumului 28, Cluj-Napoca, Romania
bogdan.gherman@mep.utcluj.ro

[2] Digital Twin, Bd. Mircea Voda 24, Bucharest, Romania

Abstract. Quality of life [QOL] is a powerful tool used overwide to measure self-perception about life offering valuable information in various domains. One of effectiveness methods used to analyze QOL is based on fuzzy system, since fuzzy numbers are more suitable with this type of evaluation considering the ambiguous nature of the answers. In this paper a fuzzy logic system was developed to analyze QOL for seniors in order to assess the positive outcomes of a digital mentoring platform-WisdomofAge. The results demonstrated that fuzzy system developed is superior to conventional methods in the analysis of quality of life and could be implemented with successful. Furthermore, the AHP analyses revealed that psychological aspects of the life such the reducing symptoms of depression are closely related with the utilization of the platform and the utilization of robots in medical treatment and recovery.

Keywords: Fuzzy logic system · Mentoring platform · Quality of Life · Health of seniors

1 Introduction

The increased life expectancy of people worldwide could be viewed as a direct result of the advance of our society, many studies revealing that in the past century, there have been more people over 60 than at any other time in history [1, 2]. However, this positive aspect of our society brought with it a series of concerns, many of them being regarded to the psychological condition of elderly [3], considering that disorders such as depression and anxiety are very often met at old people [4].

Because one of the major causes of depression at this age is represented by poor interactions and the inactivity of individuals [3], a possible solution for this difficult situation could be the reintegrating of seniors into a healthy work environment, thus assuring a superior quality of life (QOL).

Wisdom of Age (WOA) [5, 6], is a mentoring platform, developed to bring together the elderly people with a background in domains like engineering, IT or management and companies which need an expert in such fields. The platform offers adequate support

D. Tarnita et al. (Eds.): MESROB 2023, MMS 133, pp. 50–59, 2023.
https://doi.org/10.1007/978-3-031-32446-8_6

for those seniors who want to be in touch with the new discoveries of the field in which they have the expertise and want to share a vast experience, ensuring an additional source of income.

Even though WoA represents a viable solution to improve the psychological condition of individuals, reintegrating them into a suitable work environment, the platform's aim is to offer a superior experience for users so, a quality-of-life survey based on fuzzy logic was introduced, to analyze the impact of the platform on the seniors and to examine how in which way their life is impacted by the platform.

There are different methods used to evaluate QOL, the most known being Likert scale [7], where every item received a score from 1–5 or 1–7. Using this tool, data analysis can be performed at the ordinal level or the interval level. For the ordinal level, the central tendency is typically measured by the median or mode, while for the interval level, the analysis of variance (ANOVA) or Pearson's correlation is used. Even though this tool presents a series of advantages such as user friendliness or the ability to operationalize complex topics, there are some drawn backs that should be mentioned like the predisposition for bias or the possibility of subjective interpretations.

As a response for the weaknesses presented above, recently a new approach based on fuzzy set theory (FST) was proposed. Incorporating FST in traditional scales, this method shows obvious advantages including the improvements in validation of clinical applications, providing a large quantity of information about the psychology of the patients and reduce the bias in self questionnaire [8]. Compared with standard logic where all values are 0 and 1, fuzzy systems can handle complex situations where the statements can have value of partial truth (0.4, 0.7 etc.).

The aim of this paper is to develop a fuzzy logic system for WoA platform, which will be eventually implemented to analyze the quality of life for seniors involved in surgery or recovery procedures performed with robotics systems. The same architecture, using a different survey, can be used for other applications as well, i.e. automatic analysis and prioritization of patients waiting in the emergency reception unit.

Following the introduction section, Sect. 2 describes the methodological aspects involved in both the quality-of-life surveys and the fuzzy system developing. Section 3 presents the results of the system, followed by Sect. 4 where the results and the possibility to reintegrate the system in medical robots' procedure are discussed. In Sect. 5 the final ideas about the paper are presented.

2 Methodology

2.1 Quality of Live Surveys

Many quality-of-life scales developed over the time, each of them being able to highlight status of different aspects of life such as physical condition, economic situation or social aspects. For this study QOL developed by World Health Organization (WHO) in 2012 was chosen, this scale targeting six domains (Physical health, Psychological health, Level of Independence, Social relationships, Environment Spirituality/Religion/Personal beliefs) [9].

Since spiritual beliefs don't provide a meaningful perspective inside the WisdomofAge platform, only the first five domains from the entire number were maintained for the purposes of this paper.

The survey was developed in cooperation with a specialist in psychology and contains 15 questions (three for each analyzed area). For each question, there are five items on a 5-point scale ranging from 1 to 5 (with respect for WHO quality of life model), as can be seen in Table 1. This question is just an example from surveys [10] and refers to the capacity to perform everyday activities being part of physical health. Other questions are related to the desire to experience positive feelings (psychological health), to the possibility of sustaining a decent life (economic), to aspiration of having more friends (social health) and to feeling of being safe and independent in the current environment (environment).

Table 1. Examples of question from QOL survey

Question	Answer
In your opinion, in what capacity can you perform everyday activities? (Physical health)	A Completely impaired capacity (1 p) B Severely impaired capacity (2 p) C Moderate capacity (3 p) D Good capacity (4 p) E Excellent capacity (5 p)

2.2 Fuzzy Logic System

Fuzzy Logic Designer provided by MATLAB framework [11] was used to develop the fuzzy system employing Mamdani system. This system is often used to create fuzzy systems in different domains, having a simple and easy understandable configuration based on three main stages:

1. **Fuzzification process** where the inputs are transformed from crisp values fuzzy membership functions.
2. **Defining and executing fuzzy rules**
3. **Defuzzification process** which involves the conversion of outputs in crisp values

The fuzzy system proposed is described in Fig. 1. The system is composed of 15 inputs (each for every question) and 5 outputs (one output for every domain).

In the first stage membership functions for inputs were constructed to correlate with all possible answers from every question (Fig. 2). For this aim, the interval of member function was defined from 0 to 5 and all member functions was set to be Gaussian, this function returning fuzzy membership values using the function presented in Eq. (1).

$$f(x, \sigma, c) = e^{\frac{-(x-c)^2}{2\sigma^2}} \quad (1)$$

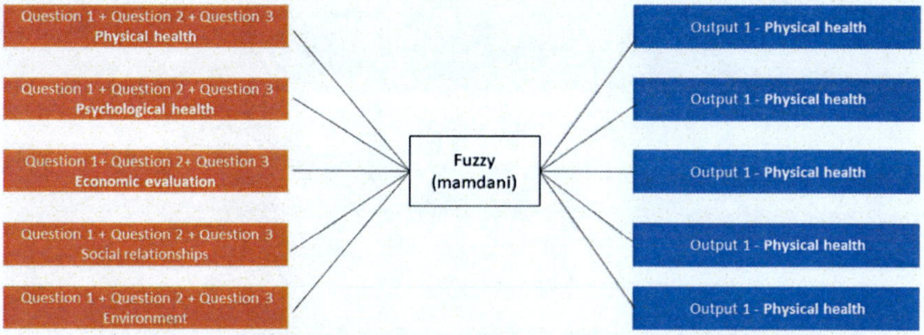

Fig. 1. QOL Fuzzy logic system developed for WoA platform.

where x are the input values, σ is the standard deviation and c is the mean.

Every question contains three functions named:

- PoorQn (**n** being the **no** of the question) function's input values [1 0];
- AverageQn function's input values [1 2.5];
- GoodQn function's input values [1 5];

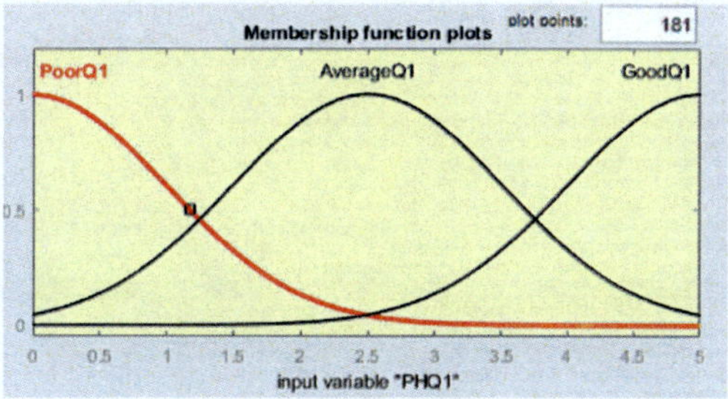

Fig. 2. Membership functions defined as input

For outputs the constructed membership outputs (Fig. 3) are defined on a scale from 0 through 15, using a triangular membership function presented in Eq. (2).

$$f(x, a, b, c) = \max\left(\min\left(\frac{x-a}{b-a}, \frac{c-x}{c-b}\right), 0\right) \tag{2}$$

where x represents the input parameters, a and c are defined as the base of membership and b its defined as the peak of the function.

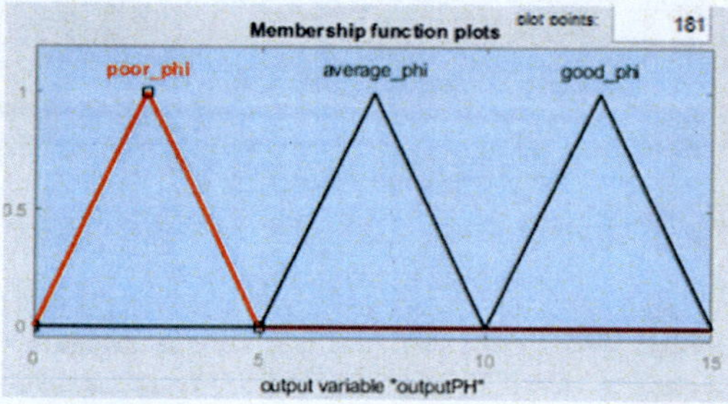

Fig. 3. Membership functions defined as output

For every output are defined three membership functions:

- Poor – function's input values [0 2.5 5]
- Average – function's input values [5 7.5 10]
- Good- function's input values [10 12.5 15]

Since the fuzzy systems are based on IF-THEN rules, the **stage two** consists in creation of a rule's set to cover every possible scenario (Fig. 4). For every domain six rules were created, resulting a total of 30 rules, every rule having a weight equal with 1.

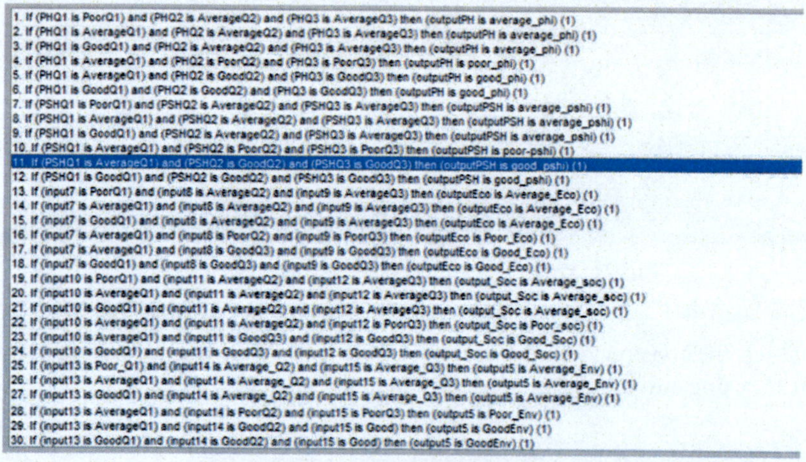

1. If (PHQ1 is PoorQ1) and (PHQ2 is AverageQ2) and (PHQ3 is AverageQ3) then (outputPH is average_phi) (1)
2. If (PHQ1 is AverageQ1) and (PHQ2 is AverageQ2) and (PHQ3 is AverageQ3) then (outputPH is average_phi) (1)
3. If (PHQ1 is GoodQ1) and (PHQ2 is AverageQ2) and (PHQ3 is AverageQ3) then (outputPH is average_phi) (1)
4. If (PHQ1 is AverageQ1) and (PHQ2 is PoorQ2) and (PHQ3 is PoorQ3) then (outputPH is poor_phi) (1)
5. If (PHQ1 is AverageQ1) and (PHQ2 is GoodQ2) and (PHQ3 is GoodQ3) then (outputPH is good_phi) (1)
6. If (PHQ1 is GoodQ1) and (PHQ2 is GoodQ2) and (PHQ3 is GoodQ3) then (outputPH is good_phi) (1)
7. If (PSHQ1 is PoorQ1) and (PSHQ2 is AverageQ2) and (PSHQ3 is AverageQ3) then (outputPSH is average_pshi) (1)
8. If (PSHQ1 is AverageQ1) and (PSHQ2 is AverageQ2) and (PSHQ3 is AverageQ3) then (outputPSH is average_pshi) (1)
9. If (PSHQ1 is GoodQ1) and (PSHQ2 is AverageQ2) and (PSHQ3 is AverageQ3) then (outputPSH is average_pshi) (1)
10. If (PSHQ1 is AverageQ1) and (PSHQ2 is PoorQ2) and (PSHQ3 is PoorQ3) then (outputPSH is poor-pshi) (1)
11. If (PSHQ1 is AverageQ1) and (PSHQ2 is GoodQ2) and (PSHQ3 is GoodQ3) then (outputPSH is good_pshi) (1)
12. If (PSHQ1 is GoodQ1) and (PSHQ2 is GoodQ2) and (PSHQ3 is GoodQ3) then (outputPSH is good_pshi) (1)
13. If (input7 is PoorQ1) and (input8 is AverageQ2) and (input9 is AverageQ3) then (outputEco is Average_Eco) (1)
14. If (input7 is AverageQ1) and (input8 is AverageQ2) and (input9 is AverageQ3) then (outputEco is Average_Eco) (1)
15. If (input7 is GoodQ1) and (input8 is AverageQ2) and (input9 is AverageQ3) then (outputEco is Average_Eco) (1)
16. If (input7 is AverageQ1) and (input8 is PoorQ2) and (input9 is PoorQ3) then (outputEco is Poor_Eco) (1)
17. If (input7 is AverageQ1) and (input8 is GoodQ3) and (input9 is GoodQ3) then (outputEco is Good_Eco) (1)
18. If (input7 is GoodQ1) and (input8 is GoodQ3) and (input9 is GoodQ3) then (outputEco is Good_Eco) (1)
19. If (input10 is PoorQ1) and (input11 is AverageQ2) and (input12 is AverageQ3) then (output_Soc is Average_soc) (1)
20. If (input10 is AverageQ1) and (input11 is AverageQ2) and (input12 is AverageQ3) then (output_Soc is Average_soc) (1)
21. If (input10 is GoodQ1) and (input11 is AverageQ2) and (input12 is AverageQ3) then (output_Soc is Average_soc) (1)
22. If (input10 is AverageQ1) and (input11 is AverageQ2) and (input12 is PoorQ3) then (output_Soc is Poor_soc) (1)
23. If (input10 is AverageQ1) and (input11 is GoodQ3) and (input12 is GoodQ3) then (output_Soc is Good_Soc) (1)
24. If (input10 is GoodQ1) and (input11 is GoodQ3) and (input12 is GoodQ3) then (output_Soc is Good_Soc) (1)
25. If (input13 is Poor_Q1) and (input14 is Average_Q2) and (input15 is Average_Q3) then (output5 is Average_Env) (1)
26. If (input13 is AverageQ1) and (input14 is Average_Q2) and (input15 is Average_Q3) then (output5 is Average_Env) (1)
27. If (input13 is GoodQ1) and (input14 is Average_Q2) and (input15 is Average_Q3) then (output5 is Average_Env) (1)
28. If (input13 is AverageQ1) and (input14 is PoorQ2) and (input15 is PoorQ3) then (output5 is Poor_Env) (1)
29. If (input13 is AverageQ1) and (input14 is GoodQ2) and (input15 is Good) then (output5 is GoodEnv) (1)
30. If (input13 is GoodQ1) and (input14 is GoodQ2) and (input15 is Good) then (output5 is GoodEnv) (1)

Fig. 4. List of rules for QOL fuzzy system

To complete stage number three the defuzzification method was used named centroid described in Eq. (3)

$$xCentroid = \frac{\sum_i \mu(x_i)x_i}{\sum_i \mu(x_i)} \tag{3}$$

3 Results

Based on the rules defined in stage two, and the inputs taken from the survey a graphical representation of the outcome resulting from the fuzzy process is presented in Fig. 5.

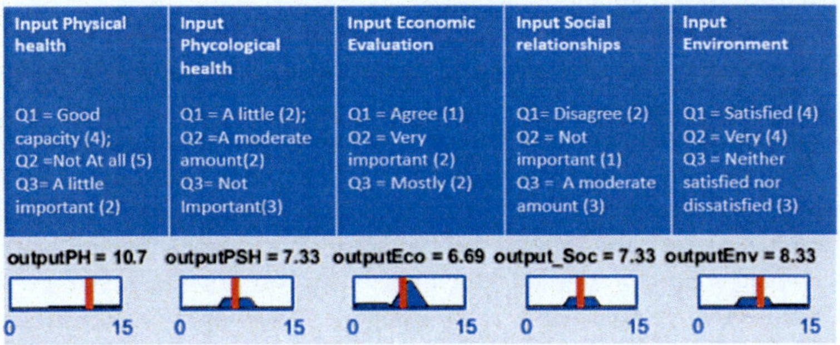

Fig. 5. Graphical representation of defuzzification process based on given inputs.

In order to test the system, a group of seniors from the end-user group of WoA platform was asked to complete the survey. The study group consisted in 38 participants (6 females and 34 males) from Switzerland, Belgium and Romania, the average age being 55 +. This survey was conducted in English. The answers were introduced as inputs data for the fuzzy system (like in Fig. 5) for a first analysis and then these answers were also analyzed with a conventional method (Median), in order to validate the system.

The results can be observed in Fig. 6.

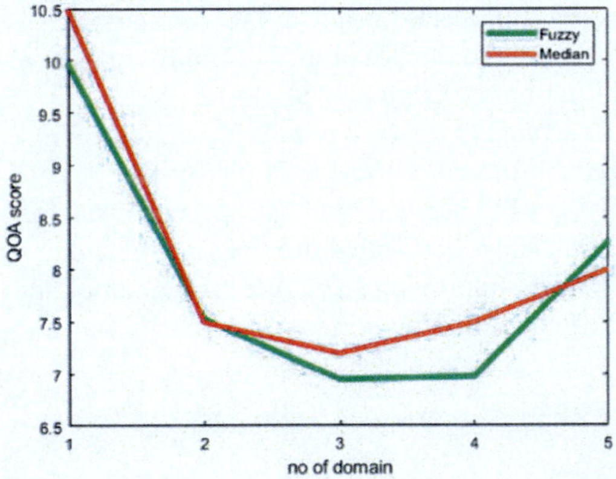

Fig. 6. A comparation between FST and median method.

As can be seen these two methods offered similar general information, this fact validating the fuzzy system. The difference between methods consists in the way the fuzzy system is built, which can provide more detailed information about the score, considering that there are many situations in which a value belongs more to one interval than to another, and this information can only be revealed using a fuzzy system (considering that FST is defined by ambiguous boundaries).

The results were analyzed by a specialized sociologist (from In4Care-Happy ageing organization from Belgium), who validated the results and confirmed that system could be used to analyze with success QOL for elderly.

To highlight those factors considered to be important for the elderly, both platform users and beneficiaries of treatments involving medical robots, such as rehabilitation. [12–14], two groups of seniors (10 users from platform and 10 patients in the motor rehabilitation phase) were asked which aspects of the platform, respectively of the robotic treatment are more important. Based on their responses two Analytic hierarchy process (AHP) analyses were performed (Fig. 7 a,b) using the following characteristics:

- **Ergonomics** refers to how comfortably and easily the robot can be used for rehabilitation purposes, as well as how easily users can operate the platform.
- **Increased self-esteem** refers to the evaluation of the impact on self-esteem aspect as a result of rehabilitation treatment/platform usage.
- **Continuous evolution** refers to the importance of continuous evolution process in rehabilitation/using the platform.
- **Depression** represents the factor that can be treated in rehabilitation process (if depression is caused by medical condition) or using the platform (if depression is caused by inactivity and lack of purpose).

Increased motivation refers to the importance of increasing motivation in rehabilitation treatment/utilization of the platform.

Improved social life refers to the possibility of improving social relationships as a result of medical rehabilitation/ utilization of platform.

Improved economic situation refers to possibility of improving economic situation as a result of medical rehabilitation/ utilization of platform.

Based on AHP analyses can observed that the aspects considered most important in both cases (WoA utilization and robotic rehabilitation) are related to reducing symptoms of depression and respectively improving social life, as the same time the less important aspects are related to the economic situation.

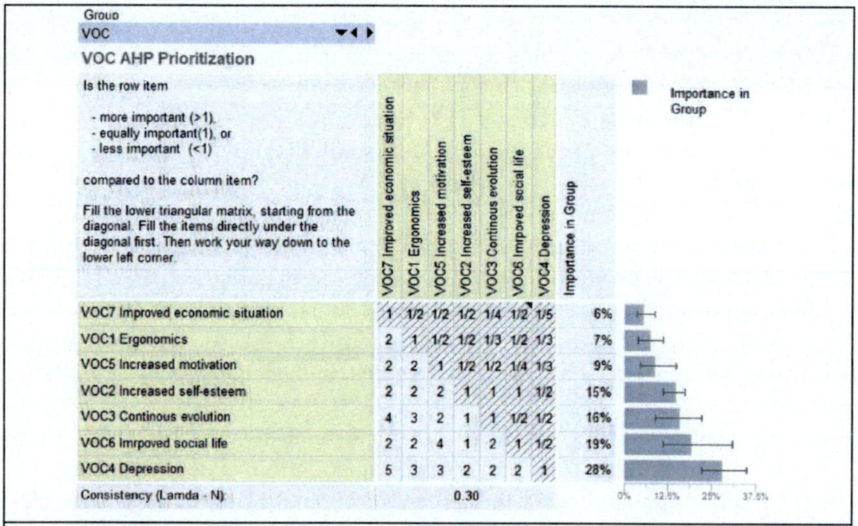

a) AHP analysys of mentoring platform users

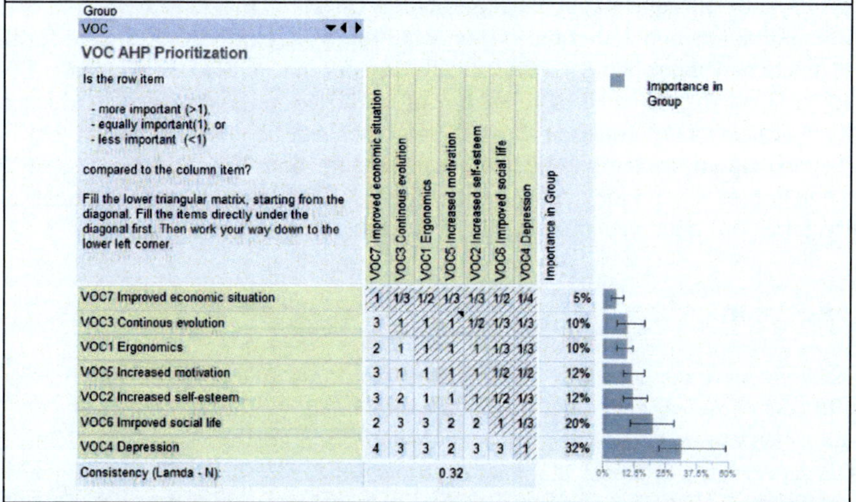

b) AHP analysys of rehabilitation treatment patients

Fig. 7. a) AHP analysys of mentoring platform users. b) AHP analysys of rehabilitation treatment patients

4 Discussion

Quality of life measure is a tool very useful when the perception of a person about his life could influence results for important aspects of life such as social relationships, financial decisions, medical treatment, or medical recovery.

Considering the impact of self-perception about life in medical treatment its critical [15, 16], QOL could provide valuable information in more medical subdomains where this method wasn't introduced yet.

Though medical robotics systems [17] became more popular and are being used more often [18, 19], there have been relatively few studies on how psychological factors may affect procedures with robots. A brief analysis of the subject revealed that self-perception could influence some aspects that are tangent with medical robots, especially in medical rehabilitation process, with emphasis on surgery post-operative follow-up recovery or rehabilitation of neuro-motor deficit. Because the effectiveness of the robots [16] for these applications is often analyzed based on recovery process, a deprecated perception about life could influence the recovery of patient. In this context, for an adequate evaluation of medical robots, psychological and social aspects should as part of the evaluation.

The fuzzy system developed to measure QOL could be easily implemented in pre- and post-operative patient analysis or in post-stroke rehabilitation, taking into account that psychology condition could influence the perception about the procedure, and implicitly on the way in which the procedure was done (with or without robots), mostly because some patients are still reticent about using robotics system in medicine.

It is important to notice that the system used for WoA platform is suitable for the patients mentioned above being it's designed for seniors and studies revealed that people who suffered from strokes and medical treatment are those people who are at an advanced age [20]. Furthermore, comparing the AHP analyses can be easily observed that the psychological situation seems to be very important for both group of seniors, so the implementation of a superior quality of life survey in robotic medical treatment and recovery, based on implementation in WoA platform, is more than useful.

5 Conclusion

The measurement of quality of life is particularly beneficial in many areas and provides insightful data on people regarding their perception on the quality of their life.

A fuzzy system using 30 rules has been developed to analyze assess the results of the QOL survey used to assess the positive impact of the WoA platform, designed to improve the life of retired seniors based on their valuable experience shared through the platform.

This analysis can be applied both to the WoA platform, which targets elderly people, and to the pre- and post-operative analysis of people who were subjected to medical procedures involving robots, offering a superior perception of how valuable robots in the medical domain are and how they could improve patient life.

Exploiting a topic rarely addressed in medical robotic area, an analysis about the importance of psychological condition in medical robotic treatment has been performed in this paper. Based on the idea that seniors using the platform and seniors involved in robotic rehabilitation have the same interest related to the improving the psychological condition a system that could be used to measure QOL for seniors was developed starting from the mentoring platform.

Acknowledgments. This work was supported by a grant of the Romanian Ministry of Research and In-novation, CCCDI - UEFISCDI and of the AAL Programme with co-funding from the European Union's Horizon 2020 research and innovation programme project number AAL-CP-AAL-2020–7-83-CP-WisdomOfAge within PNCDI III.

References

1. Partridge, L., Deelen, J., Slagboom, P.E.: Facing up to the global challenges of ageing. Nature **561**(7721), 45–56 (2018)
2. Beard, J.R., et al.: The World report on ageing and health: a policy framework for healthy ageing. The Lancet **387**(10033), 2145–2154 (2016)
3. Cosco, T., et al.: Healthy ageing, resilience and wellbeing. Epidemiology and Psychiatric Sciences **26**(06), 579–583 (2017)
4. Liu, L., Gou, Z., Zuo, J.: Social support mediates loneliness and depression in elderly people. J. Health Psychol. **21**(5), 750–758 (2014)
5. Gherman, B., et al.: WisdomOfAge: designing a platform for active and healthy ageing of senior experts in engineering. ICT for Health, Accessibility and Wellbeing. IHAW 2021. Communications in Computer and Information Science **1538** (2021)
6. Doina, P., et al.: Development of a learning management system for knowledge transfer in engineering. Acta Technica Napocensis - series: Applied Mathematics, Mechanics, and Engineering, [S.l.], **64**(3) (2021)
7. Bhandari, P., Nikolopoulou, K.: What Is a Likert Scale? | Guide & Examples. Scribbr. Retrieved January 7, 2023 (2022)
8. Chen, P.-Y., Yao, G.: Measuring quality of life with fuzzy numbers: in the perspectives of reliability, validity, measurement invariance, and feasibility (2015)
9. Programme on mental health-WOOQOL- user manual,2012
10. https://c8tbckvja0r.typeform.com/to/WFgEqYW9
11. Mathworks https://www.mathworks.com/products/fuzzy-logic.html. Accessed 5 Jan 2023
12. Major, Z.Z., et. al.: The impact of robotic rehabilitation on the motor system in neurological diseases. a multimodal neurophysiological approach. Int. J. Environ. Res. Public Health **17**, 6557 (2020)
13. Tucan, P., et al.: Optimization of the ASPIRE spherical parallel rehabilitation robot based on its clinical evaluation. Int. J. Environ. Res. Public Health, **18**, 3281.plitea (2021)
14. Pisla, D., et al.: Parallel robot with torque monitoring for brachial monoparesis rehabilitation tasks. Appl. Sci. **11**, 9932 (2021)
15. Britteon, P., Cullum, N., Sutton, M.: Association between psychological health and wound complications after surgery. Br. J. Surg. **104**(6), 769–776 (2017)
16. Panzeri, A., et al.: Interventions for psychological health of stroke caregivers: a systematic review. Frontiers in Psychology **10** (2019)
17. Gherman, B., et. al.: Singularities and workspace analysis for a parallel robot for minimally invasive surgery. In: 2010 IEEE International Conference on Automation, Quality and Testing, Robotics (AQTR), pp. 1–6
18. Plitea, N., et al.: Innovative development of surgical parallel robots. Acta Electronica, Mediamira Science, Cluj-Napoca **4**, 201–206 (2007)
19. Tucan, P., et al.: Used in single incision laparoscopic surgery, symposium on robot design, dynamics and control. ROMANSY-2022, CISM, **606**, pp. 115–122
20. Béjot, Y., et al.: Epidemiology of stroke and transient ischemic attacks: current knowledge and perspectives. Revue Neurologique **172**(1), 59–68 (2016)

Design of Medical Devices

Grip-Type Pseudo Force Display with Normal and Tangential Skin Stimulation

Mayuka Kojima(✉), Shunsuke Yoshimoto, and Akio Yamamoto

The University of Tokyo, Kashiwanoha 5-1-5, Kashiwa, Chiba, Japan
kojima@aml.t.u-tokyo.ac.jp
https://www.aml.t.u-tokyo.ac.jp/

Abstract. A device has been developed to present pseudo-force sensations by applying pressure stimulation to a palm. The device is equipped with a stimulator to apply normal pressure to a palm, which can be rotated within a 180° opening on the device's surface. The normal pressure can invoke pseudo-force sensations as if an external force is applied to the hand through the device. In previous devices, the direction of the pressure presentation was limited, but the new device can produce the pressure in various directions using a rotation mechanism. This enables the presentation of pseudo-force sensation in various directions. The rotation also allows skin stretch stimulation on the palm. These new features are expected to expand the range of scenarios experienced in virtual reality environments. As a demonstration, a simple VR fishing system was developed using the device, which could virtually present a force sensation from a fish on a hook.

Keywords: pseudo-haptics · normal pressure · skin stretch · palm

1 Introduction

It is known that the presentation of force perception enhances the sense of presence and intuition, and improves operation efficiency [1,2]. Therefore, its application has been studied in various fields such as teleoperation [3], virtual training [4], remote simulated surgery [5], and entertainment [6]. Pseudo-force presentation is one of the simple methods to provide force sensation. Pseudo force is often presented by visual stimuli, for example, by changing the speed of a pointer in a screen. However, the range of force that can be presented through such visual stimuli is limited. Another method for providing pseudo-force perception is tactile stimulation, in which mechanical stimulation to the skin creates the illusion of force [7]. Skin stimulation devices used for pseudo-force presentation do not need to be grounded, like typical haptic devices, and can thus be mobile. Such a feature makes it an ideal force presenting devices in immersive virtual reality environments.

Recently, grip-type controllers have been widely used in immersive virtual reality. Therefore, incorporating a pseudo-force presentation function into grip-type devices is essential. In order to present skin stimulation on a grip-type

D. Tarnita et al. (Eds.): MESROB 2023, MMS 133, pp. 63–70, 2023.
https://doi.org/10.1007/978-3-031-32446-8_7

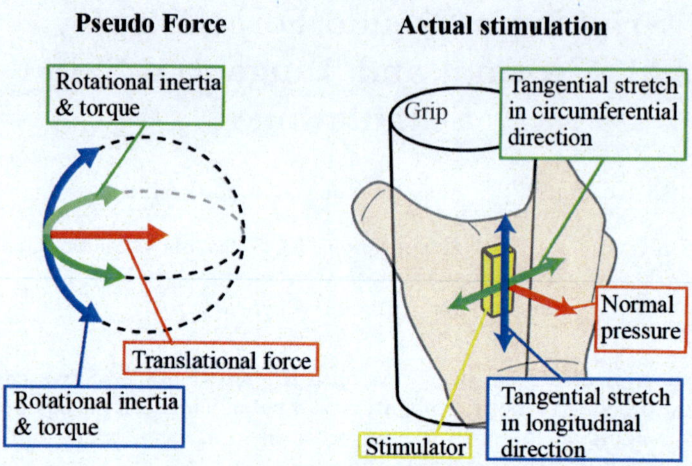

Fig. 1. Three types of cutaneous stimuli on a palm that may induce pseudo-force perception. Blue is the tangential force stimulus along the grip's longitudinal direction, green is along the circumferential direction, and red is the normal pressure stimulus. This work targets a combination of green and red stimuli.

controller, the most realistic target area is the palm, which is in direct contact with the grip. In the literature, tangential stimulation (skin stretch) [8] and normal stimulation (pressure) [9] for fingertips have been widely studied, but stimulation to the palm has not been extensively studied.

Three different stimulations are possible against a palm, which is normal pressure and tangential skin stretch in two directions, as shown in Fig. 1. When normal pressure is applied, the user feels as if he/she is being pushed by an external force through the grip [10]. On the other hand, tangential skin stretch can present rotational inertia and torque [11]. The tangential stretch along the longitudinal direction of a grip has already been demonstrated in [11], but the one along the circumferential direction (the direction from the thumb to the other fingers) has not been widely studied.

This work develops a grip-type device that can present two of the above three stimulations against a palm, which are normal pressure stimulation and tangential skin stretch in the circumferential direction, as in Fig. 2. The device is based on a normal pressure stimulation device developed in previous studies [10,12]. In the past, there have been studies on the presentation of pseudo force sensation to a palm using normal pressure [10,12–14]. Asada et al. [10] developed a one-degree-of-freedom pseudo-force presentation grip that can present pressure stimuli in the normal direction like the left one in Fig. 2. Nakamura et al. [12] developed a game-controller-type device that can present a pseudo-force sensation to both hands, which was applied for the operation of a tank in a virtual environment. However, those previous devices can present normal pressure only in a pre-defined direction (such as in the left illustration of Fig. 2). This work extends the degrees of freedom to enhance user experiences in virtual reality

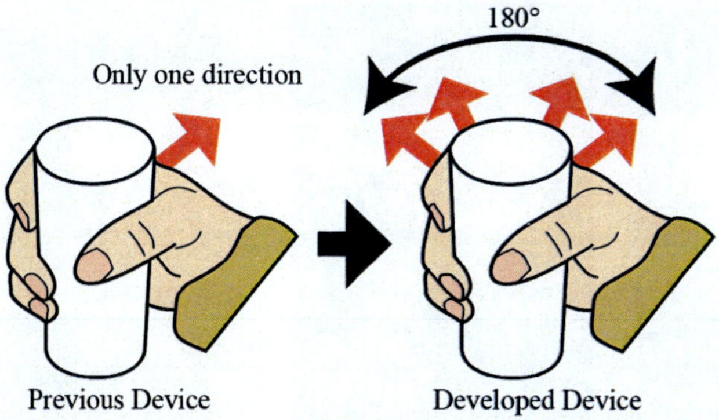

Fig. 2. Differences between previously developed devices and the device of this work. The previous devices can provide pressure only in one direction, but the new device can provide pressure within a 180° opening on the device.

(VR) and other applications. The device enables pseudo-force presentation in various directions on a palm using a rotation mechanism.

2 Device

2.1 Overview

Figure 3(a) shows the developed device. A user grasps the black gripping area covered with a low elastic rubber sheet, as in Fig. 3(b). The mechanism shown in Fig. 3(c) is installed under the black rubber, which pops out and rotates a stimulator. The device has two motors, which are used to pop out and rotate the stimulator, respectively. A combination of the DC gear motor and the lever pops out the stimulator. When the stimulator pops out, it provides normal pressure to the palm, which results in a pseudo-force sensation; due to the pressure, the user feels as if the device is pushing the palm. The servo motor rotates the whole mechanism to change the direction of popping out. This allows pseudo-force presentation in various directions, as well as skin stretch along the circumferential direction. Although the skin stretch in the circumferential direction has not been studied extensively, it would realize pseudo-force sensations such as torsion.

2.2 Device Design and Production

The developed device has a stepped cylindrical shape with diameters of 50 mm and 90 mm. The outer cover was made of PLA and was fabricated using a 3D printer. The lever and the cam were made of polyacetal and were machined using Roland MODELA PRO II MDX-540.

Figure 4 shows an exploded view of the device without the rubber sheet. The cavity opening in the cover is the area where the stimulator pops out and rotates. The rubber sheet covers the opening to reduce discomfort during grasping.

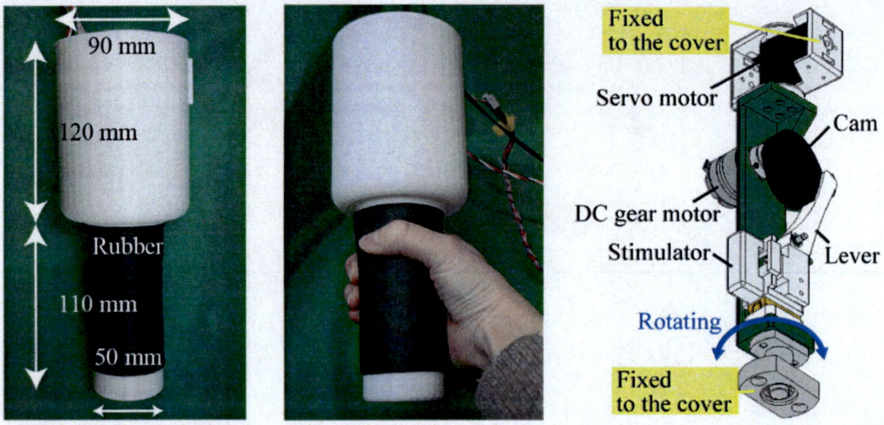

(a) Developed device. (b) The device gripped. (c) Device without cover (CAD).

Fig. 3. (a) Developed device. (b) The device gripped (c) CAD image of the internal mechanism.

It also smooths the contact surface and reduces friction between the stimulator and the palm during the rotation of the stimulator.

To provide normal pressure against the palm, a DC gear motor (FAULHABER, 2619S024SRIE2-16 112:1) rotates a cam to push a lever. The other end of the lever is connected to the stimulator through four springs (MiSUMi, WM3-10). The contraction of the springs is monitored using a reflective photo-interrupter (SG-105) for force measurement. Based on the measured contraction length, the rotation of the DC gear motor is controlled in the same manner as series elastic actuators (SEA).

A block diagram of the control is shown in Fig. 5(a). The pressure stimulus presentation unit was controlled by a microcomputer (Mbed LPC1768). A cascaded controller was programmed in the microcomputer, as in the figure. The maximum force at the stimulator was 15 N. As the contact area of the stimulator was 270 mm^2, the resulting normal pressure to the palm reached approximately 56 kPa.

The rotation is realized by a servo motor (Kondo Kagaku, KRS-3204R2 ICS). The servo motor is fixed to the cover of the device. The stimulator, the lever, and the DC gear motor are all installed on a single plate, which is shown using a green color in Fig. 3(c). This plate is connected to a rotary shaft and the servo motor, such that the servo motor can rotate it, as shown in Fig. 5(b). The servo motor is controlled by a microcomputer (Waves, ESP32-DevKitC V4), through a dedicated interface board (Kondo Kagaku, ICS conversion board). The angle of the opening on the grip surface, in which the stimulator rotated, was 180°.

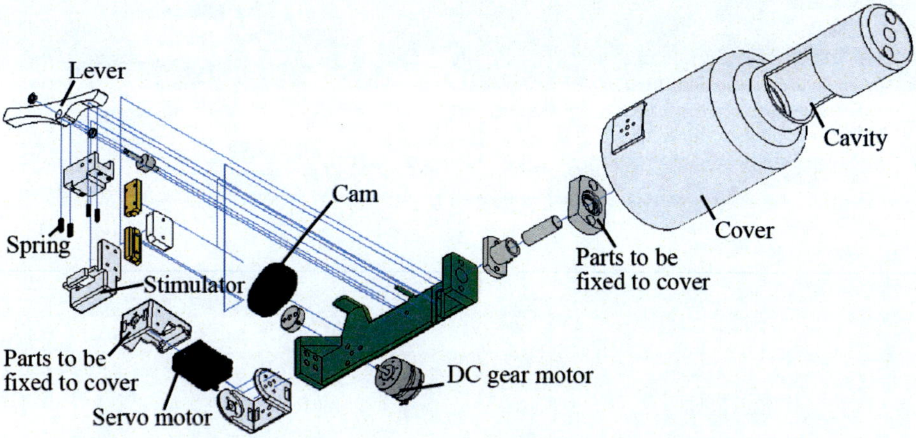

Fig. 4. Exploded view of the developed device.

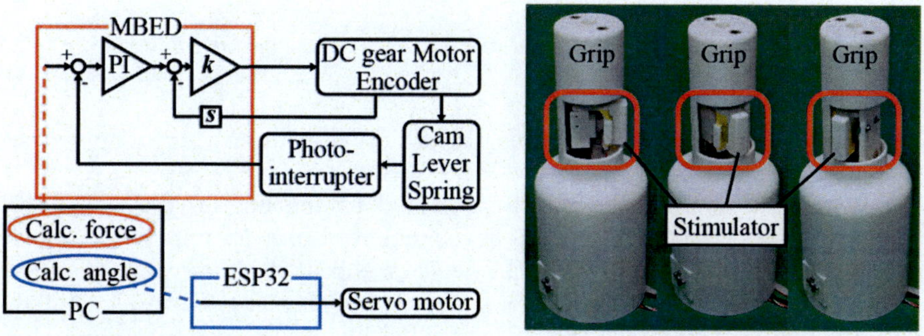

(a) Block diagram of control. (b) Stimulator is rotating.

Fig. 5. Block diagram of control and how the stimulator is rotated by the control.

3 Applications

The device can provide two different types of pseudo-force sensations: (1) normal force from the device by normal pressure and (2) rotational torque by skin stretch. Using these two types of sensations, various tools or experiences could be presented in a VR environment, such as operating a steering wheel of a car, operating a handle grip of a motorbike, and manipulating the oars or paddles of a boat.

In this article, we introduce VR fishing, in which a user operates a fishing rod, perceiving force in various directions. The demonstration focuses on the ability of the device to present pressure in various directions and the skin stretch was not demonstrated. The VR environment was implemented on a PC (Windows 11) using Unity, and communication with the device was done by serial communication on both ESP32 and Mbed. To simplify the implementation, the VR scene

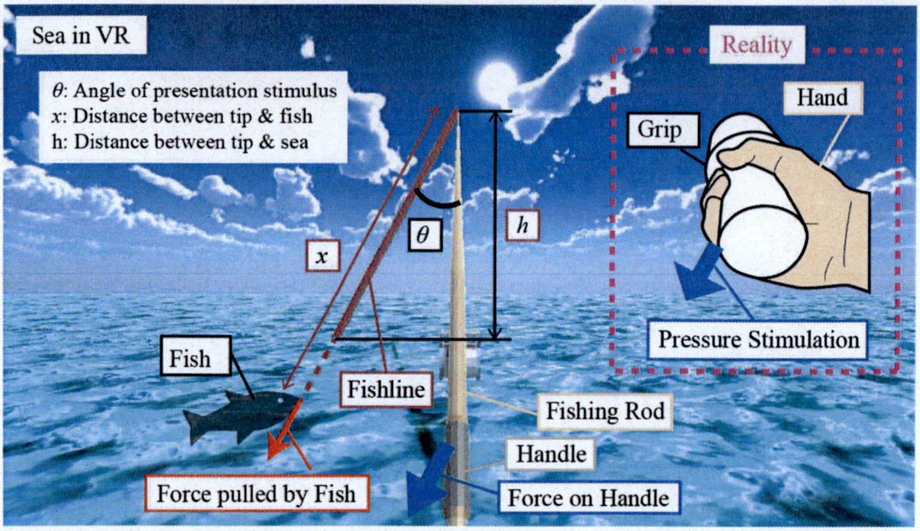

Fig. 6. A system that presents the force felt from a fishing rod while fishing.

was rendered on a typical 2D computer display; a VR head-mounted display was not utilized.

As shown in Fig. 6, a fishing rod and a red fishing line are shown in the computer display. Although in future development, a user is supposed to move the device to operate the fishing rod, the device was kept stationary for this time. This is because the motion tracking for the device was not yet implemented. Instead, the fish hooked at the end of the fishing line was moved by a computer mouse. As the fish moves, the fishing line is pulled by the movement of the fish, and the user feels as if the fishing rod is pulled in the direction of the fishing line.

The stimuli were calculated using x, h, and θ shown in the figure. The normal pressure applied to the palm was roughly proportional to the length of the fishing line, but with some offset. The height of the fishing rod, h, was used as the offset. As a result, the pressure was proportional to $x - h$. The direction of the pressure was decided by the angle θ. In such a way, the device simulated the sensation of a fishing rod being pulled by a fish from various directions.

4 Conclusion

This paper reported on a pseudo-haptic device that can apply pressure stimulation to a wide range of areas in the palm by rotating the stimulator. The pressure given by the stimulator invokes pseudo-force sensations in the user, whose direction can be changed within an opening of 180°. Such a rotation capability considerably expands the range of scenarios that can be experienced using the device. As an example, the paper reported on a VR fishing system that simulates the force felt from a fishing rod when a fish on a hook is moving. Future plans include an evaluation of the dynamic performance of the device, implementation of the system in immersive VR environments, and subjective studies to confirm the effectiveness of the pseudo-force sensation.

References

1. Stone, R.J.: Haptic feedback: a brief history from telepresence to virtual reality. In: Brewster, S., Murray-Smith, R. (eds.) Haptic HCI 2000. LNCS, vol. 2058, pp. 1–16. Springer, Heidelberg (2001). https://doi.org/10.1007/3-540-44589-7_1
2. Hayward, V., Astley, O.R., Cruz-Hernandez, M., Grant, D., Robles-De-La-Torre, G.: Haptic interfaces and devices. Sens. Rev. **24**(1), 16–29 (2004). https://doi.org/10.1108/02602280410515770
3. Artigas, J., et al.: KONTUR-2: force-feedback teleoperation from the international space station. In: Proceedings of the 2016 IEEE ICRA, pp. 1166–1173 (2016). https://doi.org/10.1109/ICRA.2016.7487246
4. Gibo, T.L., Bastian, A.J., Okamura, A.M.: Grip force control during virtual object interaction: effect of force feedback, accuracy demands, and training. IEEE Trans. Haptics **7**(1), 37–47 (2014). https://doi.org/10.1109/TOH.2013.60
5. Abdi, E., Kulić, D., Croft, E.: Haptics in teleoperated medical interventions: force measurement, haptic interfaces and their influence on user's performance. IEEE Trans. Biomed. Eng. **67**(12), 3438–3451 (2020). https://doi.org/10.1109/TBME.2020.2987603
6. Shim, Y.A., Park, K., Lee, S., Son, J., Woo, T., Lee, G.: FS-Pad: video game interactions using force feedback gamepad. In: Proceedings of the ACM UIST 2020, pp. 938–950 (2020). https://doi.org/10.1145/3379337.3415850
7. Ujitoko, Y., Ban, Y.: Survey of pseudo-haptics: haptic feedback design and application proposals. IEEE Trans. Haptics **14**(4), 699–711 (2021). https://doi.org/10.1109/TOH.2021.3077619
8. Schorr, S.B., Okamura, A.M.: Three-dimensional skin deformation as force substitution: wearable device design and performance during haptic exploration of virtual environment. IEEE Trans. Haptics **10**(3), 418–430 (2017). https://doi.org/10.1109/TOH.2017.2672969
9. Prattichizzo, D., Pacchierotti, C., Cenci, S., Minamizawa, K., Rosati, G.: Using a fingertip tactile device to substitute kinesthetic feedback in haptic interaction. In: Kappers, A.M.L., van Erp, J.B.F., Bergmann Tiest, W.M., van der Helm, F.C.T. (eds.) EuroHaptics 2010. LNCS, vol. 6191, pp. 125–130. Springer, Heidelberg (2010). https://doi.org/10.1007/978-3-642-14064-8_19
10. Asada, T., Nakamura, T., Yamamoto, A.: Investigation on substitution of force feedback using pressure stimulation to palm. In: Proceedings of IEEE Haptics Symposium 2016, pp. 389–390 (2016)
11. Guinan, A.L., Montandon, M.N., Doxon, A.J., Provancher, W.R.: Discrimination thresholds for communicating rotational inertia and torque using differential skin stretch feedback in virtual environments. In: Proceedings of the 2014 IEEE Haptics Symposium (HAPTICS), pp. 277–282 (2014). https://doi.org/10.1109/HAPTICS.2014.6775467
12. Nakamura, T., Nemoto, S., Ito, T., Yamamoto, A.: Substituted force feedback using palm pressurization for a handheld controller. In: Hasegawa, S., Konyo, M., Kyung, K.-U., Nojima, T., Kajimoto, H. (eds.) AsiaHaptics 2016. LNEE, vol. 432, pp. 197–199. Springer, Singapore (2018). https://doi.org/10.1007/978-981-10-4157-0_34

13. Yoshimoto, S., Yamamoto, A.: Pressure stimulus to the palm substitutes and augments force sensation. IEEE Trans. Haptics **14**, 930–935 (2021). https://doi.org/10.1109/TOH.2021.3087230
14. Kojima, M., Yoshimoto, S., Yamamoto, A.: Evaluation of point of subject equality using constant method in pseudo force sensation by pressure stimulation to the palm. In: Proceedings of the 2022 31st IEEE International Conference on Robot and Human Interactive Communication (RO-MAN), pp. 205–210 (2022). https://doi.org/10.1109/RO-MAN53752.2022.9900745

Design of a Surgical Stapler for Laparoscopic Colectomy

Dhruva Khanzode[1,2], Ranjan Jha[1,2], Alexandra Thomieres[3], Emilie Duchalais[3], and Damien Chablat[4](✉)

[1] CSIR-Central Scientific Instruments Organisation, Chandigarh 160030, India
{khanzode.dhruva,ranjan.jha}@csio.res.in
[2] Academy of Scientific and Innovative Research (AcSIR), Ghaziabad 201002, India
[3] CHU Nantes, Centre hospitalier universitaire de Nantes,Nantes, France
{alexandra.thomieres,emilie.dassonneville}@chu-nantes.fr
[4] Nantes Université, École Centrale Nantes, CNRS, LS2N, UMR 6004, 44000 Nantes, France
damien.chablat@cnrs.fr

Abstract. In this article, a flexible surgical stapler mechanism is designed to serve as a basis for laparoscopic rectal cancer surgery in which conventional tools cannot be easily accessed. The mechanism is designed by implementing a stacked tensegrity mechanism with a flexible beam as the central spine. The workspace analysis for the stapler was done by studying collaborative data of CT scans of the surgical site from the Axial, Coronal, and Sagittal planes at different intervals. The kinematic equations for the mechanism were synthesized using Hooke's law with a rotational spring and bending moment. For the tensegrity mechanism, singularities and simulations of the mechanism were also analyzed incorporating the eyelet friction parameter. The results of the study signify that the friction parameter can modify the radius of curvature of the mechanism and needs to be analyzed correctly.

Keywords: Surgical stapler · anastomosis · laparoscopy · tensegrity mechanism

1 Introduction

The field of medical science has grown by leaps and bounds during the last two decades. Minimally invasive surgical procedures have emerged as one of the preferred alternatives for most conventional surgeries. Minimally invasive surgical procedures require very small incisions over the body and specialized slender tools that have miniature tools are inserted through those incisions. These miniature tools have also been modified and modernized over the period of time. Previously, these tools were manually controlled and operated, but nowadays, these tools are being operated using robotic systems. Also, nowadays, robotic systems are also being used in various fields of medical science, like diagnosis, drug delivery, and therapy.

D. Tarnita et al. (Eds.): MESROB 2023, MMS 133, pp. 71–80, 2023.
https://doi.org/10.1007/978-3-031-32446-8_8

One such procedure is colectomy, wherein all or some part of the colon is removed due to numerous reasons like infection, cell death, tumor, etc. During this procedure, the damaged part of the colon is separated and the rest of the healthy colon tissues or segments are joined together. The joining of the colon segments or any tubular segment is called anastomosis. To perform colon anastomosis, a specialized surgical tool is required known as a "surgical stapler" [1].

The first surgical stapler was invented in 1908 by Victor Fischer and Hümér Hültl. This device was initially developed to prevent the risk of infection due to spillage of Gastro-Intestinal contents on the wounds of patients undergoing abdominal surgeries. The idea was to seal and shut the hollow organs before their division, hence preventing spillage. The surgical stapler was then called a "mechanical stitching device" [2] but later, the design was known as the "Fischer-Hültl stapler". The first modern stapler was invented in 1964 by Mark Ravitch, Leon Hirsch, and Felicien Steichen under the banner of the United States Surgical Corporation (USSC). The USSC products became so popular that their acronyms are still used as a part of surgical vocabulary such as TA, thoracoabdominal, GIA, GI anastomosis. With such success, a competitor named Ethicon appeared in 1997, which was then and still is a subsidiary of the Johnson & Johnson brand and USSC itself successively became Covidien, which is now a part of medical & healthcare giant Medtronics.

In today's surgeries, generally, five kinds of staplers are used, namely TA, Thorasic-Abdominal; GIA, Gastro-Intestinal Anastomosis; Endo GIA, Endoscopic Gastro-Intestinal Anastomosis; EEA, End-End Anastomosis and Skin Stapler. The TA stapler is not equipped with a knife to cut the tissue after the firing of stapler pins and hence the tissue needs to be separated manually. The EEA stapler provides circular staples and the skin stapler is used to close superficial wounds. The TA stapler is most prominently used in veterinary surgical procedures [3]. GIA and Endo GIA are the most used staplers for abdominal surgeries and the Endo GIA staplers are specifically used for minimally invasive surgical procedures [4]. Presently, the Endo GIA staplers are available in 3 forms: passive articulated wrist type (PAW), active articulated wrist type (AAW), and radial reload type staplers (RR). In PAW, the desired bending of the wrist is achieved by pressing the jaw upon the abdominal wall, whereas in AAW, a lever is provided to articulate the wrist into pre-determined bending angles. RR comes with a fixed "U" shape jaw and has been proven to be very useful for pulmonary surgeries [5]. The RR-type stapler is only commercialized by Covidien Inc. The main drawback of the RR type stapler is that it requires a very large incision to enter the body and hence defeats the purpose of "minimally invasive surgery" [6]. Hence there is a dire need for a surgical stapler that can enter through the laparoscopic openings but can work as an RR-type of stapler inside the body.

To solve the positioning and maneuverability issue of an endoscopic surgical stapler [7], this article discusses the design and development of a hyper-redundant flexible surgical stapler for laparoscopic procedures [8]. The envisioned surgical stapler possesses the capability to flexibly orient itself in complex surgical sites. Its flexibility helps achieve the positioning and orientation of the stapler over the tissue which will seal and bisect the tissue more efficiently as compared to current conventional endoscopic surgical staplers. The envisioned stapler will have four major parts, namely, the upper jaw, lower jaw, stapling cartridge, and wrist. The upper jaw and the lower jaw will encapsulate the stacked tensegrity mechanism which will enable both jaws to bend in the same plane. The bending will be actuated by pushing or pulling of tendons engaged in the tensegrity mechanism [9,10]. The stapling cartridge will house the surgical staple pins and the cutting knife. The firing mechanism of the cartridge will enable the stapling pins to engage with the tissue as well as actuate the knife to separate the tissue simultaneously. The wrist attached to the base of the jaw will also have a flexible structure able to move in the same plane as the upper and lower jaws. The bending of the wrist will have another couple of tendons for its actuation and the opening and closing of the jaws will be actuated separately. So overall, for the complete operation of the flexible surgical stapler, a total of 4 actuators will be required, (i) for bending of the wrist, (ii) for the firing of staple pins and knife, (iii) for opening and closing of jaws, and (iv) for bending of the upper and lower jaw, which will be actuated synchronously and by a combined single actuation.

2 Workspace Analysis

In the field of design and modeling, the first step is to analyze the problem statement provided, followed by determining the limitations and constraints that the design will encounter. Therefore, the first constraint for the design is the available workspace. For viably designing a flexible surgical stapler it is required to investigate how much workspace is available for the stapler to maneuver. Many times, it happens that the total area available is very limited and it is hard to maneuver the surgical tool inside the intended surgical site. Therefore, while developing a new minuscule surgical tool, it is required to analyze the actual space available for the tool move. Typically, computed tomography (CT) scans are used to estimate available space. For our analysis, we collected data for patients who were admitted for colon surgery. The abdominal workspace volume is highly dependent on the age, sex, weight, and physiology of the patient. To illustrate our research, we have the data of a male patient aged 65 years, measuring 1.66 m and weighing 55 kg. This patient was particularly selected as his physiological characteristics provided the smallest workspace volume for the flexible surgical stapler. We proceeded to record the data in the form of CT scans of the generalized surgical site along the three anatomical planes, namely Axial, Coronal, and Sagittal at the interval of 3.33 mm for all the planes respectively. The data was then marked by an experienced surgeon for dimensional parameters of the surgical site, represented by red and blue markings in Fig. 1 for each plane respectively using CARESTREAM software. This data was first analyzed to estimate the highest volume of workspace available for the flexible stapler. Second, we can identify the smallest cross-sectional area present at the surgical site. A 3D model is created to simulate stapler placement and laparoscopic insertion. Thus, we can determine the size of the tool that can be used in this smallest available area.

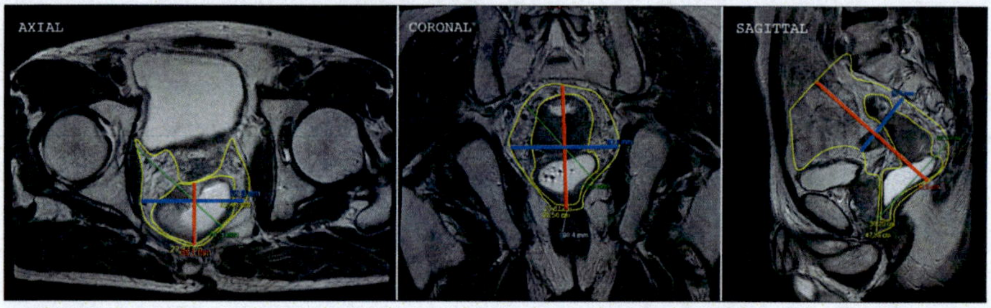

Fig. 1. Sample CT scan data for workspace evaluation in Axial, Coronal, and Sagittal planes. The red and blue markings represent the available dimension (mm) in each plane.

3 Mechanism Design of Surgical Stapler

For a flexible mechanism, usually, large deflections or deformations are nonlinear in nature, therefore, for simplification in kinematic modeling, the constant curvature technique is adopted. Constant curvature mechanisms have a finite number of curved segments. These segments are described by a quantitative set of arc parameters which could be modified into analytical frame transformations. The piece-wise constant curvature approximation (PCCA) presented in the prior art helps us provide the direct kinematics of the mechanism taking the tendon or cable tension as input and giving posture as an output. Sometimes, the flexible mechanism can have a singular flexible spine for all of its segments, but in that case, too, the PCCA can be applied [11]. The constant curvature approximation technique has been successfully applied to various flexible mechanisms, some of which also serve in the medical science and surgery [12].

In this article, the mechanism under study comprises three trapezoidal segments Ⓐ, Ⓑ and Ⓒ, stacked one above the other, as depicted in Fig. 2. This is a new formulation of the tensegrity mechanism defined in [13]. For connecting the base to the mobile platform of each segment, a continuous flexible beam is incorporated capable of deformation in the plane, but with good stiffness in the plane (Fig. 2). The link A_0J_0 is a continuous beam from the base to the tip of the mechanism. But, for the sake of analysis, we are taking into consideration only a section of it, i.e. A_0D_0, and are analyzing by using the piecewise constant curvature approximation (PCCA). The base platform and the moving platform are attached with the help of two cables/tendons ρ_1 and ρ_2, present on either side of the central spine and two springs of stiffness k_1 and k_2 between $(A_1\ D_1)$ and $(A_2\ D_2)$, respectively.

The contraction of the cables will stimulate angular displacement in the flexible beam of the central spine and replication of this phenomenon in each of the three segments will eventually facilitate the bending of the mechanism. The length of the cable is measured as ρ_i.

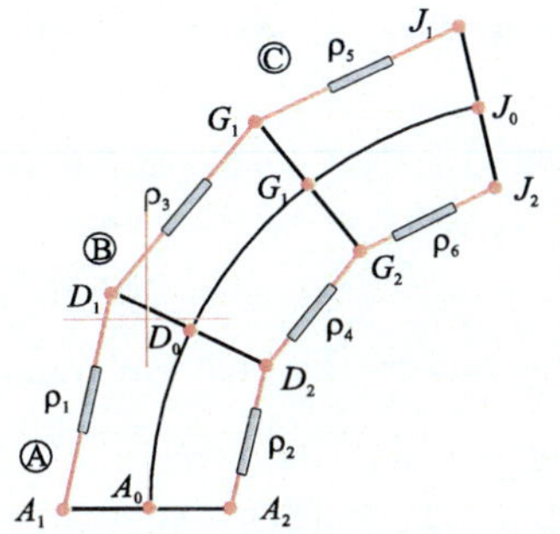

Fig. 2. The tensegrity mechanism understudy with three segments stacked, named Ⓐ, Ⓑ, Ⓒ with a flexible beam

3.1 Kinematics Equations of the Tensegrity Mechanism

To establish the positions of the points of the mobile platform, it is necessary to study the deformation of a beam subjected to torsion. We assume that the distance between A_0 and D_0 is h_1. The coordinates of the fixed points are:

$$\mathbf{a}_1 = \begin{bmatrix} -l_1 & 0 \end{bmatrix}^T \quad \mathbf{a}_2 = \begin{bmatrix} l_1 & 0 \end{bmatrix}^T \tag{1}$$

To map cable tensions and spring forces for one segment to its radius of curvature, we use a lumped parameter model. For a beam, the springs and cables apply forces on its end that generate a torsional torque:

$$\mathcal{T}_1 = \mathcal{T}_{f1} + \mathcal{T}_{f2} + k_1(\rho_1 - l_{01})l_2 - k_2(\rho_2 - l_{02})l_2 \tag{2}$$

where $\mathcal{T}_{f1} = -f_1 l_2$ and $\mathcal{T}_{f2} = f_1 l_2$. Equation 3 is a Hooke's law with a rotational spring and the bending moment where K_θ is an effective bending stiffness (in N· m/rad), h_1 is the arc length between A_0 and D_0, f_1 and f_2 the forces applied by the two cables and r_1 is the radius of curvature (see Fig. 3). For one section, we have

$$h_1/r_1 = \mathcal{T}_1/K_\theta \tag{3}$$

Beam characterization may be expressed by its bend radius r_1 and the angle θ_1

$$r_1 = h_1/\theta_1 \quad \text{and} \quad \theta_1 = \tau_1/K_\theta \tag{4}$$

This definition stands when we bend in one direction, either left or right and it allows us to perceive the position of D_0.

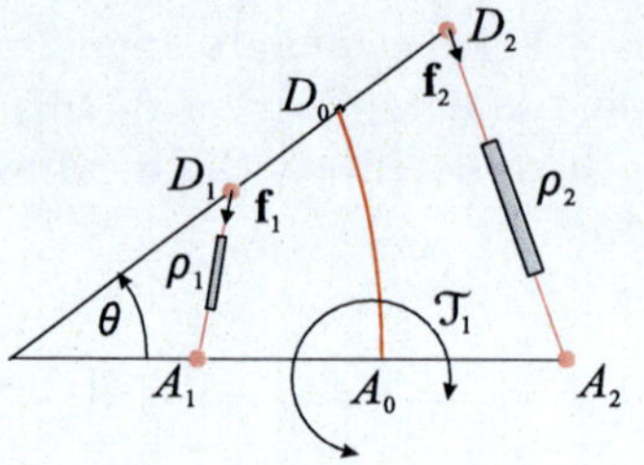

Fig. 3. Bending moment equilibrium [12] when two forces f_1 and f_2 are applied to generate the torque $\mathcal{T}_1$.

The segment (D_1D_2) is normal to the beam at point D_0 and the coordinates of these points are

$$d_0 = \begin{bmatrix} r_1 - r_1\cos(\theta_1) \\ r_1\sin(\theta 1) \end{bmatrix} \tag{5}$$

$$d_1 = \begin{bmatrix} r_1 - r_1\cos(\theta 1) - l_2\cos(\theta 1) \\ R\sin(\theta 1) + l_2\sin(\theta 1) \end{bmatrix} \tag{6}$$

$$d_2 = \begin{bmatrix} r_1 - r_1\cos(\theta 1) + l_2\cos(\theta 1) \\ R\sin(\theta 1) - l_2\sin(\theta 1) \end{bmatrix} \tag{7}$$

The inverse kinematic model for a mechanism with a flexible beam is as follows:

$$||\mathbf{a}_1 - \mathbf{d}_1|| = \rho_1, \quad ||\mathbf{a}_2 - \mathbf{d}_2|| = \rho_2 \tag{8}$$

These equations can also be expressed as functions of the lengths of the springs, therefore

$$(-l_1 - r_1 + r_1\cos(\theta 1) - l_2\cos(\theta_1))^2 + (-r_1\sin(\theta_1) + l_2\sin(\theta_1))^2 = \rho_1^2 \tag{9}$$

$$(l_1 - r_1 + r_1\cos(\theta_1) + l_2\cos(\theta_1))^2 + (-r_1\sin(\theta_1) - l_2\sin(\theta_1))^2 = \rho_2^2 \tag{10}$$

Similar to previous assumptions, for sections Ⓑ and Ⓒ, we can write the equations in the same way for the positions of the joints. The inverse kinematic model of the sections is given by

$$||\mathbf{d}_1 - \mathbf{g}_1|| = \rho_3, \quad ||\mathbf{d}_2 - \mathbf{g}_2|| = \rho_4, \quad ||\mathbf{g}_1 - \mathbf{j}_1|| = \rho_5, \quad ||\mathbf{g}_2 - \mathbf{j}_2|| = \rho_6 \tag{11}$$

To know the position of the mobile platform due to the application of force in the tendons or cables, it is necessary for us to calculate the radius of curvature and the angle of inclination that satisfies the kinematic model. The optimization problem is written by using Eq. 8. For each segment, the bending moment and the transfer to the previous one should be evaluated. If $f_2 > f_1$, the beam will bend to the right. The cables go through the thought eyelet where there is friction μ. Figure 4 illustrates the transfer of forces before and after the cable passes through the eyelets of the mobile platform. The study of the stability of the segments by taking into account the friction of the cables in the eyelets

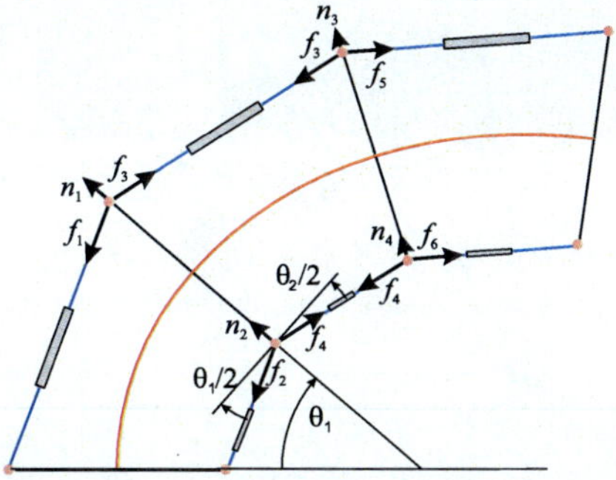

Fig. 4. Static equilibrium of three segments

enables the force transmission factors to be obtained [12]. For even values of actuators, the tensions in the cables reduce from the base to the end as

$$\frac{f_{i+3}}{f_{i+1}} = \left(\frac{1-\mu\sin(\theta_1/2)}{1+\mu\sin(\theta_1/2)}\right) \tag{12}$$

For odd values of actuators, the tensions in the cables increase from the base to the end as

$$\frac{f_{i+2}}{f_i} = \left(\frac{1+\mu\sin(\theta_1/2)}{1-\mu\sin(\theta_1/2)}\right) \tag{13}$$

3.2 Simulation and Singularities

This section promotes a simulation study to show the mechanism's behavior. Some of the model parameters cannot be defined at this time without careful selection of materials and complete knowledge of the workspace within the semi-colon. Figure 5 depicts the bending motion when $f_1 - f_2 = 0 + \epsilon$ to 17 N. A slight offset has to fix with ϵ to avoid the radius of curvature tending to infinity. If we apply the length constraints on the springs having a spring constant of 100 N/m, this movement is not entirely feasible. The extreme position is reached when one of the springs is of zero length (or its minimum length) or when the cable becomes tangent to the bent. By using the constraint into the spring lengths (40% of the spring length in the home pose), the maximal angle is 1.15 rad ($\approx 130°$).

The simulation allows us to solve the inverse kinematics from Eqs. 8, and 11 by using the same optimization algorithm as for a single segment. The simulation of the flexion of the mechanism without friction makes it possible to obtain a perfect curve, without discontinuity between each segment as shown in Fig. 6 (left). The MAPLE software optimization package resolver was used to determine the beam curvature based on cable forces and spring tensions.

When friction is added, the tensions in the two cables are no longer the same in each segment, which changes the curvature as shown in Fig. 6 (right). It is important to note that the model we use is simplified because it assumes that the angle of curvature does not vary from one segment to the next.

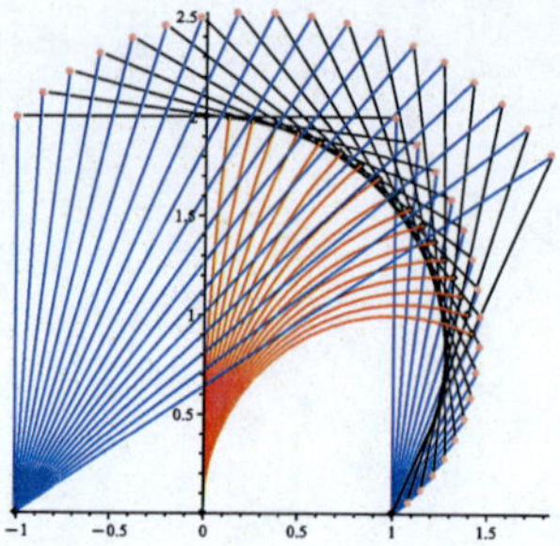

Fig. 5. Simulation of the bending of one segment with $l_1 = l_2 = 1$ cm and $h_1 = 2$ cm

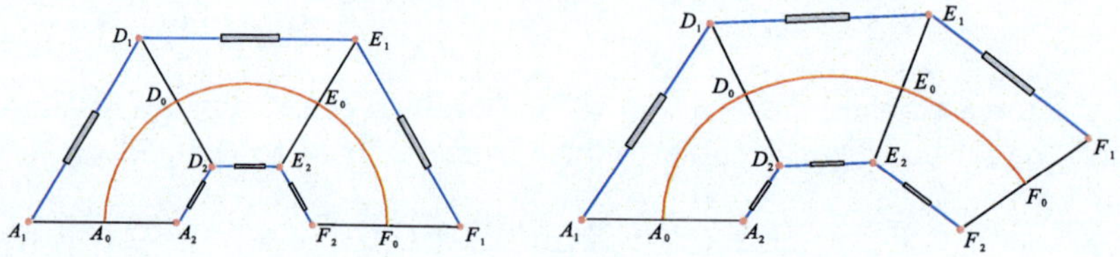

Fig. 6. Simulation of bending for three segments with $\mu = 0$ (left) and $\mu = 0.2$ (right) with $l_1 = l_2 = 1$ cm and $h_1 = 2$ cm

4 Application to the Stapler Design

The physical constraints arising due to limited and complex workspace inside the patient's body reduce the cross-section of each segment. Figure 7 illustrates how the designed tensegrity mechanism is positioned in a physical system to create a bendable stapler.

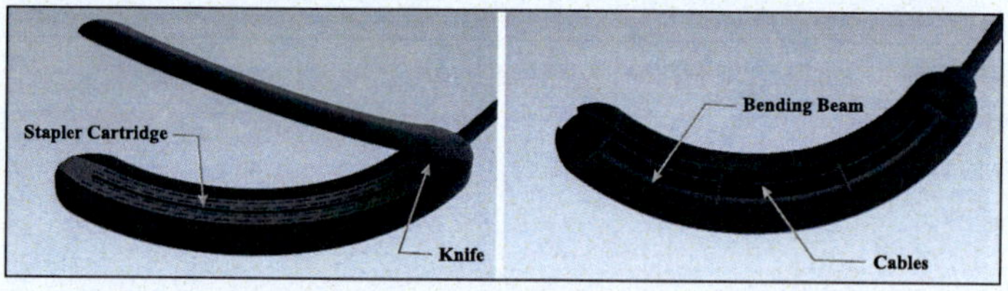

Fig. 7. Integration of the mechanism inside the stapler

The problem with this design is that, due to the smaller width of the cross-section, the folding beam reaches the actuating cables even for a smaller angle of deviation, therefore resulting in a greater radius of curvature (Fig. 8). To ensure that the patient's workspace is accessible, another joint must be added similar to a wrist before the stapler. Another solution to this problem is to increase the number of segments, but doing so will result in an increase in the number

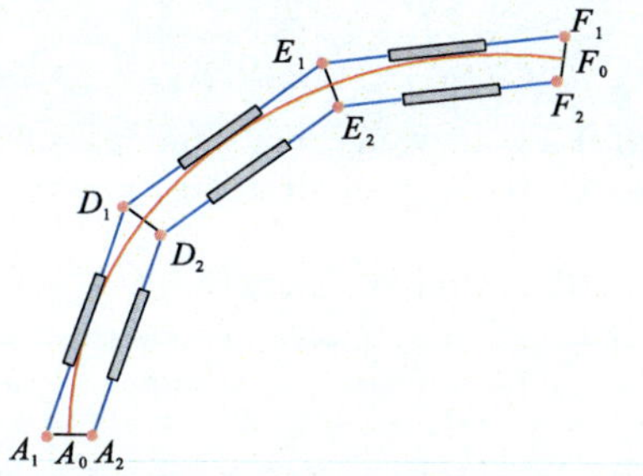

Fig. 8. Reduction of the cross-section of the mechanism to be used inside the stapler with $l_1 = l_2 = 1/5$ cm and $h_1 + h_2 + h_3 = 2$ cm

of eyelets through which the cable passes and this might lead to an increase in total friction between the eyelets and the cable.

5 Conclusions

In this article, we have studied a flexible mechanism that can be used inside a stapler during laparoscopic colectomy for rectal cancer and other coloanal procedures, where conventional tools cannot be easily accessed. This mechanism consists of a stack of three tensegrity mechanisms made with rigid bodies, linear springs, cables for actuation, and a flexible beam. The size of the stapler depends on a number of criteria that depend on the patient's anatomy and the constraints of laparoscopy. Patient scans are currently being studied to define the workspace where the surgery is performed. Using a lumped parameter model, the analysis was performed with and without the friction parameter within the eyelet of the rigid segment of each segment. It has been demonstrated that the friction parameter can modify the radius of the curvature and needs to be analyzed correctly.

Future research is underway to analyze the impact of friction between the mobile platform eyelets, through which the cable passes, and the cable itself. Evaluation is underway to find the relationship between friction and the curvature of the mechanism. It is estimated that with an increase in the number of sections, the overall friction will increase hence the curvature of the mechanism will not be as expected. The materials used are currently being evaluated to determine the influence of the sheathing covering the mechanism. The skin of the stapler will be made of elastomer to serve as a spring and ensure the sealing to improve its use as medical equipment.

Acknowledgements. This research is sponsored by the Indian Council of Medical Research, New Delhi, India under the "Senior Research Fellowship" awarded to Mr. Dhruva Rajesh Khanzode (File no. 5/3/8/46/ITR-F/2022) and supported under MoU between CSIR- Central Scientific Instruments Organisation, Chandigarh, India, and Centrale Nantes, France.

References

1. Gaidry, A.D., Tremblay, L., Nakayama, D., Ignacio, R.C.: The history of surgical staplers: a combination of Hungarian, Russian, and American innovation. Am. Surg. **85**, 563–566 (2019)
2. Akopov, A., Artioukh, D.Y., Molnar, T.F.: Surgical staplers: the history of conception and adoption. Ann. Thorac. Surg. **112**, 1716–1721 (2021)
3. Tobias, K.M.: Surgical stapling devices in veterinary medicine: a review. Vet. Surg. **36**, 341–349 (2007)
4. Schemmer, P., et al.: The Use of Endo-GIA vascular staplers in Liver surgery and their potential benefit: a review. Dig. Surg. **24**(4), 300–305 (2007)
5. Ema, T.: The experience of using Endo GIA^{TM} radial reload with Tri-Staple^{TM} technology for various lung surgery. J. Thorac. Dis. **6**(10), 1482–1484 (2014)
6. Rivadeneira, D.E., Verdeja, J.C., Sonoda, T.: Improved access and visibility during stapling of the ultra-low rectum: a comparative human cadaver study between two curved staplers. Ann. Surg. Innov. Res. **6**, 11 (2012)
7. de Calan, L., Gayet, B., Bourlier, P., Perniceni, T.: Chirurgie du cancer du rectum par laparotomie et par laparoscopie. EMC - Chirurgie **1**, 231–274 (2004)
8. Laparoscopic rectal resection for severe endometriosis of the mid and low rectum: technique and operative results. Surg. Endosc. **26**(4), 1035–1040 (2012)
9. Furet, M., Lettl, M., Wenger, P.: Kinematic analysis of planar tensegrity 2-X Manipulators. In: Lenarcic, J., Parenti-Castelli, V. (eds.) ARK 2018. SPAR, vol. 8, pp. 153–160. Springer, Cham (2019). https://doi.org/10.1007/978-3-319-93188-3_18
10. Wenger, P., Chablat, D.: Kinetostatic analysis and solution classification of a class of planar tensegrity mechanisms. Robotica **37**, 1214–1224 (2019)
11. Gravagne, I.A., Rahn, C.D., Walker, I.D.: Large deflection dynamics and control for planar continuum robots. IEEE/ASME Trans. Mechatron. **8**(2), 299–307 (2003)
12. Kato, T., Okumura, I., Song, S.-E., Golby, A.J., Hata, N.: Tendon-driven continuum robot for endoscopic surgery: Preclinical development and validation of a tension propagation model. IEEE/ASME Trans. Mechatron. **20**(5), 2252–2263 (2015)
13. Khanzode, D., Jha, R., Chablat, D., Duchalais, E.: Stapler design with stacked tensegrity mechanisms for surgical procedures. In: Proceedings of the ASME 2022 International Design Engineering Technical Conferences & Computers and Information in Engineering Conference (2022)

An Experimental Characterization of RIBOLUTION Rib Fracture Fixator

Marco Ceccarelli[1(✉)], Elaisa Consalvo[2], Matteo Russo[1], and Vincenzo Ambrogi[2]

[1] Department of Industrial Engineering, University of Rome Tor Vergata, 00133 Rome, Italy
{marco.ceccarelli,matteo.russo}@uniroma2.it
[2] Department of Surgical Sciences, University of Rome Tor Vergata, 00133 Rome, Italy
ambrogi@uniroma2.it

Abstract. The results of an experimental validation campaign of RIBOLUTION, a new rib fixator, are presented with a functional characterization at the biomechanical level in terms of motion and force transmission using samples of pork ribs. The reported results show a satisfactory functionality of the implementation of the rib fixator during a breathing simulation using a suitable experimental testbed with a set of significant statistical results.

Keywords: Biomechanics · Experimental Biomechanics · Rib Fixators

1 Introduction

Rib fracture is an important multifaced injury that very often is involved with severe conditions in chest trauma [1], whose effect is classified as third cause of death worldwide, after cardiovascular diseases and cancer, [2].

Up to now, approved surgical interventions are based on procedures with absorbable suture cables [3]. In addition, titanium plates, clamps and bicortical screws are used as fixators for appropriate mechanical stability, but they cannot be considered a definitive solution since secondary fractures have occurred in osteoporotic bones, as pointed out in [4, 5]. Example of ordinary usage are Judet's Agraphes implants, [6] with circling the rib, in a way that however can irritate the intercostal nerve with neural effects and pain consequences, [7], compromising ventilation mechanics, [8]. In addition, the major disadvantage is that a second surgery is usually required to remove the parts.

With the aim to avoid the above-indicated conditions, we have designed a mini-invasive implant for single/multiple rib fractures with a rib fixator that can be fixed by a biological glue, [9]. In addition, since rib osteosynthesis takes approximately one month, a biodegradable material can be conveniently chosen in avoiding a second thoracic surgery as to complete the design of REBOLUTION, a new rib fixator, [10].

In this paper we discuss results of a campaign of experimental validation of the functionality of the rib fixator RIBOLUTION and its implanting with a bioabsorbable glue by testing pork rib in a testing machine simulating the mechanics of respiration as a further development of previous experiences, [11].

D. Tarnita et al. (Eds.): MESROB 2023, MMS 133, pp. 81–89, 2023.
https://doi.org/10.1007/978-3-031-32446-8_9

2 RIBOLUTION Design and Functionality

In Fig. 1 the design of RIBOLUTION, [9, 10], a novel rib fixator (1), is described with a geometry designed as rectangular shape to be adaptable to a rib (3). As shown in Fig. 1 a), it is a flat plate to be flexible and to guarantee elasticity in following the motion of the anatomic bone on which is installed. It is reduced at minimum dimension in terms of width, length, and thickness to let the fixator be invasive as less as possible, overcoming the intercostal nerve lesions matters. Designed are holes (2, 3) at the extremities to let the biological glue (4) (chosen as anchor system) be inserted in and expanded as to give adhesion surface for a powerful attachment to the tissues above the periosteum (5), likewise they were nails once the glue is solidified.

Figure 1 b) shows a lab prototype that was used in lab tests made of made of a ZM31 magnesium-based alloy as per absorbable material.

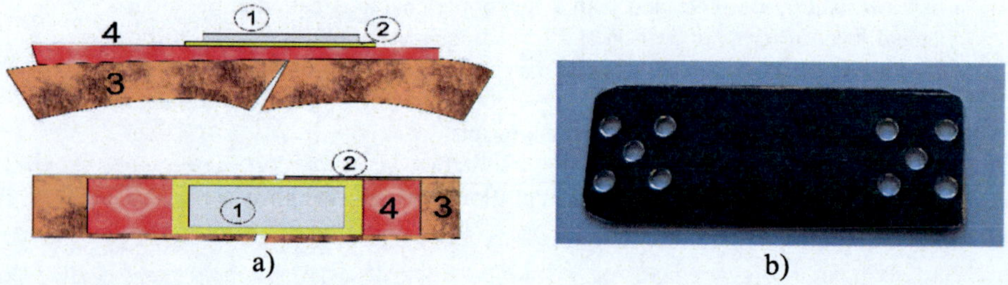

Fig. 1. RIBOLUTION design, [9]: a) conceptual scheme of implementation; b) a prototype. (1: fixator; 2 glues; 3; fractured rib; 4 tissue)

The functionality of the RIBOLUTION fixator consists in keeping the two trunks of a fractured rib connected while still allowing relative movement between them for convenient breathing. The main characteristic can be recognized in the fact that the connection of the two fractured trunks is kept aligned and close with a mechanical system constituted by the prosthetic plate without further invasive elements of the anatomical application area.

3 Testing Design

An experimental campaign for the validation and functional characterization of the application of the RIBOLUTION prosthesis was designed using samples of human-like pork ribs in the TEMARI experimentation machine, [12], in lab experience according to a rigorous protocol for statistical validity with the reported results in the following.

The experimentation was designed with a specially elaborated protocol with a sequence of activities that can ensure not only the repeatability of the tests but also a statistical validity of the results thanks to the use of TEMARI, [12], a test bed specifically developed to simulate and monitor the biomechanics of movements in both artificial and anatomical ribs. Testing is aimed to check the transmission of motion and force along a rib, comparing the results between integer and fractured conditions, only. Figure 2a) shows the testing machine TEMARI that, was designed and used at LARM2 as shown in Fig. 2 b) to simulate breathing mechanics of sample ribs. The cam follower impacts against sternal rib extremity, whereas a sensor Load Cell 1, measures the impact force. A second Load Cell 2 at the opposite site where the vertebral rib extremity is clamped, measures the transmitted force along the rib structure. Two more sensors IMU 1 and 2 (Inertial Measuring Unit) are used to monitor the follower input motion and fixator response, respectively. A linear potentiometer on the cam follower head measures the input displacement, from 0 to 4 cm as used simulating the ribcage motion.

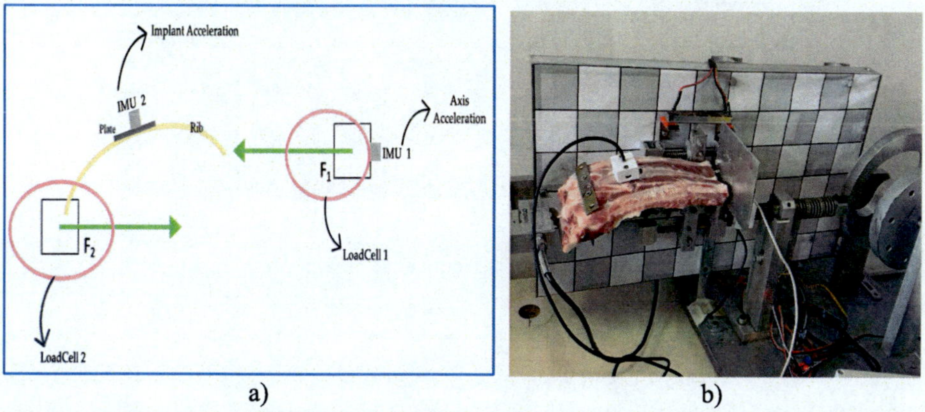

Fig. 2. Design of lab testing: a) conceptual scheme; b) lab layout with TEMARI testing machine.

In particular, the experimentation was carried out on samples of pork ribs with a specimen consisting of three ribs (III, IV and V of the ribcage), one of which (the IV one), after being fractured, is monitored in its functionality when integer, fractured and repaired with RIBOLUTION. In addition, tests were performed with two or three repetitions of a displacement that reasonably replicates the modes simulating basal breathing, maximal breathing, and coughing. Each test lasted 10 s with intact rib, broken rib and repaired rib with RIBOLUTION fixator.

The rib sample composed of three ribs is used within three hours after slaughter of the animal in order to have the tissue as more reactive as possible. Each sample is prepared by removing the superficial muscles along the fascial plane, leaving the intercostals and the serratus anterior muscle. The sternum is removed at the level of the chondrosternal joint, keeping the hemi-rachis. The vertebral pedicle is dissected to remove the vertebral arch, leaving the vertebral hemi-body. The rib specimen is fixed at its posterior end among two plates by means of two metal screws passing the tissue so that its free end faces the moving plate of the TEMARI machine, Fig. 2b). On the fourth rib, that will be broken and repaired, an IMU is installed on the posterolateral area by using a stitch silk, as visible white box in Fig. 3.

The rib fracture is obtained with a direct blow with a hammer and chisel on the external tissue of the IV rib at 8.5 cm from the parasternal free end, Fig. 3a). After testing the broke specimen, a cyanoacrylate synthetic surgical glue is used for rib fracture repair in fixing RIBOLUTION rib fixator made of Magnesium alloy on site as shown in Fig. 3b). The fixing is considered stable after 2 min and after 5 min testing is performed with the repaired rib specimen.

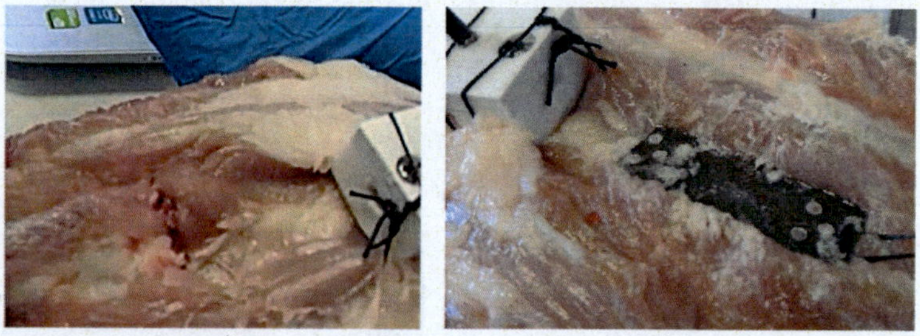

a) b)

Fig. 3. A lab testing of the pork rib specimen: a) broken rib; b) repaired rib

4 Test Results

Illustrative results of testing for an experimental characterization of the fixator operation are reported in Figs. 4, 5 and 6 from a lab campaign with several tests using TEMARI testing machine in Fig. 2. In general, the pig of the rib specimen was 10 months old and about 170 kg. Testing was run sequentially for the unbroken rib, broken rib and repaired rib repeating each test two or three times to have a statistical significance of the results. At the end of the tests, the rib fixator was pulled with a manual dynamometer to measure the force of adhesion along the direction of the rib with an average measure of more than 10 N during five minutes.

In Fig. 4 the acceleration of the rib reference point gives indication of the motion response of the unbroken rib during the three modes, and it can be noted that in the unbroken rib the value is measured with similar values reaching maximum 0.5 g and similar time history. In the repaired rib the maximum values were reduced to about 0.2–0.3 g with a time history indicating much more sensed acceleration in Figs. 4 b) and c) so that it can be interpreted that the rib fixator gives more rigidity to the rib specimen when considering that the acceleration is due to the motion dissipation among the tissues surrounding the ribs. The forces F1 and F2 measured by the load cells, Figs. 5 and 6 show the force transmission from one extremity to the other during the ribcage simulated motion of respiration. The Load Cell 2 in Fig. 5 is saturated in the test with unbroken rib but still the acquired values are useful for the analysis purposes of the testing, since those values for the repaired rib give proper indications of the force transmission. One can note in Fig. 5 a) that the transmitted force with maximum values of about 100 N is in any case reproduced in the fractured rib with the same trend and frequency but with a maximum value that is reduced to a maximum value of 40–45 N at the free end extremity and of 30–33 N at the fixed extremity. This indicates that a fracture shows a lower structural integrity despite the rib fixator is able to transmit this force beyond the fracture yet.

The transmitted acceleration with smaller values in the broken repaired rib with respect to the integer one is indicative of the fact that the rib fixator, although permit a connection of the two extremities of the broken rib, does not restore the integrity of the bone structure by limiting the motion capability of the rib. Smaller values of acceleration can be interpreted as related to smaller motion transfer. In the broken repaired rib, although the motion and force are transmitted from the free extremity to the fixed one with reduced values in acceleration and force, one can appreciate the effect of the rib fixator that permits still such a transmission ensuring both the rib functioning and keeping the fractured rib portions near to each other. The stiffer behavior of the repaired fractured rib with the implant of the RIBOLUTION rib fixator can be understood by the reduced values of the motion and force transmission that can represent a more rigid response of the rib against the actuating motion coming from the simulating sternum motion.

5 Considerations for RIBOLUTION Fixator Implementation

From the results of the experimental campaign, as summarized in its essential aspects by the example reported in Figs. 4, 5 and 6, the following aspects can be identified for an effective implementation of the RIBOLUTION rib fixator. The transmission of movement in the repaired rib while being effective, shows a stiffening with loss of flexibility of the rib movement which could be optimized by increasing the flexibility of the rib fixator with its thickness while ensuring its integrity for the necessary period of osteosynthesis; in particular, it is possible to think of reducing the dimension of the thickness even to less than 0.3 mm. The transmission of force along the rib shows efficiency of the repair in securing the structure of the ribcage despite the above mentioned stiffening criticality which in terms of force can be mitigated by increasing the longitudinal dimension of the fixator not only to increase the area of adhesion to the tissues but also for a more gradual distribution of the force in transmission; in particular, it is possible to consider increasing the longitudinal dimension from the current 3 cm up to 6 cm.

The above considerations regarding optimization of the RIBOLUTION rib fixator must be supplemented by a greater attention to the installation location and above all to the fixing by using the absorbable glue both in terms of quality and quantity.

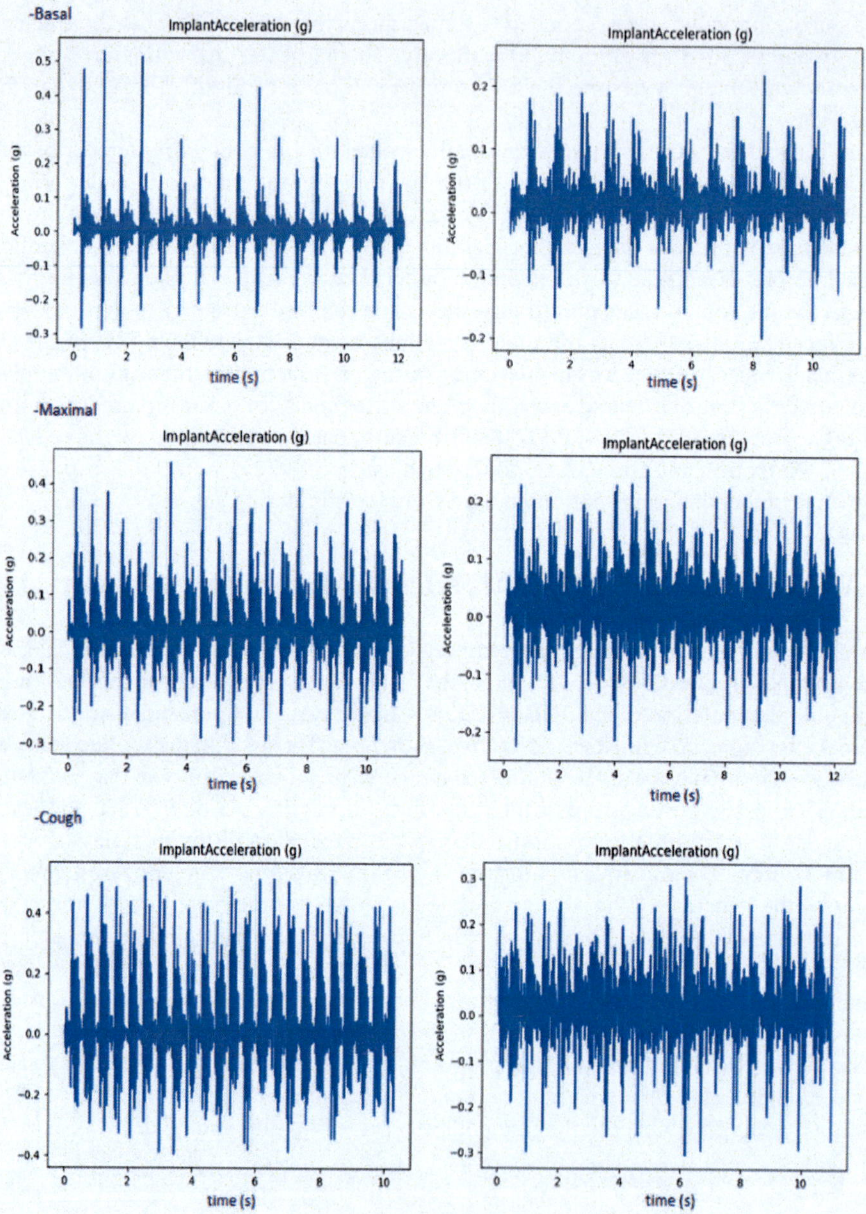

Fig. 4. Test results in terms of acceleration of the rib fixator in unbroken (left) and repaired (right) rib during: a) basal respiration; b) maximal respiration; c) coughing.

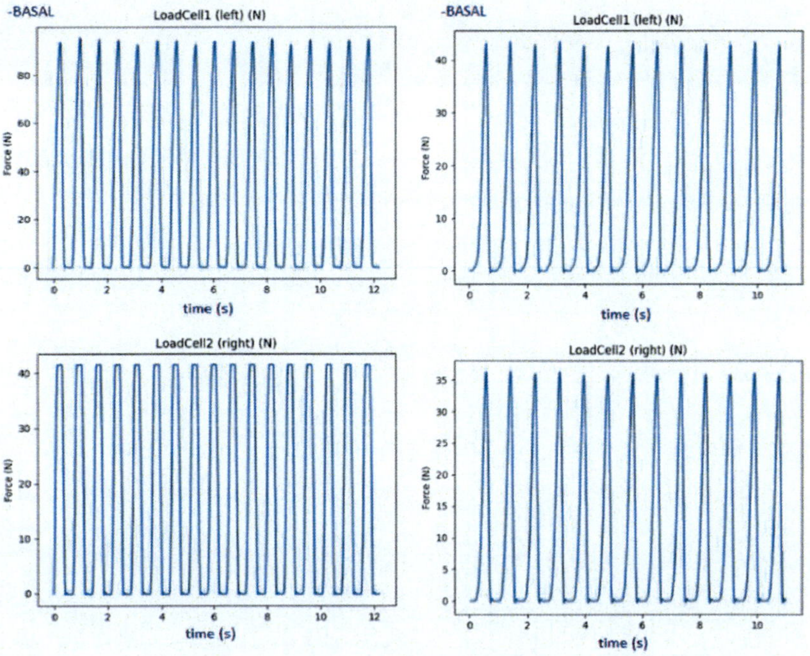

(a)

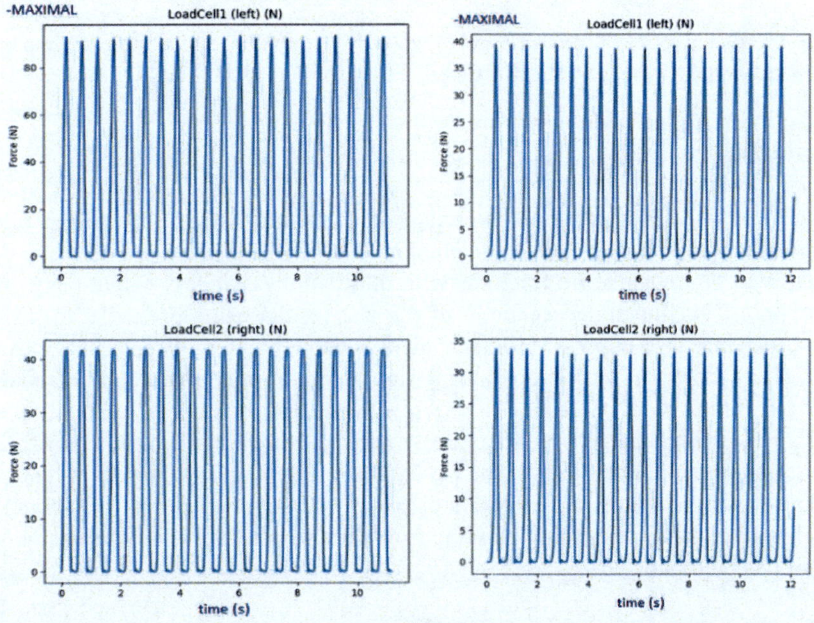

(b)

Fig. 5. Test results in terms of forces F1 and F2 at the rib extremities in unbroken /left) and repaired (right) rib during: a) basal respiration; b) maximal respiration.

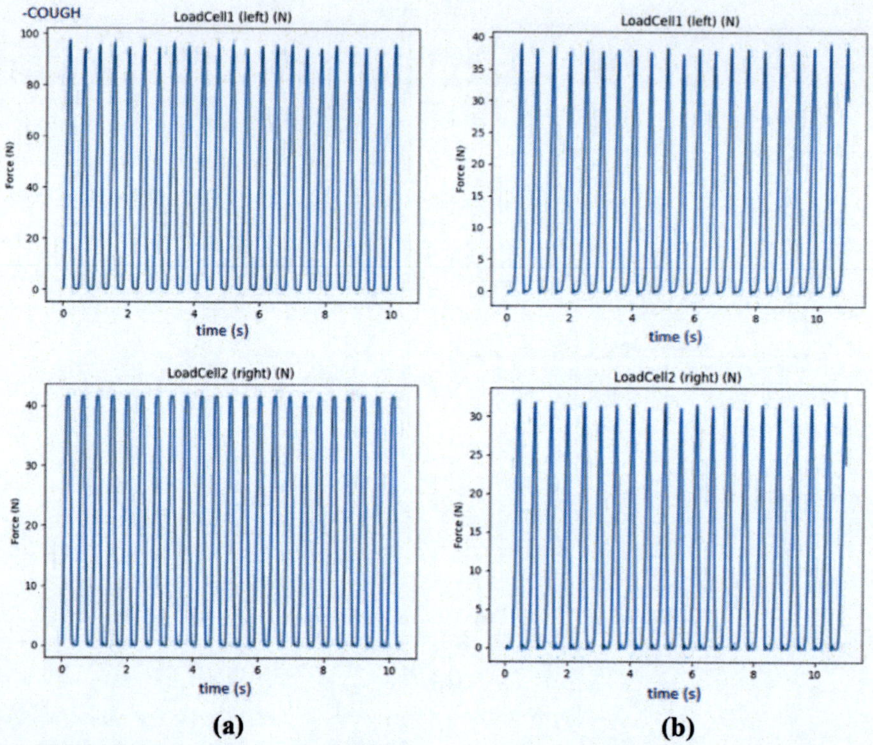

Fig. 6. Test results in terms of forces F1 and F2 at the rib extremities rib during coughing in: a) unbroken rib; b) repaired rib

6 Conclusions

The experimental campaign, whose an example of results is discussed in the paper, shows the practical feasibility and efficiency of the RIBOLUTION prosthesis and its functionality in the repair of rib fractures with minimal invasiveness without any other fixing support. The illustrative example of the test results using pork ribs in a strict protocol procedure also allows a biomechanical characterization of the efficacy of the RIBOLUTION prosthesis with good transmission of motion and force along the repaired fractured rib. Future work is planned to improve the design for surgical application and the resorbable adhesion to the tissues to increase minimally invasiveness of the prosthesis. In order to improve the flexibility of the rib fixator, future work is planned in reducing the thickness and the width of the rib fixator plate, with relative testing validation that very likely will consider also damping effects of the material involved in the design and implant of the rib fixator.

References

1. Chrysou, K., Halat, G., Hoksch, B., Schmid, R.A., Kocher, G.J.: Lessons from a large trauma center: impact of blunt chest trauma in polytrauma patients—still a relevant problem?. Scandinavian Journal of Trauma, Resuscitation and Emergency Med. **25**, 42 (2017). https://doi.org/10.1186/s13049-017-0384-y
2. Sirmali, M., et al.: A comprehensive analysis of traumatic rib fractures: morbidity, mortality and management. Eur. J. Cardiothorac. Surg. **24**(1), 133–138 (2003). https://doi.org/10.1016/S1010-7940(03)00256-2
3. Zhang, Q., Song, L., Ning, S., Xie, H., Li, N., Wang, Y.: Recent advances in rib fracture fixation, J. Thoracic Disease 11 S1070-S1077 (2019). https://doi.org/10.21037/jtd.2019.04.99
4. Engel, C., Krieg, J.C., Madey, S.M., Long, W.B., Bottlang, M.: Operative chest wall fixation with osteosynthesis plates. J. Trauma: Injury, Infection, and Critical Care **58**(1), 181–186 (2005). https://doi.org/10.1097/01.TA.0000063612.25756.60
5. Bottlang, M., Helzel, I., Long, W., Fitzpatrick, D., Madey, S.: Less-invasive stabilization of rib fractures by intramedullary fixation: a biomechanical evaluation. J. Trauma **68**(5), 1218–1224 (2010). https://doi.org/10.1097/TA.0b013e3181bb9df1
6. Vyhnánek, F., Jírava, D., Očadlík, M., Škrabalová, D., Šáber, M., Michal, P.: Innovated Judet Ribs Plates - Preclinical Study, First Clinical Experience, Acta Chirurgiae Orthopaedicae et Traumatologiae Cechoslovaca **85**(3), 226–230. PMID: 30257784. (2018, in Czech)
7. Gordy, S., Fabricant, L., Ham, B., Mullins, R., Mayberry, J.: The contribution of rib fractures to chronic pain and disability. The American J. Surgery, **207**(5), 659–62; discussion 662–3 (2014). https://doi.org/10.1016/j.amjsurg.2013.12.012
8. Dogrul, B.N., Kiliccalan, I., Asci, E.S., Peker, S.C.: Blunt trauma related chest wall and pulmonary injuries: an overview. Chin. J. Traumatol. **23**(3), 125–138 (2020). https://doi.org/10.1016/j.cjtee.2020.04.003
9. Ambrogi, V., Ceccarelli, M.: Fixing plate for osteosynthesis of fractured ribs, Patent IT102019000005638 – 03 Mar 2021. (in Italian)
10. Ceccarelli, M., Ambrogi, V.: RIBOLUTION, a minimally invasive rib fixator, International Society of Bionic Engineering: ISBE 2022 Newsletter **11**(2), 18–19 (2022)
11. Puglisi, L., Ceccarelli, M., Ambrogi, V.: An experimental study of feasibility of a mini-invasive fixator for rib osteosynthesis. ASME. J. Med. Devices. **17**(1), Paper No: MED-22–1042 (2023). https://doi.org/10.1115/1.4055861
12. Ceccarelli, M., Aguilar Perez, L.A., Torres San-Miguel, C.R.: Testing machine for artificial ribs, Patent no. IT 102017000036498 – 23 July 2019

Pre-clinical Study of a Customized Rehabilitation Device Prototype for Patients with Immobility Syndrome

T. Ribeiro[1], L. Roseiro[1], M. Silva[1], F. Santos[1], R. Bernardes[2], R. Cardoso[2], V. Parola[2], H. Neves[2], A. Cruz[2], W. Xavier[3], R. Durães[4], and C. Malça[1,2,3,4,5](✉)

[1] Polytechnic Institute of Coimbra – ISEC, Rua Pedro Nunes, 3030 Coimbra, Portugal
candida@isec.pt
[2] Nursing School of Coimbra - UICISA: E, Av. Bissaya Barreto 143, 3000 Coimbra, Portugal
[3] WISEWARE Lda., Rua 12, Zona Industrial da Mota, 3830-527 Ílhavo, Portugal
[4] ORTHOS XXI, Unipessoal LDA, Rua Santa Leocádia 2735, 4809-012 Guimarães, Portugal
[5] Polytechnic Institute of Leiria - CDRSP, Rua de Portugal, 2430 Marinha Grande, Portugal

Abstract. To reduce the dreadful consequences of immobility syndrome in the elderly population and adults and young people with some restriction of mobility or disability, an innovative device - ABLEFIT - was designed. This biomechanical device aims to provide an advanced solution to support a customized physical rehabilitation, combining a physical system to aid physical exercise, in passive and active modes, in bed and in a wheelchair, a control system for monitoring and storing biofeedback variables and motivational stimulus through interaction with gamification. After prototype construction, a preliminary usability study was carried out to evaluate the developed prototype, namely regarding its functionality, ergonomics and safety, both from the point of view of the end user and health professionals' perspectives. The results from pre-clinical studies will allow the optimization of the ABLEFIT device by developing solutions that ensure the implementation of customized physical rehabilitation programs in a controlled and interactive way.

Keywords: Immobility Syndrome · Rehabilitation Devices · Rehabilitation Customized Plan · Active/Passive Training · IoT · Gamification · Pre-Clinical Tests

1 Introduction

The Prolonged Immobility Syndrome (PIS) is characterized by a set of disorders that result in a reduction in the functional capacity of all body systems, particularly in the musculoskeletal and cardiovascular systems, due to the marked loss of muscle mass and joints stiffness [1–3]. Furthermore, the risk of developing additional physical and psychological complications significantly increases, as greater is the degree of restricted mobility and the time spent in bed or in a wheelchair [3–6]. Regardless of PIS cause, the effects of prolonged immobilization and disuse atrophy require intensive physical

D. Tarnita et al. (Eds.): MESROB 2023, MMS 133, pp. 90–98, 2023.
https://doi.org/10.1007/978-3-031-32446-8_10

reconditioning to allow the body systems to return to a normal functioning condition as soon as possible [1–10]. It is, therefore, crucial to provide technical solutions that ensure the implementation of physical rehabilitation programs in a controlled and interactive way so patients can regain their physical, psychological and social functions. The literature provides information about the development and application of technical solutions to help the physical rehabilitation process [6–10]. However, most of these solutions are limited to the physical rehabilitation of the lower limbs. Characteristics such as e.g. modularity, adaptability, versatility, hygiene, portability and flexibility, among others, have been neglected. Moreover, they do not respond effectively to the need for integrated control and evaluation of bioparameters involved in the rehabilitation process. Most rehabilitation devices do not include biofeedback systems that ensure the measurement, in real time, of those bioparameters and their availability to the medical team to increase the control of the effectiveness of rehabilitation plans. Additionally, they do not promote the emotional involvement of patients, e.g. through gamification interfaces, an approach that leads to a progressive increase in the motivation to complete the prescribed rehabilitation plan [9–11].

A recently published review reports that a plethora of plans, domains, devices and evaluated bioparameters can be found in the literature as a result of the need to adjust to the specificities and individual needs of the patients [10]. Therefore, the challenge is developing an enough versatile rehabilitation device that responds effectively to the need to establish customized and individualized rehabilitation plans. To provide an advanced solution to support physical rehabilitation, a prototype was designed and built that provides a physical support system for physical exercise, in passive and active modalities, in bed and in a wheelchair. The prototype integrates a control interface for monitoring, storage and availability of biofeedback variables, and another for motivational stimulation of the patient through interaction with gamification. The following sections describe how ABLEFIT works, as well as the results of the first usability tests carried out to the device.

2 ABLEFIT: Device Description

Based on a recent review of the literature and patents on medical devices used in rehabilitation plans, project requirements were established to proceed with the design and development of advanced rehabilitation equipment that may overcome the gaps and limitations identified in currently used equipment [7, 9, 10]. The detailed setting out of these design requirements versus user requirements can be found in [12]. Table 1 summarizes the macro requirements and the functionalities that the ABLEFIT device must respond to. To fulfil the requirement "1. Versatility of the structure, components and materials", the device is composed of a "C" shaped structure as illustrated in Fig. 1A (no. 1). The mobility of the structure is guaranteed by the 4 wheels attached to it, being the immobilization of the device also possible due to the blocking system they integrate. The structure and coupling elements, e.g. screws, are made of low density and oxidation and corrosion resistant material. The standard technical profiles that make up the structure device were selected after carrying out structural numerical calculations to guarantee the necessary: i) stability of the device, and ii) safety of the user and caregivers. The suitability of the ABLEFIT device to different types of beds and wheel- chairs is assured by the vertical movement of the horizontal bar - carriage - that integrates the device structure. This movement is controlled by an actuator that moves the threaded rod attached to the horizontal bar and ensures its up and down movement (or stop) to adapt the height of the device to the type of exercise intended, regardless of whether it is performed on a bed or in a wheelchair.

Table 1. Identification of ABLEFIT functionalities based on the establishment of design requirements vs. user requirements.

	Device Functionality
1. Versatility of structure, components and materials	Modularity: Integration of a linear module and a rotary module (adaptability to different types of movement: flexion, extension, abduction, inversion, eversion, internal and external rotation) Compactness: Adequacy to different environments of use (from hospital environments, clinics, and homes) Portability: Ease of transport (high mobility, reduced dimensions and weight) Hygiene: Ease of cleaning (adaptation of materials and geometries) Resistance: Resistant structure suitable for different movements and high weight of patients (adaptation of the cross-section of the profiles used) Adaptability: Suitability for beds and wheelchairs Low cost: Use of standard components, coupling elements and materials Safety and Ease of assembly/disassembly
2.Versatility of motions	2.1 Performing the movements of flexion, extension, abduction, inversion, eversion, internal and external rotation of the upper and lower limbs in active or passive mode 2.2 Performing linear, circular and amplitude movements 2.3 Easy and fast interchangeability between rotary linear modules 2.4 Possibility of using auxiliary immobilization devices and others

(*continued*)

Table 1. *(continued)*

	Device Functionality
3. Versatility of Man-Machine Interface	3.1 Application of different levels of load, velocity and amplitude 3.2 Definition of load, velocity, amplitude and time cycles 3.3 Definition of different load, velocity and amplitude increments 3.4 Acquisition, monitoring, registration and storage 3.5 Control of maximum values of strength, speed, amplitude and time 3.6 Wireless communication 3.7 Interoperability between systems 3.8 User-friendly operability 3.9 Safety, Autonomy and Energy savings

Depending on the type of movements to be performed in the exercises, different modules are alternatively coupled to the horizontal bar: i) the linear module that ensures the performance of linear movements (e.g. flexion, extension) and amplitude (linear movements with curvilinear paths, such as adduction and abduction), as represented in Fig. 1A (no. 2); or ii) the rotary module, which ensures rotary movements (e.g. internal and external rotation), as represented in Fig. 1A (no. 3). An easy-fit mechanism has been specially designed to allow the easy switching between the two modules. Any of these modules is activated by an actuator that allows the exercises to be performed in an active mode, i.e., the machine moves the user, or alternatively, the patient makes the machine move (passive mode). Additionally, an interface was adapted to each of these modules allowing not only the adaptation of the use of the module either by the feet or by the hands, i.e., any of the modules can be used for rehabilitation plans to be applied either to the upper limbs or to the lower limbs, but also the possibility of using immobilization aids and fixing parts of the limbs. Figure 2 illustrates, as an example, the adaptation of a orthosis (walker) to the linear module to perform lower limb flexion movements for adductor rehabilitation. The use of this auxiliary device helps avoid ankle and hip injuries. In this way, the fulfilment of requirement "2. Versatility in the type of movements" is ensured. A more detailed description of the elements that make up the rotary and linear modules, as well as their particular functions, can be found in [13].

Figure 3A outlines the fulfilment of requirement "3. Versatility of the Human-Device interface", (see also Fig. 1A, no. 4). The developed Human-Device interface includes: i) a microcontroller that integrates BLE and WiFi interfaces and receives set-point definitions for a customized rehabilitation plan, acting as the brain of the system; ii) sensors for measuring forces, velocities and times, as well as the acquisition of biofeedback parameters, i.e. user's vital signs and cadence, such as blood pressure (BP), heart rate (HR) and oxygen saturation (SPO2); iii) actuators that make up the linear and rotary modules controlling their performance; iv) a database that parameterizes, monitors, registers and

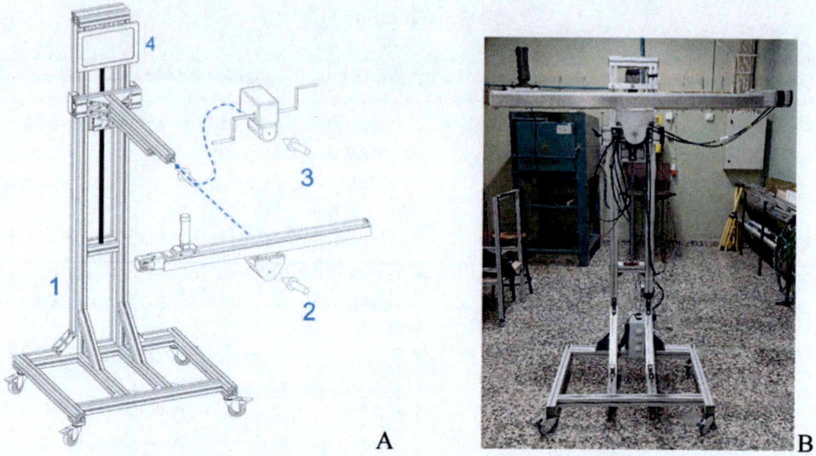

Fig. 1. ABLEFIT Representation: A. The virtual CAD model; B. The physical model

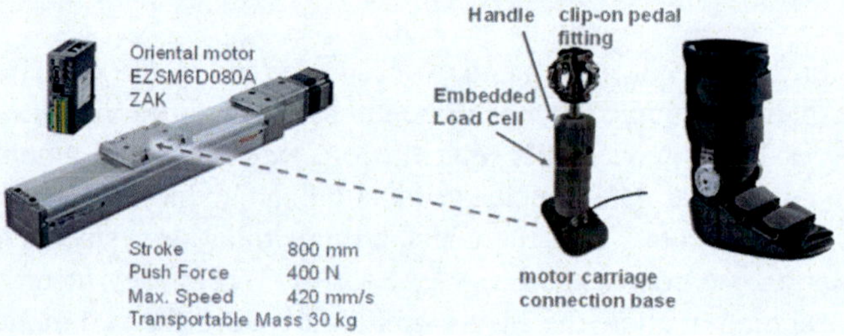

Fig. 2. Coupling of fixation and immobilization aids to the linear module of ABLEFIT

stores, for each patient, the parameters that characterize each rehabilitation plan (forces, velocities, times, repetition cycles) and the biofeedback parameters during the exercise, allowing the generation and availability of automatic reports and, if necessary, sending them remotely to medical teams or caregivers; and v) a tablet, whose function is to allow the configuration and visualization, of real time or stored values, of the parameters of the rehabilitation plan and biofeedback, through the integrated graphics interface (Android APP) as shown in Fig. 3B.

The use of a tablet also allows the implementation of a methodology that takes advantage of the use of games to enrich different contexts - gamification. In this case, the use of games will allow the patient to be motivated to carry out a certain re- habilitation plan during a certain period of time. It should be noted that the Human-Device interface was developed internally using a classic closed-loop control configuration to ensure, for safety reasons, that the patient never exceeds his physical limitation, a condition initially set by the health professional, by the caregiver or by the user. A detailed description of the Human-Device interface implemented in ABLEFIT and the interoperability between all the systems that constitute it has been recently published [14].

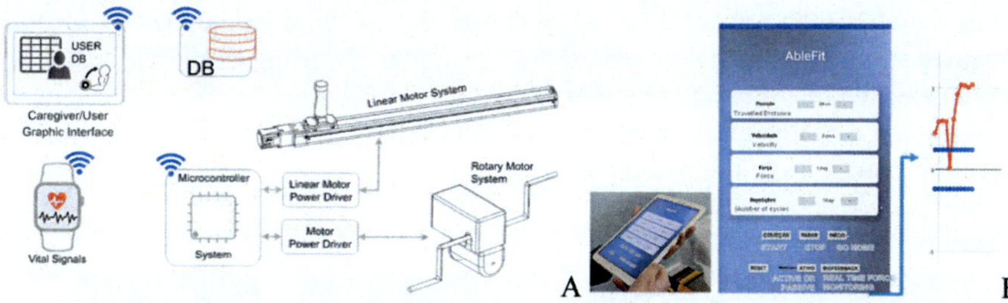

Fig. 3. Interfaces of ABLEFIT: A. The Human-Device interface; B. The Graphical interface

3 ABLEFIT: Pre-clinical Study

The development of new medical devices implies confronting their characteristics with a group of specialists' theoretical and practical knowledge [15]. As such, after the construction of the prototype, a pre-clinical study was carried out using the user-centered multimethod approach (User and Human-Centered Design) to evaluate the usability of the developed prototype, namely concerning its safety, functionality and ergonomics. The pre-clinical study started with a sample of 12 healthcare professionals (who manipulated the device's functions) and 10 end users (who used the device). Data were analyzed and treated using a mixed methodology: quantitative analysis of empirical instruments (such as surveys) and qualitative analysis of testimonies from interviews. Detailed information on how this pre-clinical study was conducted can be found in [16]. As previously described, ABLFEFIT's structure features the option to include modules, which are highly dependent on the therapeutic goals determined by the healthcare professional. Figures 4A and 4B show an example of the performance of a linear movement, in this case, the extension and flexion of the knee along a linear axis. For the efficiency of the exercise, apart from the distance and direction of movement, the healthcare professional, together with the patient, should also determine movement velocity and any resistance (force) applied to the module. Figures 4A and 4B also illustrate the need to apply an orthosis to the ABLFEFIT device, ensuring the mobilization of the lower limbs and, thus, the patient's safety and comfort. For upper limbs, the same criteria should be applied. Figures 4C and 4D illustrate the combined movement of the extension/flexion of the shoulder and elbow.

Safety assessment is mandatory for any new medical device [17]. In this study, end users felt safe with the ABLEFIT device and no adverse effects were observed. However, health professionals reported that the existing wires required by the equipment may pose a risk of accidental falls. Health professionals also highlighted the importance of continuous monitoring of vital signs, namely BP, HR and SpO2, the definition of maximum and minimum values for these bioparameters, and the possibility of triggering an alarm whenever these values are reached, thus ensuring the patient's safety. Additionally, they praised that ABLEFIT allows upper and lower limb exercises, actively and passively, to train the musculoskeletal and cardiovascular domains in their fullness. They pointed out the possibility of generating and implementing personalized rehabilitation plans as an additional advantage of the device. However, almost half of the professionals were concerned with limitations in the amplitude of upper limb exercises. Although any amplitude is better than none, this is an issue that requires in depth analysis for future implementation [18]. It was also reported as an added value the fact that ABLEFIT includes a gamification interface to motivate the user to complete the prescribed rehabilitation plans and a biofeedback interface that allows the health professional to monitor the status and evolution of the patient at all times.

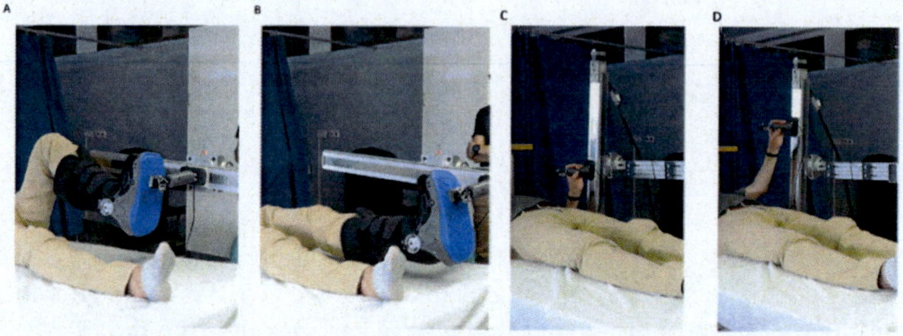

Fig. 4. Usability tests using the linear module of ABLEFIT

Regarding the ergonomics and comfort of the ABLEFIT device, most participants re- ported that they felt comfortable using it. However, both end-users, professionals and the research team pointed out the need for better fixation and positioning of the hand, wrist and foot. Thus, it becomes necessary to use and/or specifically develop technical aids that guarantee joint stability and correct positioning of the limbs for a safer, more comfortable and effective use of the ABLEFIT device, complying with the usability principles and ergonomic design [17, 19]. In addition, one of the most negative points mentioned by both end users and professionals was the size and flexibility of the device, making transport, storage and handling of the device difficult, particularly in hospital wards. In fact, the level of use of a device can be affected by its location and the surrounding conditions in which the device is used [20]. Professionals were also concerned with cleaning requirements and the noise produced as a result of the device operation. Another concern of professionals and end-users was the need for proper training to use the ABLEFIT device. Finally, it is crucial that the device meets ergonomic requirements and presents a friendly design [17]. The technical limitations reported in this pre-clinical study will be taken into account in the optimization phase of the developed prototype optimization.

4 Conclusions

To contribute to a significant reduction in morbidity and mortality associated with complications resulting from prolonged inactivity or even from a sedentary lifestyle that can be seen both in the elderly population and in young people with some mobility restriction or disability, a rehabilitation device was designed and built: the ABLEFIT device. A pre-clinical study was carried out that addressed different dimensions of the advanced rehabilitation system prototype built such as safety, functionality and ergonomics, both from the point of view of the end user and of the professional. Both end users and practitioners found ABLEFIT useful and an added value in caring for people suffering from PIS. Some professionals even claimed that ABLEFIT could help fill the shortage of professionals. In addition, they mentioned that it is one of the few devices that allows the exercise of the upper limbs. ABLEFIT enables the of the upper and lower limbs, actively and passively, and training the musculoskeletal and cardiovascular domains. Other advantages pointed out to the ABLEFIT device were the inclusion of a gamification component to motivate the user and a biofeedback system that allows the health professional to follow the user's evolution over time, namely in terms of vital signs and strength. The ABLEFIT device is thus a technical rehabilitation solution that ensures the implementation of physical rehabilitation programs in a personalized, controlled and interactive way. Even though the advantages reported above, some restrictions and limitations were raised during the pre-clinical study as regards software and hardware issues. These drawbacks and corresponding improvement proposals will be analyzed and their implementation constitutes the (next) phase of the developed prototype.

Funding:. This research was co-financed by the European Regional Development Fund (ERDF) through the partnership agreement Portugal 2020-Operational Programme for Competitiveness and Internationalization (COMPETE2020) under the project POCI-01–0247-FEDER-047087ABLEFIT: Desenvolvimento de um Sistema avançado para Reabilitação.

References

1. Arai, H., et al.: Association between skeletal muscle mass index and convalescent rehabilitation ward achievement index in older patients. Prog. Rehabil. Med., **7** (2022)
2. Guedes, L.P.C.M., et al.: Deleterious effects of prolonged bed rest on the body systems of the elderly. Rev. Bras. Geriatr. Gerontol. **21**, 499–506 (2018)
3. Li, J., et al.: Nursing resources and major immobility complications among bedridden patients: a multicenter descriptive study in China. J. Nurs. Manag. **27**, 930–938 (2019)
4. Wu, X., et al.: The association between major complications of immobility during hospitalization and quality of life among bedridden patients: a 3 month prospective multi-center study. PLoS ONE **13**, e0205729 (2018)
5. Marshall, R.N., et al.: Nutritional strategies to offset disuse-induced skeletal muscle atrophy and anabolic resistance in older adults: from whole-foods to isolated ingredients. Nutrition **12**, 1533 (2020)
6. Aqel, M.O.A., et al.: Review of recent research trends in assistive technologies for rehabilitation. In: Proceedings - 2019 International Conference Promising Electronic Technologies ICPET, pp. 16–21 (2019)
7. Bernardes, R.A., et al.: Innovative Devices for Bedridden Older Adults Upper and Lower Limb Rehabilitation: Key Characteristics and Features, p. 1185 (2020)
8. Jiang, C., Xiang, Z.: A novel gait training device for bedridden patients' rehabilitation. J. Mechanics in Med. Bio. **5**, 20 (2020)
9. Campos, A., Cortés, E., Martins, D., Ferre, M., Contreras, A.: Development of a flexible rehabilitation system for bedridden patients. J. Braz. Soc. Mech. Sci. Eng. **43**(7), 1–19 (2021)
10. Cardoso, R., et al.: Review physical rehabilitation programs for bedridden patients with prolonged immobility: a scoping review. Int. J. Environ. Res. Public Health, **19** (2022)
11. Fernandes, J., et al.: Rehabilitation workforce challenges to implement person centered care. Int. J. Environ. Res. Public Health **19** (2022)

12. Malça, C., et al.: Design of a customized rehabilitation device for patients with prolonged immobility syndrome. Submitted to: X Congress of the Portuguese Biomechanical Society, Figueira da Foz, Portugal (2023)
13. Roseiro, L., et al.: Development of a Biomechanical System for Rehabilitation Purposes of Bedridden Patients with Prolonged Immobility-Prototype and Preliminary Results. Submitted to: 11st World Conference on Information Systems and Technologies, Pisa, Italy (2023)
14. Santos, F., et al.: Biomechanical System Prototype with Advanced Biofeedback for Rehabilitation of Bedridden Patients. Submitted to: 16th International Joint Conference on Biomedical Engineering Systems and Technologies, Lisbon, Portugal (2023)
15. Dumas, J.S., Fox, J.E.: Usability testing. human-computer interact. Handb. Fundam. Evol. Technol. Emerg. Appl. Third Ed., 1221–1241 (2012)
16. Neves, H., et al.:Ablefit: development of an advanced system for rehabilitation, submitted to BioMedInformatics (2022)
17. Bitkina, O.V., Kim, H.K., Park, J.: Usability and user experience of medical devices: an overview of the current state, analysis methodologies, and future challenges. Int. J. Ind. Ergon. **76** (2020)
18. Winnard, A., Debuse, D., Wilkinson, M., Samson, L., Weber, T., Caplan, N.: Movement amplitude on the functional re-adaptive exercise device: deep spinal muscle activity and movement control. Eur. J. Appl. Physiol. **117**, 1597–1606 (2017)
19. Koppelaar, E.: Use and Effect of Ergonomic Devices in Healthcare (2017)
20. Zamzam, A.H., Abdul Wahab, A.K., Azizan, M.M., Satapathy, S.C., Lai, K.W., Hasikin, K.: A systematic review of medical equipment reliability assessment in improving the quality of healthcare services. Front. Public Heal. **9**, 1–12 (2021)

A Step Towards Obtaining an Innovative Smartbath for Shower in Bed of Disabled and Elder's People

Karolina Bezerra[1,2], José Machado[2(✉)], Vítor Carvalho[3,5], Demétrio Matos[4], and Filomena Soares[5]

[1] NUTES/UEPB, Center for Strategic Technologies in Health, State University of Paraiba, Campina Grande 58429-500, Brazil

[2] MEtRICs Research Center, School of Engineering, University of Minho, 4800-058 Guimarães, Portugal
jmachado@dem.uminho.pt

[3] 2Ai-EST-IPCA, Polytechnic Institute of Cávado and Ave, 4750-810 Barcelos, Portugal

[4] ID+-ESD-IPCA, Research Institute for Design, Media and Culture, School of Design, Campus do IPCA, 4750-810 Barcelos, Portugal

[5] ALGORITMI Research Centre, School of Engineering, University of Minho, 4800-058 Braga, Portugal

Abstract. Every project that obtained good results in the research needs to continue its development and start the process go-to-market. In the specific case related in this paper, the Smartbath, a shower system takes a new step towards its technological evolution becoming an intelligent shower system that promotes better features that the previous system was not fulfilling. Therefore, during the research it was defined that it is essential to make the system more portable and easier to use. In the context that will be used, this technology whereas, it represents an important contribution to the quality of life of caregivers. Considering an increase in the share of the elderly population and the related problems arising in daily care, this project intends to be beneficial and contemporarily. The bathing system is according to the needs of users who need to have really effective and technological systems, with a safety dynamic use with the water temperature to guarantee a quality bath and systems of checking heart rate and body temperature. In this sense, the development of technology moves to a new phase of product design, thinking about solving real problems with real products following a design project methodology.

Keywords: Shower · Disabilities · Bedridden · Portable System · Medical Device

1 Introduction

Currently, the contribution of science in advancing the development of technology through the creation of an innovative system is of paramount importance to address

D. Tarnita et al. (Eds.): MESROB 2023, MMS 133, pp. 99–108, 2023.
https://doi.org/10.1007/978-3-031-32446-8_11

real problems in real environments, specifically, in everyday healthcare. The growth of incentives for the development of assistive technologies indicates the high potential of market needs, which come with the objective of minimizing the social needs of the population, which indicates rates of gradual increase in population aging worldwide [1–3].

For the development of this project, it is used a design methodology that shapes world culture and influences the quality of life and improves aspects of daily life for users [2].

For professional performance, the activity of the product development team uses specifications that optimizes functions, creates shapes and emphasizes appearance, raise value and design systems to benefit integration with users. Therefore, to help multidisciplinary teams in the development of new products, the authors suggest using five criteria in the execution of tasks and in the creation of products. Each of them is exemplified below:

- Utility: The product's interface must be secure, easy to use and intuitive, with each requirement being generated in order to convey the product's function to the user;
- Appearance: The use of elements such as shape, line, proportion and color have an influence in order to create a product with a pleasant appearance;
- Ease of maintenance: Product designs must be carried out in a way that conveys how they should be preserved and repaired;
- Low cost: Shapes and functions are responsible for budgetary impacts on production and tooling costs, so they should be considered by the product development team;
- Communication: The visual qualities of the product must communicate the philosophy and corporate mission, an activity that is the responsibility of the Product Design team [2, 3].

In order to meet the bathing needs of elderly and bedridden people, the development of a solution of great relevance for the area of care and health was initiated [5]. Therefore, the system is now designated by the Smartbath brand, with the meaning: intelligent and portable bathing system. This solution has a proposal that seeks to improve the quality of life of caregivers and their patients in the bathing activity, and also minimize critical processes such as: different environments, different physical limitations, time limit and caregivers' exhaustion; and it focuses on helping a single caregiver to care for bedridden people [6, 7].

It is fundamental that the process of raising awareness, followed by intervention in the practice of bathing, instigates and promotes a new vision in daily care to be carried out in any environment and that can be performed by any individual.

The first solution was prototyped in 2018, and was successful both in functions and in tests performed in real environments [7]. The Smartbath project had as a definition some hypotheses to carry out as future work, which are the result of the understanding and need for improvement in some formal and functional aspects analyzed during the tests. In this moment, were defined some new requirements to develop and increase the reliability of needs, thus defining to the version of final prototype and makes the validations in real ambience. This process would be very important for the system developers for reaching new levels of technology transfer with the new solution product design.

The first water supply system gave rise to the built prototype. Tests were carried out to validate its functionality. The system has a capacity of 80 L of water storage, idealized for home care and can also be used in a hospital environment. Therefore, it is considered that this concept has the capacity to give more than one bath per day, without the caregiver needing more time in the procedure of filling the reservoirs and heating the water [6, 7].

During the development of this project technical tests and usability tests were carried out by the caregiver in a real environment with the prototype developed in 2018 [7], which ensured its use in any environment, such as the bedroom, as this guarantees control of the water temperature and water storage, which facilitates the various tasks and reduces this need relatively.

The prototype 1 was developed considering the project requirements (see Fig. 1).

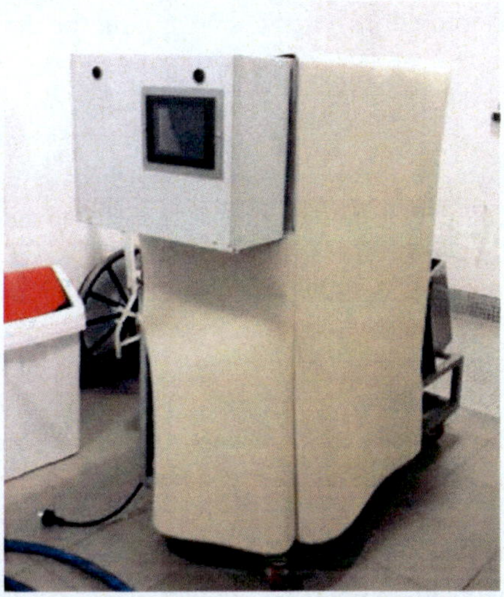

Fig. 1. Prototype 1 of the water supply system [7]

The system has a robust structure due to the dimensioning that considers a high amount of water and, also, because a posture was adopted, with regard to the development of this concept, of choosing existing components that, not always, are suitable for equipment that is intended to be specific and innovative [8–11]. There is no other device for bathing with suction system integrated and using the same equipment.

Although the concept is capable of holding all the components, it demonstrates a clearly oversized robust structure, where the worst scenarios of transport and use in environments with reduced dimensions and without accessibility were considered.

In this context, the development of concept 2 began, to demonstrate the possibility of meeting other requirements not met with concept 1. The improvements were made in order to make it possible for this system to adjust the function and form of the system to the needs of the users, giving rise to concept 2. The details of the project are listed below:

- Designed to be used at home and with a capacity of 20 L of water, which means it can only be used for a shower;
- Its shape facilitates mobility (avoiding problems with different types and sizes of doors) and has a retractable handle to reduce clutter when not in use;
- The developed concept has a base diameter 500 mm and height of 1000 mm;
- Designed for ease of use by a formal caregiver or an informal caregiver in both home and hospital settings;
- The simple structure idealized in Stainless Steel;
- Wheels with multidirectional movement and safety braking;
- Modular concept provides for user disassembly and maintenance.

This paper is organized in 4 sections. Section 2 presents the new step on the development of the existing Smartbath system; Sect. 3 is devoted to present the components – both hardware and software – that compose the new Smartbath system; and, finally, in Sect. 4, there are presented some final remarks concerning the developed work.

2 Design of the New Step of Smartbath

In this new step in the development of the new Smartbath solution, it is extremely important to take into account that patients in a state of dependence have important restrictions regarding bathing. In this way, Smartbath provides bedridden patients at home and in hospitals around the world with a new experience of well-being, comfort and safety [6].

The equipment can be used in any domestic environment, having in its structure a height support designed to allow ergonomic and comfortable handling.

The Smartbath has a capacity of 20 L of water, which is four times less than the capacity of concept 1. In these terms, concept 2 does not invalidate concept 1, it only demonstrates that specific equipment can be developed that fulfills all initial requirements. For this, components that do not exist on the market have to be developed, such as, for example, the development of the reservoirs themselves with shapes suitable for the intended equipment.

This requirement can be easily met if the prototype designed in concept 2 is built, therefore, in the next section will be show which functional aspects were implemented in the new step of the project.

To show the arrangement of all the parts, Fig. 2 represents the view of the components of the water supply system concept with all the integrated parts.

The mechanical system is completely built-in 306 stainless-steel material. It is divided into three parts, which are the heating and water tank, suction tank and the fixing structure. The entire system is fixed on 306 stainless steel metal support, reservoirs are willing to be removable. A structural advantage is to promote the easy removal of the fixing structure reservoirs as it effectively provides easy maintenance of the structure. Considering the modular structuring of all physical components promotes the assembly and disassembly of the physical parts and electronic components.

The electronic components are implemented separately and effectively do not contact water. The mechanical system supports the system's general operation, the functions are activated from the user interface on the 10.1 in. LCD monitor.

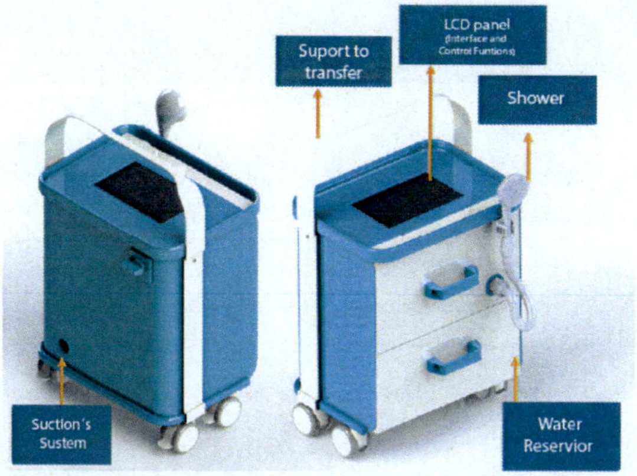

Fig. 2. Detailed image of the second concept to prototype parts (LCD control panel, water tank, transfer stand, shower and suction system)

In the construction of the mechanical part of the prototype, the operation was validated through the filling and automated water discharge procedure.

The system under development aims to meet the demand for bathing and suctioning residual water in the care environment. The two reservoirs are for water supply and suction, with a capacity of 20 L each. And based on the needs explored in several scientific studies, [4–12]. At this moment, some parameters are presented as need for the implementation of health care and bath activities. Below, there are presented some parameters being implemented in this product:

- Connectivity, with data transmission via Wi-Fi or Bluetooth, and offline use is also possible.
- Low cost, as it is a national technology that should cost something around 5 to 10% of the systems currently commercialized;
- Low energy consumption enabling prolonged use;
- Prototype development, aiming to provide speed and flexibility in the creation of more compact and resistant formats;
- Portability, allowing use in any environment;
- Temperature safety for water outlet;
- Biomedical sensors included;
- Checks and indicates the ambient temperature.

In addition to the various functions that are being implemented in this new concept, a flow was developed for the shape system that performs the simplified function [14–17]. The flow of devices implemented in the system is tested and enabled to exercise its functionalities, see Fig. 3.

The operating flow takes into account the extreme need to use a filter right after the beginning of the supply to ensure that no residue enters the device. The solenoid valve is used to ensure the opening of the system at the water inlet of the reservoir. So that the filling of the reservoir is under control, the level sensors are used and, in this way,

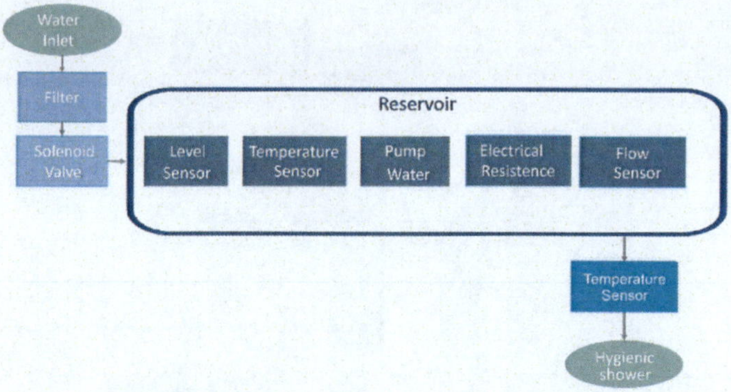

Fig. 3. Flow of devices implemented within the second prototype

the user knows when the device is full and when it is emptying, the whole process is accessed through the interface. The electrical resistance has the function of ensuring that the water is heated, but for safety the temperature sensor is used.

As important as the other components, the water pump is responsible for the water outlet and to ensure that the water flow is controlled, a flow sensor is used and is directly linked to the extreme need for this solution. The system has several settings to ensure user's safety, as well as the temperature sensor at the final outlet of the water system. The components were simplified in relation to the first project, which means that the Smartbath is in the process of being improved in relation to the initial idea and, at this moment, it is intended to move forward to increase the technological maturity (TRL 6).

Therefore, the main focus of the development of the new prototype and the performance of new concept tests, in the related institutions, and this validation will bring us new results both scientifically and for the market [6, 7].

3 Smartbath Hardware and Software Systems

3.1 Hardware System

The hardware system has had its development with several sensors with different objectives to secure the use of equipment. Which one will be described one by one with the specific's requirements.

This part of product has the water flow sensor that will be pumped after leaving the reservoir. The purpose of this sensor is to provide some data to the system, such as the energy required to heat the mass of water being pumped; how many liters per minute are being used in the bath; based on the water level you have in the reservoir, how long you have a bath available.

The most important to guarantee the security about temperature, is the temperature sensors, two sensors are installed, one that measures the temperature at which the water is leaving the tank, with the aim of calculating, together with the water flow, the amount of energy that must be supplied to the resistance to water reaches the desired temperature. The second temperature sensor is used to verify that the water coming out of the resistance has the desired characteristics. And thus, being able to release or not the flow of water for the bath shower.

Another component applied is Hygrometer with thermometer. The objective of that component is to measure the temperature and relative humidity of the air, so that it can stipulate a more suitable temperature for the bath, always thinking about the patient's thermal comfort. It must have sensors that check for current leakage in the equipment in addition to an emergency stop button. It must contain solenoid valve-type actuators that change the water flow, if it does not have the desired characteristics and conditions.

The radiator implemented in the circuit serves to cool the already heated water and make a return of the same water, trying in this way to homogenize the temperature of the water system.

The overall diagram of the system, that was created, can be seen in Fig. 4.

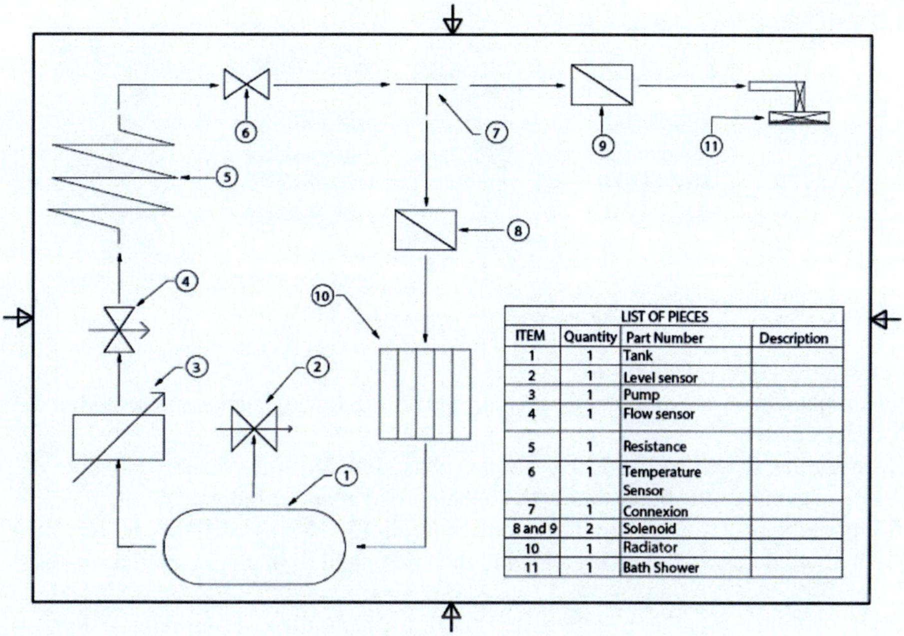

LIST OF PIECES			
ITEM	Quantity	Part Number	Description
1	1	Tank	
2	1	Level sensor	
3	1	Pump	
4	1	Flow sensor	
5	1	Resistance	
6	1	Temperature Sensor	
7	1	Connexion	
8 and 9	2	Solenoid	
10	1	Radiator	
11	1	Bath Shower	

Fig. 4. Overall diagram of the System.

3.2 Software System

There must be a software system for the equipment and to be used on mobile devices such as smartphones and tablets in which the two must communicate and exchange data and drive commands, using cloud computing that promotes to access all tools with just the registered login and password, on any device connected to the internet, scaling business through cloud solutions.

The software for mobile devices can serve as a kind of medical record, storing all data related to the patient and the bath (whether through machine sensors, photographs or filling out forms), in addition to what it´s contain POPs (standard operational procedure), bathing recommendations and other technical information that can help nurses, caregivers and patients. As referred the user communicates with the system throught the Human Machine Interface (HMI) 10.1 LCD monitor where specific software was developed (Fig. 5).

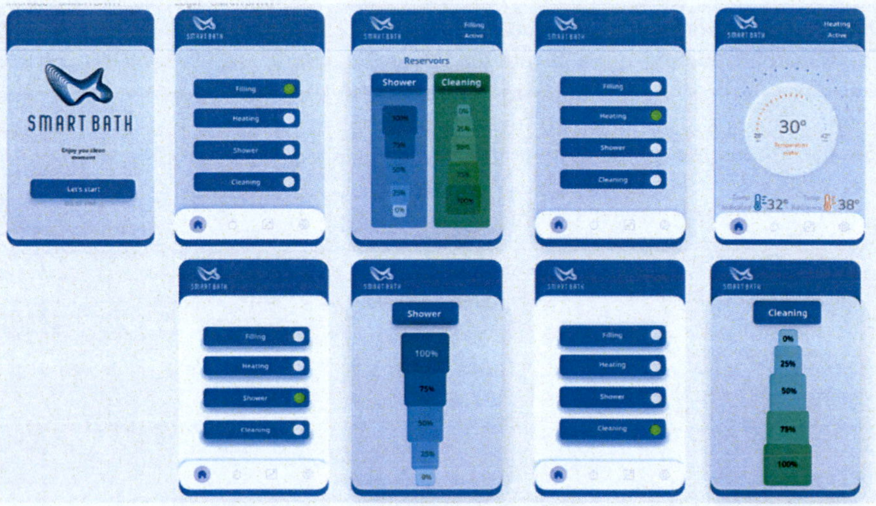

Fig. 5. Interface implemented

The sequence of use of the system is through the following steps represented in the HMI interface:

Turn on the device to the 230 V single -phase power grid – 50 Hz; Conduct the hydraulic network of the bathroom with the help of an adapter; Indicate in the interface the filling of the reservoirs; Turn off the device to the 230 V Single Phase - 50 Hz; Turn off the hydraulic network adapter, allowing the equipment to be transported to the bath site.

Start water heating; Choose the temperature for bath, through the interface of the system; Check the light (yellow) signal, when active the system ended the heating process; Start the bath; Start the bath manually, by driving the shower; Start in parallel with tasks that are related to the device functions and follow the patient's care. Organize the environment with the following activities: take the clothes out of the bed; Change the bedding; The surface must be mounted on a horizontal plane.

Start the bath, using the equipment shower; Wash the front of the body; Washing of the side parts (back); Head washing; Washing of the feet. Surface cleaning of the environment with the suction system; Turn off the bath system, start the suction function at the controller interface; Perform the complete suction of surface water and the environment; Perform mechanical drying of the user with a towel; Perform the surface mechanical drying with a towel; Turn off the served water suction system; Travel to a place where it can promote the emptying of water reservoirs; Termination of the bath procedure.

4 Final Remarks

Every project that obtained good results in research and development and resulted in the first prototype has been presented, but we understand that the market needs a solution that simplifies the activity and also the level of wear and tear, thus being an added value. The development continued and, in this case, the second version of the bathroom system takes a new step from its technological evolution, the Smartbath, an intelligent bathroom system that promotes better functionalities and is involved in a more portable, safer and more user-friendly system.

The supply system prototype integrates the mechanical system and the electronic system (controller), as well as the user interface LCD monitor. The software embedded in the machine must be able to read data from the different sensors and be able to calculate bathing needs, and must work independently of the software for mobile devices. It should identify, record and feed the patient's medical record, monitor the time and bathing conditions, evaluate the bath quantitatively and qualitatively according to the nurse and the patient as well as being able to communicate with other platforms.

Therefore, in view of the need pointed out above, the adequacy of a support system for multifunctional and multi-articulated bathing is tolerated in order to reduce the influence of the low mobility of bedridden patients on periodic bathing when accompanied by a caregiver in your residence or institutions. This bathing system supports not only the hygiene of the bedridden, but also due to the long stay in beds, as well as to increase their protection and quality of life. Continuing with the future work, the health assessment record will be implemented, the biomedical sensor system to ensure monitoring at the time of bathing.

References

1. World Health Organization: A contribution of the WHO to the second united nations world assembly on ageing. In: 2 United Nations World Assembly on Ageing; United Nations, Madrid, Spain, pp. 12–31 (2002)
2. Eppinger, S., Ulrich, K.: Product Design and Development. McGrawHill Inc., New York (1995)
3. Carlos Pereira, J.: Metodologia De Projeto Aplicada À Concepção De Sistemas Mecatrónicos a Partir Da Elaboração De Um Modelo Prescritivo De Desenvolvimento. Tese de Doutoramento, UFCS (2016)
4. Fonseca, E.F.: Cuidados de higiene - Banho: significados nos cuidados de enfermagem. Perspectiva dos enfermeiros. In: Dissertação de Mestrado, Instituto de Ciências Biomédicas Abel Salazar da Universidade do Porto (2013)
5. AAL Strategy 2014–2020 for the Active and Assisted Living Programme. http://www.aal-europe.eu/wp-content/uploads/2015/11/20151001-AAL-Strategy_Final.pdf. Accessed 10 May 2015
6. Bezerra, K., et al.: Bath-ambience—a mechatronic system for assisting the caregivers of bedridden people. Sensors **17**(6), 1156 (2017)
7. Bezerra, K., et al.: A new methodology for use by a single caregiver to bathe bedridden elderly persons using advanced mechatronic systems. Healthcare (2019)
8. Bruno, S., José, M., Filomena, S., Vítor, C., Demétrio, M., Karolina, B.: The conceptual design of a mechatronic system to handle bedridden elderly individuals. Sensors **16**(5), 725 (2016)

9. Hybs, J.: An evolutionary process model of design. Des. Stud. **13**(3), 273–290 (1992)
10. Bezerra, K., Machado, J., Leão, C.P., Soares, F., Carvalho, V., Matos, D.: Requirements for the development of medical devices - caregivers perspectives survey. In: ASME International Mechanical Engineering Congress and Exposition, Proceedings (IMECE), vol. 2 (2016)
11. Bezerra, K., et al.: System for assistance on bath of bedridden elderly people. In: ASME International Mechanical Engineering Congress and Exposition, Proceedings (IMECE), vol. 3 (2014)
12. Golding-Day, M., Whitehead, P., Radford, K., Walker, M.: Interventions to reduce dependency in bathing in community dwelling older adults: a systematic review. Syst. Rev. **6**(1), 198 (2017)
13. Yukiko, K., McIntosh, J., Thomas, G.: Bathroom design for assisted showering that improves the quality of life of the elderly. J. Aging Soc. Change **8**(3), 69–89 (2018)
14. Yukiko, K., McIntosh, J.: Housing design and the quality of life for older people with care needs: gaps in knowledge. J. Aging Soc. Change **12**(1), 49–74 (2022)
15. Pierce, D.: The Accessible Home: Designing for All Ages and Abilities. Edited by Alan Walker and Catherine Hagan Hennessy. The Taunton Press, Newtown, (2012)
16. Aanand, N., Concato, J., Gill, M.T.: Bathing disability in community-living older persons: common, consequential, and complex. J. Am. Geriatr. Soc. **52**(11), 1805–1810 (2004)
17. Ángel, O., Yébenes, M., Rodríguez-Laso, Á., Zunzunegui, M.: Unmet home care needs among community-dwelling elderly people in Spain. Aging Clin. Exp. Res. **15**(3), 234–242 (2003)

Lab Experiences for a Driver Monitoring System

María Garrosa[1(✉)], Marco Ceccarelli[2], Matteo Russo[2], and Daniele Cafolla[3]

[1] University Carlos III of Madrid, 28911 Madrid, Spain
mgarrosa@ing.uc3m.es
[2] University of Rome Tor Vergata, 00133 Rome, Italy
{marco.ceccarelli,matteo.russo}@uniroma2.it
[3] Robotics and Intelligent Systems Lab, Department of Innovation in Engineering and Physics, IRCCS Neuromed, Pozzilli, IS, Italy
contact@danielecafolla.eu

Abstract. This paper presents the aspects to be taken into account when analyzing the risk of injury to the neck of vehicle occupants as a consequence of an impact. To carry out the analysis, a low-cost driver monitoring system is designed and prototyped, consisting of wearable head, neck and torso units in which acceleration sensors are installed. Two distance sensors are placed inside the vehicle to know the displacement of the head and neck in addition to acceleration sensor. The results of the lab experiments have made it possible to characterize the biomechanical response of the neck. Considerations of the results are used to formulate a new criterion for assessing the risk of neck injury due to impact.

Keywords: Biomechanics · Testing Design · Injury Criteria · Experimental Tests

1 Introduction

Nowadays, nonfatal injuries are a worldwide public health problem. Impact injury investigation and the analysis of experimentally based biomechanics play a key role in the mitigation of injuries caused by traffic crashes. In general, in low-speed rear-end crashes, the head of the impacted vehicle occupant moves relative to the torso causing distortion of the neck, which makes the cervical spine the most vulnerable area and can lead to minor (sprains/strains), moderate (intervertebral disc derangement) and severe (fractures, dislocations and spinal cord injuries) injuries. The frequency of these injuries is inversely proportional to their severity, so that the most common and least severe are musculoligamentous strains which are known as whiplash. Less common are disc injuries and vertebral fractures, and the least common are spinal cord injuries [1]. The analysis of the mechanisms of whiplash is complicated by the complex structure of the cervical spine and the various impact conditions. Numerous investigation reports can be found in the literature that have been attempted to characterize the cervical spine biomechanical response. Many of these investigations have tested animals [2], human volunteers [3], human cadavers [4], crash test dummies [5], and computational models [6]. Most authors agree that the cause of whiplash injuries is due to the "S-shaped" deformation of the neck in an impact. This deformation occurs when the seat back pushes

D. Tarnita et al. (Eds.): MESROB 2023, MMS 133, pp. 109–116, 2023.
https://doi.org/10.1007/978-3-031-32446-8_12

the occupant forward and the head, moving due to inertia, retracts backward without rotation in the lateral axis. The head moves to a plane behind the torso, forcing the upper cervical spine into flexion and the lower cervical spine into extension. To analyze the risk and severity of cervical injuries in vehicle impacts different injury criteria are proposed such as NIC (Neck Injury Criterion) [2], N_{km} (Neck Protection Criterion) [7], N_{ij} (Neck Injury Criterion) [8], LNL (Lower Neck Load Index) [9], Intervertebral Neck Injury Criterion (IV-NIC) [10], Neck Displacement Criterion (NDC) [11] and Whiplash Injury Criterion (WIC) [12]. In this paper, test results of lab experiences are presented to evaluate $NHIC_2$ as an improvement of NHIC [13] and to characterize the biomechanics of a car crash in a driver using a specific low-cost monitoring system with features of comfort easy-wearing requiring design and operation of specific testing system.

2 Problems and Requirements

Problems for analyzing car impacts and their consequences in the occupants can be summarized in:

- Experiments with human volunteers involving a loading situation that can cause injury are not permitted;
- Sensors cannot be often installed in the desired locations, e.g., at the center of gravity of the head and neck, and it can be difficult to have them properly fixed on a driver;
- A large number of possible mechanisms of injury and injuries that could occur.

Consequently, requirements for a proper experimental testing can be identified as:

- During an experiment, head and neck displacements must be monitored to determine the biomechanical response of the cervical spine even during a low-speed rear-end impact;
- A driver monitoring system must be designed consisting of wearable units for head, neck and torso in which acceleration sensors are properly installed;
- Suitable sensors can be used to measure head, neck and torso displacement as well as head, neck and torso acceleration during an impact;
- The design and operation should be at low-cost levels to be included in the common safety car systems.

The problems and requirements for characterizing experimentally the human biomechanical response to a vehicle impact can be summarized as in Fig. 1.

The here-in proposed monitoring system is designed to evaluate the biomechanics of car impacts in a driver by referring to the specific injury criterion $NHIC_2$ that considers neck displacement as an improvement of the expression in [13],

$$NHIC_2 = \frac{(m_v + m) \cdot a_v}{m \cdot (V_v)^2} \cdot \frac{a_{hmax}}{a_{nmax}} \cdot \left(\left(X_{hf} - X_{hi}\right) + \left(X_{nf} - X_{ni}\right)\right) \cdot 1000 \tag{1}$$

where m_v is the vehicle weight, m is the occupant weight, a_v is the maximum vehicle acceleration, V_v is the vehicle speed at the moment of the experiment, a_{hmax} is the maximum head acceleration, a_{nmax} is the maximum neck acceleration, X_{hf} is the position of the head after the test, X_{hi} is the initial position of the head, X_{nf} is the position of the neck after the test and X_{ni} is the initial position of the neck.

Design requirements for a proper risk analysis of car impacts can be identified referring to a numerical evaluation of injury criteria. The design and operation problems attached in this work refer to designing a monitoring system that can also give data for $NHIC_2$ evaluation.

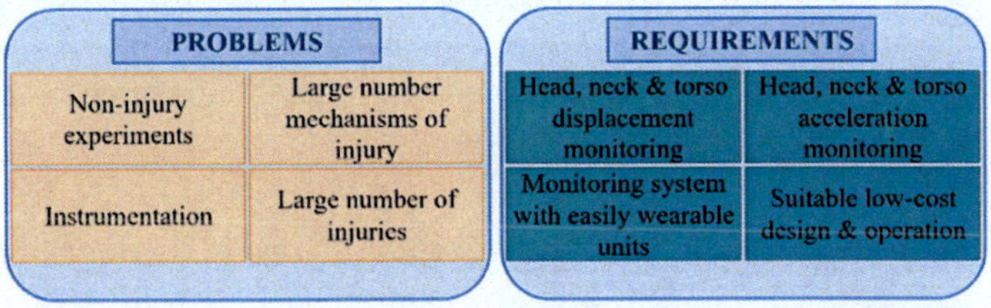

Fig. 1. A scheme of problems and requirements for analyzing injuries in vehicle impacts

3 Conceptual Design

The experiment proposed in this work consists of a test to analyze the risk of injury mainly to the neck of a vehicle occupant as a consequence of an impact. A low-cost solution is proposed for lab experiences with market components, in order to build and use a prototype that can be operated in the lab frames as summarized in Fig. 2 and Fig. 3 as improvement of previous design in [13, 14].

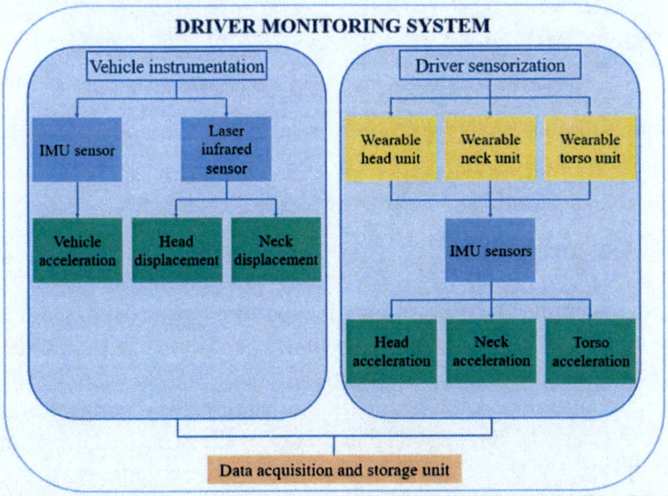

Fig. 2. A conceptual design of a system monitoring driver condition in a vehicle setup

The main objective is to characterize the biomechanical response of the neck in terms of acceleration and displacement. Figure 2 shows a conceptual scheme of the system design for monitoring a driver. The monitoring device is composed of four IMU (Inertial Measurement Units) sensors and two laser infrared distance sensors. In the vehicle, the IMU is placed at the center of gravity, horizontally and oriented with the main direction of car motion, to acquire the acceleration of the car. Two high-precision laser infrared sensors are strategically placed one on the top of the steering wheel and one on the dashboard, in order to track the trajectory and movement of head and neck points. For driver monitoring, easily wearable units can be designed on suites with IMU sensors to obtain head-forehead, neck, and torso acceleration measurement.

Figure 3 shows a CAD design with indication of suitable location of the above-mentioned sensor in a testing frame of a driver in a car.

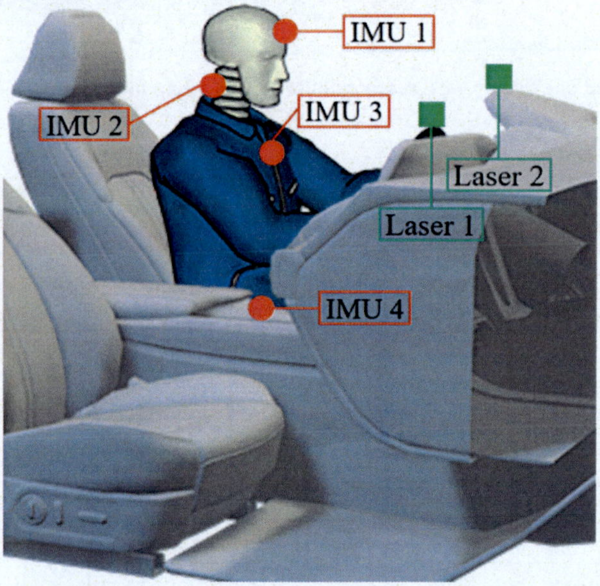

Fig. 3. Sensor location of the monitoring system in Fig. 2 in a testing car frame

4 Prototype Assembly

The here-in proposed monitoring system for lab experiments consists of four MPU6050 IMU sensors and two VL53L0X laser infrared sensors. Additionally, the TCA9548A I2C multiplexer is used to expand the I2C bus ports to connect I2C sensors with the same address to the microcontroller. Data acquisition is achieved by connecting the above components to an Arduino MEGA 2560. The design of the proposed driver monitoring system is shown in Fig. 4 with the circuit connections to the components.

In order to fix properly the IMUs on driver's body, 3D printed box houses are installed with IMU inside on a wearable suit unit as shown in Fig. 5.

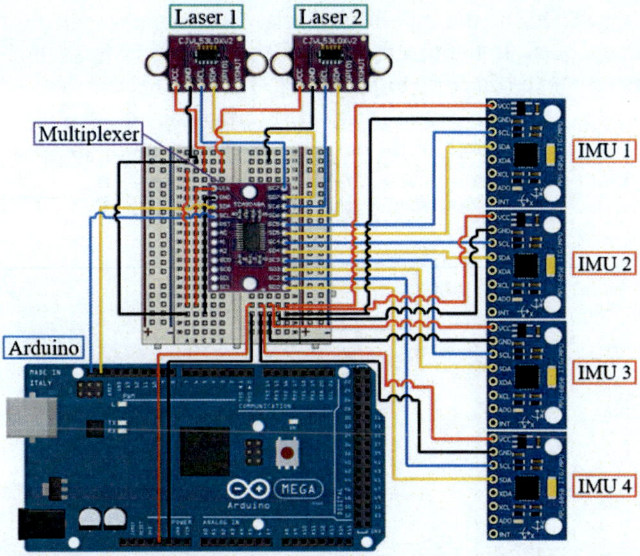

Fig. 4. Electronic layout of the driver control system design

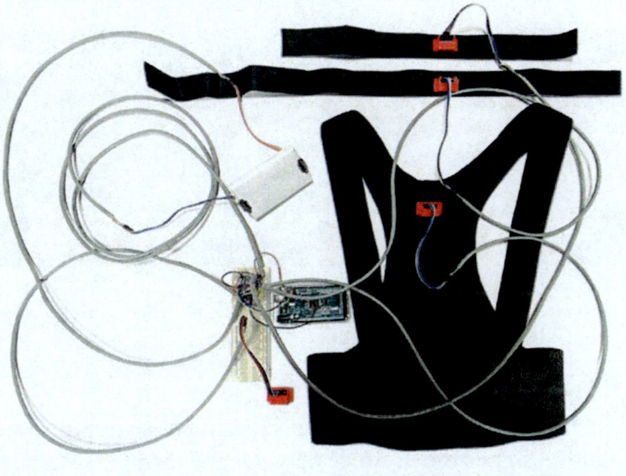

Fig. 5. The lab prototype of the driver control system design

5 Lab Tests and Results

Testing activity has been worked out in a lab frame by using the low-cost prototype with market components as shown in Fig. 5.

In particular tests are planned to compute neck and head displacements with an approximation as in the models in Fig. 6. P_h and P_n correspond to the reference points of the head and neck respectively, before the experiment begins, from which the sensor measures the distance. During the experiment these points are changed due to the movement of the head and neck. In the first step of the experiment the head moves backward and the sensor measures the distance to P'_h and P'_n. Then the head is moved forward and in this case the values of the distance to P''_h and P''_n are obtained.

Figure 7 shows the snapshots of the movement performed by the subject during a lab test with a typical movement of head and neck in a car impact.

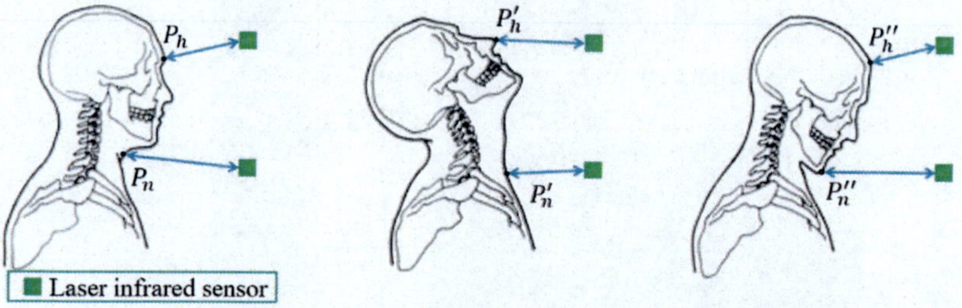

a) b) c)

Fig. 6. A scheme of data evaluation of neck/head displacements from laser infrared sensors: a) home configuration; b) backward; c) forward

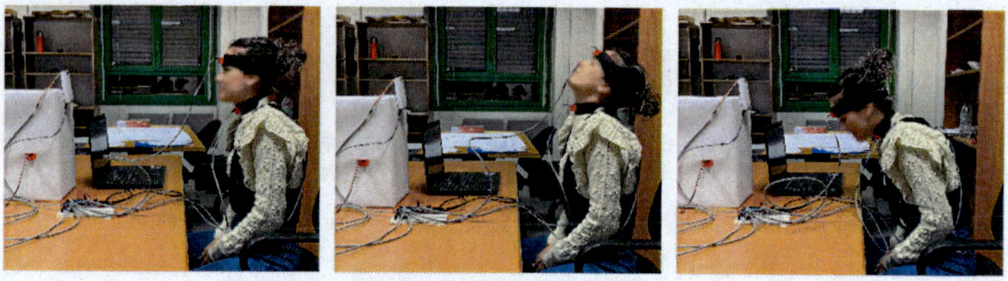

a) b) c)

Fig. 7. Snapshot of a lab test

Illustrative results from all sensors during an experiment as in Fig. 7 are reported in Fig. 8 and Fig. 9. Figure 8 shows the distance between the infrared laser sensors and the subject's head and neck. The head displacement is 0.836 m ($P_h{}' = 1.098$ m and $P_h{}'' = 0.262$ m) and the neck displacement is 0.779 m ($P'_n = 1.046$ m and $P_n{}'' = 0.267$ m). Figure 9 shows the acceleration of the head, neck and torso obtained from the IMU sensors. The maximum acceleration is experienced by the head at 9.27 m/s^2, followed by the torso at 6.05 m/s^2 and finally the neck at 4.69 m/s^2.

The two laser infrared sensors allow to obtain an approximation of the head and neck displacement to give an approximate evaluation of the $NHIC_2$.

However, the test results show the efficiency of the designed monitoring system in indicating the main biomechanics parameters of the sudden motion in a car occupant simulating a car impact.

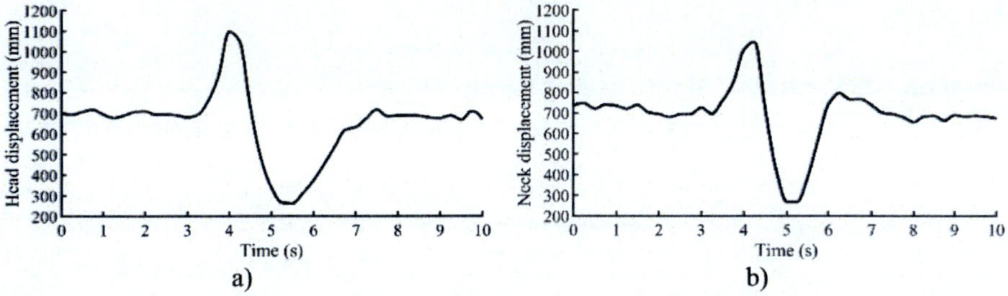

Fig. 8. Results of a lab test as in Fig. 7 from laser sensor as displacement of: a) head; b) neck

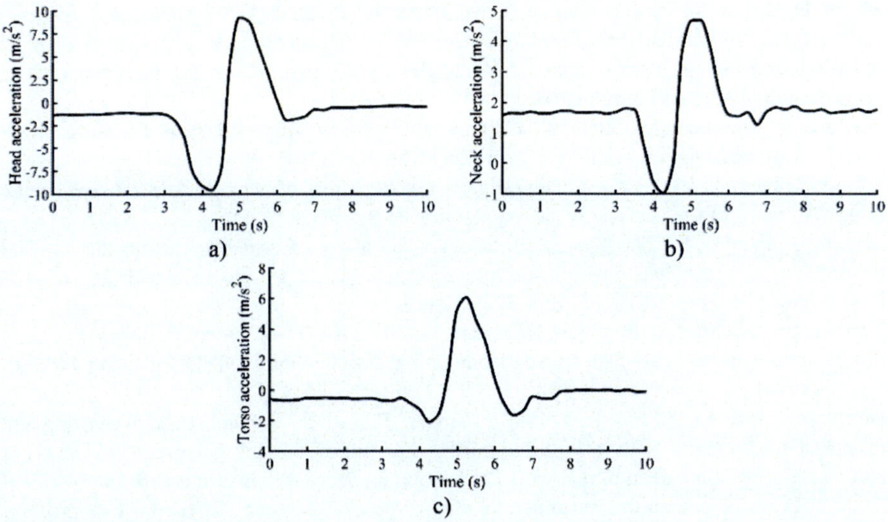

Fig. 9. Results of a lab test as in Fig. 7 from IMU sensors in term of acceleration of: a) head; b) neck; c) torso

6 Conclusions

Lab experiences are discussed to present a new driver monitoring system for analysis and risk evaluation of car impacts focusing on neck motion. A low-cost solution is designed for driver wearing to be used successfully for a campaign of testing in order to characterize the system operation and to attempt numerical evaluation of a new injury criterion with a measurement approximation of head and neck displacements.

Acknowledgments. The first author wishes to gratefully acknowledge Universidad Carlos III de Madrid "Ayudas para la movilidad de investigadores/as de la UC3M en centros de investigación nacionales y extranjeros en su modalidad: estancias de jóvenes doctores/as" for permiting her period of stay at the LARM2 of the University of Tor Vergata in 2022–23.

References

1. Freeman, M.D., Leith, W.M.: Estimating the number of traffic crash-related cervical spine injuries in the United States; an analysis and comparison of national crash and hospital data. Accid. Anal. Prev. **142**, 105571 (2020)
2. Boström, O., et al.: A new neck injury criterion candidate-based on injury findings in the cervical spinal ganglia after experimental neck extension trauma. In: Proceedings of the 1996 International Ircobi Conference on the Biomechanics of Impact, Dublin, Ireland, pp. 123–136 (1996)
3. Ono, K., Kaneoka, K., Wittek, A., Kajzer, J.: Cervical injury mechanism based on the analysis of human cervical vertebral motion and head-neck-torso kinematics during low speed rear impacts. SAE Trans., 3859–3876 (1997)
4. Meyer, F., Humm, J., Purushothaman, Y., Willinger, R., Pintar, F.A., Yoganandan, N.: Forces and moments in cervical spinal column segments in frontal impacts using finite element modeling and human cadaver tests. J. Mech. Behav. Biomed. Mater. **90**, 681–688 (2019). https://doi.org/10.1016/j.jmbbm.2018.09.043
5. Mallory, A., Stammen, J., Zhu, M.: Cervical and thoracic spine injury in pediatric motor vehicle crash passengers. Traffic Inj. Prev. **20**(1), 84–92 (2019)
6. Yan, Y., Huang, J., Li, F., Hu, L.: Investigation of the effect of neck muscle active force on whiplash injury of the cervical spine. Appl. Bionics Biomech. (2018)
7. Kumar, S., Ferrari, R., Narayan, Y., Jones, T.: The effect of seat belt use on the cervical electromyogram response to whiplash-type impacts. J. Manip. Physiol. Ther. **29**(2), 115–125 (2006). https://doi.org/10.1016/j.jmpt.2005.12.008
8. Kleinberger, M., Sun, E., Eppinger, R., Kuppa, S., Saul, R.: Development of improved injury criteria for the assessment of advanced automotive restraint systems. NHTSA Docket **4405**(9), 12–17 (1998)
9. Heitplatz, F., Sferco, R., Fay, P., Reim, J., Kim, A., Prasad, P.: An evaluation of existing and proposed injury criteria with various dummies to determine their ability to predict the levels of soft tissue neck injury seen in real world accidents. In: Proceedings of the 18th International Technical Conference on the Enhanced Safety of Vehicles, Nagoya, Japan, pp. 1–7 (2003)
10. Panjabi, M.M., Wang, J.L., Delson, N.: Neck injury criterion based on intervertebral motions and its evaluation using an instrumented neck dummy. In: Proceedings of the International Research Council on the Biomechanics of Injury conference, vol. 27, pp. 179–190. International Research Council on Biomechanics of Injury (1999)
11. Viano, D.C., Davidsson, J.: Neck displacements of volunteers, BioRID P3 and Hybrid III in rear impacts: implications to whiplash assessment by a neck displacement criterion (NDC). Traffic Inj. Prev. **3**(2), 105–116 (2002)
12. Munoz, D., Mansilla, A., Lopez-Valdes, F., Martin, R.: A study of current neck injury criteria used for whiplash analysis proposal of a new criterion involving upper and lower neck load cells. In: Proceedings of the 19th Experimental Safety Vehicles Conference, pp. 6–9 (2005)
13. Garrosa, M., Ceccarelli, M., Díaz, V.: Propuesta de un nuevo criterio para cuantificar las lesiones en impactos de vehículos. In: XV Congreso Iberoamericano de Ingeniería Mecánica, Madrid, España (2022). https://doi.org/10.5944/bicim2022.248
14. Ceccarelli, M., Cafolla, D., Russo, M., Garrosa, M., Díaz, V.: Vehicle driver monitoring device, Italy. Patent No. 102022000022092, 26 October 2022

Wire Actuation Mechanism for Wrist Exoskeleton

Narcis-Graţian Crăciun and Erwin-Christian Lovasz(✉)

Politehnica University of Timisoara, Timişoara, Romania
narcis.craciun@student.upt.ro, erwin.lovasz@upt.ro

Abstract. This paper has as main subject the mechatronic exoskeleton devices used in the rehabilitation applications of the wrist for the patients who are in the recovery period after suffering a stroke. The number of people who have suffered a stroke is constantly increasing and reaches alarming figures. People who have suffered a stroke need a long recovery period, and in most cases permanent care. There are many methods of recovering the mobility and strength of the affected limb, but along with the technological progress, the interest in mechatronic exoskeleton devices has also increased. These devices can replace human assistance, thus allowing a higher level of independence for the patient. In the paper is presented a short review from the literature with the main types of exoskeleton devices existing on the market with a short description. From this review it can be seen that most of the existing devices treat mainly the flexion/extension movement of the joint, while the abduction/adduction movement is less approached. This is due to the fact that the adduction/abduction movement is harder to generate from a kinematic point of view, but this movement is absolutely necessary for the patient to perform the necessary movements in performing daily activities. For this reason, the work presents in the second half a model of exoskeleton device seems capable of generating the abduction/adduction movement.

Keywords: wrist exoskeleton · rehabilitation device · wire actuation · adduction-abduction

1 Introduction

Stroke affects approximately 800,000 Americans annually, thus becoming one of the main causes of the increase in the number of people with locomotor disabilities in the US. People who survive a stroke face semi-paralysis in the upper and lower limbs, with a decrease in their strength, thus becoming unfit for work and often unable to perform their daily activities [1–3]. Traditional therapy methods are based on physical exercises to increase dexterity, control and strength of the affected limb. These therapy sessions must be carried out with the help of a specialized person to permanently monitor the patient's progress and generally take place in authorized treatment centers [4, 5]. A large majority of people who suffer from stroke have locomotor deficiencies at the level of the wrist joint. This joint has the role of directing and orienting the hand in the execution of various movements [6]. Even if the wrist joint has an essential role in

D. Tarnita et al. (Eds.): MESROB 2023, MMS 133, pp. 117–124, 2023.
https://doi.org/10.1007/978-3-031-32446-8_13

carrying out everyday activities, this joint enjoys much less attention from researchers than the shoulder and elbow joints. The use of exoskeleton type devices started to be more and more widespread in the rehabilitation area. These exoskeletons can be defined as mechatronic devices, which can be worn by the patient with the main role of providing support and assistance for the realization of various movements and actions within the rehabilitation sessions [7]. The use of these devices has many advantages, such as: a) much more correct realization of the rehabilitation exercises, b) the possibility to monitor the patient's evolution through exact data transmitted by the exoskeleton, c) the possibility for the patient to perform the rehabilitation exercises from the comfort own home [8, 9].

2 Background

Along with the technological advance, various models of exoskeletons for the wrist joint have been created. These are identified either by the number of possible degrees of freedom (DOFs) rendered, by the way in which the actuation is carried out, passive or active, or by the type of actuation mechanisms used. In the following, the latest models of exoskeletons used for rehabilitation applications of the wrist joint that can be found on the market will be briefly presented.

The most common exoskeletons for the wrist joint are those with a single DOF, intended for flexion/extension movements of the wrist. Such devices are presented in [10, 11], both devices are driven by electric motors through wires, which greatly reduces the weight of the device. Another exoskeleton that reproduces all flexion/extension was developed at Seoul National University [12] being driven by direct current motors.

Another exoskeleton with a single DOF is the eWrist [13]. It is intended for use at the patient's home, being able to record the progress made by the patient. The device uses the Myo armband [14] which uses surface electromyography sensors to determine the electrical signals generated by the patient's muscles when he intends to make a movement. In [15] an exoskeleton for flexion/extension movements using pneumatic artificial muscles (PMAs) is presented. The artificial pneumatic muscles are controlled using a force and pressure controller. Exoskeletons that are not actuated by external forces have also been developed, they are called passive exoskeletons and are presented in [16, 17]. These devices use springs that are tensioned by the patient's movement, and by releasing the tension they help to achieve the desired movements, flexion/extension in this case.

There are also exoskeletons designed for the entire arm, or just the wrist and forearm. Such examples are the InteliArm exoskeleton [18], which has six DOFs, four active and two passive. It can reproduce the flexion/extension of the wrist joint respectively the pronation/supination of the forearm respectively the BRAVO exoskeleton [19], which also has a DOF for the wrist and a DOF for the forearm.

In [20, 21] two prototypes of exoskeletons with two DOFs for the wrist are presented, one for the flexion/extension movement and one for the abduction/adduction movement. Both devices are driven by motors, in [20] a single geared motor is used, and in [21] three electric motors are used, because the device uses three tendons to transmit the movement. A similar device with two DOFs for hand joint movements is presented in

[22]. It uses two elastic elements actuated by two linear motors to transmit the movement. Two exoskeleton devices using artificial pneumatic muscles are presented in [23, 24]. Both have two DOFs for the wrist and reproduce its specific movements by the contraction/extension of certain pneumatic muscles at the same time. In [25] a device with 2 DOFs for the wrist is presented that uses Shape Memory Alloy based actuators to transmit the movement. This approach has the main advantages of low weight and noiseless operation, and the attachment of the device is done through a glove, which increases the patient's comfort while using the device.

ETS-MARSE [26] is an exoskeleton for the upper limb with seven DOFs, two of which are intended for flexion/extension and adduction/abduction movements of the wrist and one for pronation/supination movements of the forearm. Other devices that present two DOFs for the wrist and one DOF for the forearm are presented in [27]. In [28] a device called soft exoskeleton is presented due to the low weight materials used with the aim of developing a device as ergonomic as possible to increase the comfort of the patient during use.

3 Mechanical Design of the Proposed Exoskeleton

As could be seen from the previous chapter, most wrist exoskeleton devices used for rehabilitation applications only allow flexion/extension movement of the joint. This is because this movement is much easier to achieve from an engineering point of view with a mechatronic device. Unfortunately, the abduction/adduction motion of the wrist joint is essential for performing daily activities and leading a normal life.

The wrist joint is an ellipsoid synovial joint that has a very large range of motion (ROM) and is incredibly resistant to external stress [29]. The general ROM of the abduction/adduction movement of this joint is approximately 20° for radial deviation and approximately 26° for ulnar deviation. These values differ from men to women and especially in different age categories [29].

Next is presented a possible model of an exoskeleton type device that can reproduce the movement of radial deviation/ulnar deviation for the wrist joint of patients who are recovering after suffering a stroke.

3.1 3D Model of the Proposed Structure

The prototype presented in Fig. 1 is made up of the following component elements: a support for the thumb, which also wraps the palm, a bracelet for the joint area of the wrist, a bracelet for the forearm area, a band-type element that joins the two bracelets, two cables for transmitting the movement and a servo motor that drives the two cables.

The device is attached to the upper part of the patient's palm and forearm respectively. The support for the thumb a) is fixed in the patient's palm by means of elastic bands and has the role of preventing the device from sliding during the abduction/adduction movement. The bracelet of the wrist b) joint is fixed at the level of the wrist joint, the bracelet to which the servomotor is fixed c) is fixed on the forearm. Both bracelets are adjusted in the lower part by means of elastic bands mounted through the mounting holes f). The brand-type element d) connects the two bracelets and blocks the flexion/extension movement, its length being permanently constant. The focus is on ergonomics and on using the device as easily as possible.

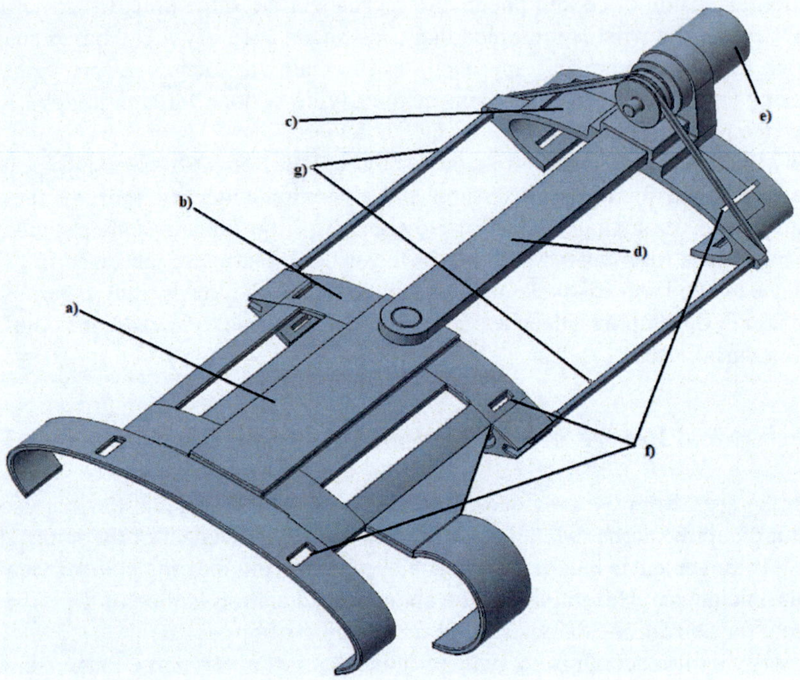

a) Support for the thumb; b) Bracelet of the wrist; c) Bracelet of the forearm; d) Brand-type elements; e) Servomotor; f) Mounting holes; g) Wires

Fig. 1. 3D model of the exoskeleton prototype

3.2 Kinematics of the Mechanism

Figure 2a shows the kinematic schema of the wrist exoskeleton designed to realize the adduction-abduction motion. There are three rotation couplers on the bracelet in the area of the wrist joint. One coupler for each of the two cables and the third coupler for the band-type element. The cables are wound on the pulley of the servomotor in opposite directions, so that when the servomotor tightens one cable, the other is de-tensioned. The length of the cables between the two bracelets changes during the abduction/adduction movement, thus the length with which one cable is tensioned is equal to the length with which the other cable is de-tensioned. The band-type element has the role of blocking the flexion/extension movement and allowing only the abduction/adduction movement through the rotation coupler located at the level of the bracelet fixed on the wrist. The support for the thumb fixes the entire mechanism in the palm area to prevent it from sliding during operation.

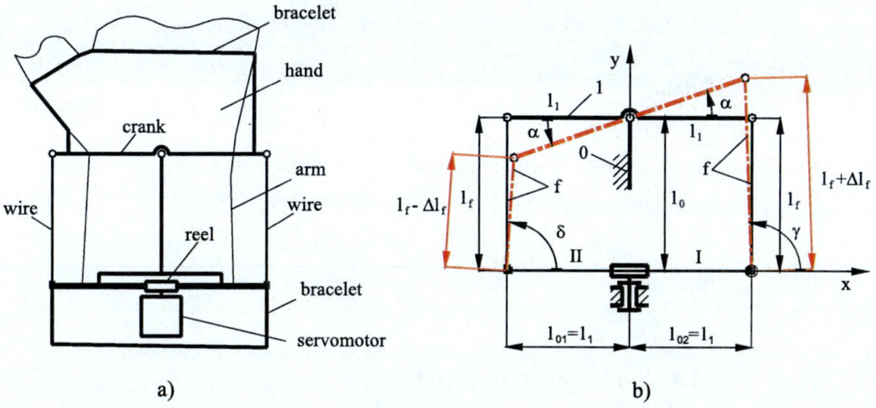

Fig. 2. Kinematic schema of the wrist exoskeleton (a) and the actuating mechanism (b)

The kinematic analysis of the exoskeleton motion is described by using the Fig. 2b. The length of the bracelet-type element is represented by l_1, the length of each free wire length by l_f, respectively the length of the brand-type element by l_0. The full wire length contains the two free wire lengths and the constant wire length used for enveloping and developing from the pulley. The adduction-abduction angle is given by α.

The vectorial equation in complex numbers for the two closed loops are given below:

$$l_1 + (l_f + \Delta l_f) \cdot e^{i\gamma} = i \cdot l_0 + l_1 \cdot e^{i\alpha}, \tag{1}$$

$$-l_1 + (l_f - \Delta l_f) \cdot e^{i\delta} = i \cdot l_0 - l_1 \cdot e^{i\alpha}. \tag{2}$$

By separating the term $(l_f + \Delta l_f) \cdot e^{i\gamma}$ in one side in the Eq. 1 and multiplying with the complex conjugate term results the relationship for computing the variation of the wire length in the first closed loop I:

$$\Delta l_f = \sqrt{{l_0}^2 + 2 \cdot {l_1}^2 - 2 \cdot {l_1}^2 cos\alpha + 2 \cdot l_0 l_1 sin\alpha} - l_f \tag{3}$$

Applying the same procedure for the Eq. 2 results the relationship for computing the variation of the wire length in the second closed loop II.

$$\Delta l_f = \sqrt{{l_0}^2 + 2 \cdot {l_1}^2 - 2 \cdot {l_1}^2 cos\alpha - 2 \cdot l_0 l_1 sin\alpha} - l_f \tag{4}$$

The rotation angle of the servomotor φ can be computed with the relationship:

$$\varphi = \Delta l_f / r \tag{5}$$

where: r is the radius of the reel.

3.3 Numerical Example

For the numerical example are chosing the geometrical parameters, given in the Table 1. The values are close to the human hand and arm dimmensions.

Table 1. Geometrical parameters of the wrist exoskeleton

Parameter	Symbol	Value
Frame lenght	l_0	100 mm
Frame lenght	$l_{01} = l_{02}$	50 mm
Free wire lenght	l_f	100 mm
Crank lenght	l_1	50 mm
Reel radius	r	15 mm

The variation of the wire length in the two loops is computed by using the relationships (3) and (4). The adduction-abduction angle α is chosen in the range of $[-15°, 40°]$. The wire length variation is represented in the Fig. 3a.

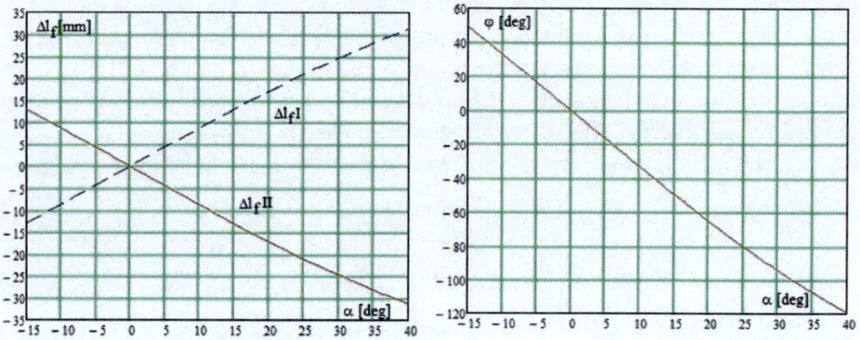

a) b)

Fig. 3. The variation of the wire length in the two loops (a) and the angular variation of the servomotor reel (b)

It is shown that the both wires length variations are simmetrical to the initial position ($\Delta l_f = 0$), that confirms the initial hypotesis to have the enveloped and developed wire length approximately equal with the maximum deviation around 1 mm. This properties of the actuation wire mechanism allows to use one servomotors. Figure 3b shows that the angular variation of the servomotor reel $\varphi \in [50°, 120°]$.

4 Conclusions

The paper deals with a mechatronic exoskeleton device used for the rehabilitation applications required for patients who have suffered a stroke. A series of the latest devices available on the market for such applications are briefly presented. From this study it could be observed that most of these devices are created to reproduce the flexion/extension movement of the wrist in general, the abduction/adduction movement being much less addressed. For these reasons, this paper presented the 3D model of a possible mechanism for an exoskeleton capable of reproducing the abduction/adduction movement. The emphasis was placed on ergonomics and on the lowest possible weight, for this reason, the bracelets and the bar-type device can be made of plastic, the transfer of the movement is done through wires by a single servomotor precisely to reduce the weight of the device as much as possible. Future improvements of this device will focus on trying to integrate the flexion/extension movement in this structure, in order to obtain an exoskeleton that can reproduce both movements of the hand joint.

References

1. Benjamin, E.J., et al.: Heart disease and stroke statistics. Circulation **137**(12), e67–e492 (2018)
2. Lang, C.E., et al.: Observation of amounts of movement practice provided during stroke rehabilitation. Arch. Phys. Med. Rehabil. **90**(10), 1692–1698 (2009)
3. Bernhardt, J., Dewey, H., Thrift, A., Donnan, G.: Inactive and alone: physical activity within the first 14 days of acute stroke unit care. Stroke **35**(4), 1005–1009 (2004)
4. Palmer, A.K., Werner, F.W., Murphy, D., Glisson, R.: Functional wrist motion: a biomechanical study. J. Hand Surg. **10**(1), 39–46 (1985)
5. Ashford, S., Slade, M., Malaprade, F., Turner-Stokes, L.: Evaluation of functional outcome measures for the hemiparetic upper limb: a systematic review. J. Rehabil. Med. **40**(10), 787–795 (2008)
6. Lambelet, C., Temiraliuly, D., Siegenthaler, M., et al.: Characterization and wearability evaluation of a fully portable wrist exoskeleton for unsupervised training after stroke. J. Neuro Eng. Rehabil. **17**(1), 132 (2020)
7. Olar, M., Leba, M., Risteiu, M.: Exoskeleton - wearable devices. In: Literature review, MATEC Web of Conferences, vol. 342 (2021)
8. Ward, N.S., Brander, F., Kelly, K.: Intensive upper limb neurorehabilitation in chronic stroke: outcomes from the queen square programme. J. Neurol. Neurosurg. Psychiat. **90**(5), 498–506 (2019)
9. Zollo, L., Rossini, L., Bravi, M., Magrone, G., Sterzi, S., Guglielmelli, E.: Quantitative evaluation of upper-limb motor control in robot-aided rehabilitation. Med. Biol. Eng. Comput. **49**(10), 1131–1144 (2011)
10. Song, Z., Guo, S.: Design process of exoskeleton rehabilitation device and implementation of bilateral upper limb motor movement. J. Med. Biol. Eng. **32**(5), 323–330 (2011)
11. Ates, S., Mora-Moreno, I., Wessels, M., Stienen, A.: Combined active wrist and hand orthosis for home use: lessons learned. In: Conference: Rehabilitation Robotics (ICORR), vol. 2, no. 4, pp. 227–241 (2015)
12. Nam, H.S., et al.: Biomechanical reactions of exoskeleton neurorehabilitation robots in spastic elbows and wrists. IEEE Trans. Neural Syst. Rehabil. Eng. **25**(11), 2196–2203 (2017)
13. Lambelet, C., Lyu, M., Wenderoth, N., Woolley, D., Gassert, R.: The eWrist - a wearable wrist exoskeleton with sEMG-based force control for stroke rehabilitation. In: IEEE International Conference on Rehabilitation Robotics 2017, pp. 726–733 (2017)
14. Visconti, P., Gaetani, F., Zappatore, G.A., Primiceri, P.: Technical features and functionalities of Myo armband: an overview on related literature and advanced applications of myoelectric armbands mainly focused on arm prostheses. Int. J. Smart Sens. Intell. Syst. **11**(1), 1–25 (2018)
15. Meng, W., Sheng, B., Klinger, M., Liu, Q., Zhou, Z., Xie, S.Q.: Design and control of a robotic wrist orthosis for joint rehabilitation. In: IEEE/ASME (AIM) International Conference on Advanced Intelligent Mechatronics, vol. 31, pp. 132–145 (2015)

16. Ates, S., Lobo-Prat, J., Lammertse, P., vad der Koji, H., Stenen, A.H.A.: SCRIPT passive orthosis: design and technical evaluation of the wrist and hand orthosis for rehabilitation training at home. In: IEEE International Conference on Rehabilitation Robotics 2013, p. 6650401 (2013)
17. Ates, S., Haarman, C.J.W., Stienen, A.H.A.: SCRIPT passive orthosis: design of interactive hand and wrist exoskeleton for rehabilitation at home after stroke. Auton. Robot. **41**(3), 711–723 (2017). https://doi.org/10.1007/s10514-016-9589-6
18. Ren, Y., Kang, S.H., Park, H.S., Wu, Y.N., Zhang, L.Q.: Developing a multi-joint upper limb exoskeleton robot for diagnosis, therapy, and outcome evaluation in neurorehabilitation. IEEE Trans. Neural Syst. Rehabil. Eng. **21**(3), 490–499 (2013)
19. Troncossi, M., Mozaffari Foumashi, M., Mazzotti, C., Zannoli, D., Castelli, V.P.: Design and manufacturing of a hand-and-wrist exoskeleton prototype for the rehabilitation of post-stroke patients. Quaderni del DIEM – GMA. Atti della Sesta Giornata di Studio Ettore Funaioli, 111–120 (2012)
20. Xiao, Z.G., Menon, C.: Towards the development of a portable wrist exoskeleton. In: 2011 IEEE International Conference on Robotics and Biomimetics, Karon Beach, Thailand, pp. 1884–1889 (2011)
21. Dragusanu, M., Lisini, T., Iqbal, M.Z., Prattichizzo, D., Melvezzi, M.: Design, development, and control of a tendon-actuated exoskeleton for wrist rehabilitation and training. In: IEEE International Conference on Robotics and Automation (ICRA), pp. 1055–1062 (2020)
22. Higuma, T., Kiguchi, K., Arata, J.: Low-profile two-degree-of-freedom wrist exoskeleton device using multiple spring blades. EEE Robot. Autom. Lett. **3**, 305–311 (2017)
23. Andri Kopoulos, G., Nikolakopoulos, G., Manesis, S.: Motion control of a novel robotic wrist exoskeleton via pneumatic muscle actuators. In: 20th IEEE International Conference on Emerging Technologies and Factory Automation (ETFA), pp. 1–8 (2015)
24. Al-Fahaam, H., Davis, S., Nefti-Meziani, S.: Wrist rehabilitation exoskeleton robot based on pneumatic soft actuators. In: Proceeding of International Conference for Students on Applied Engineering (ICSAE), pp. 491–496 (2017)
25. Serrano, D., Copaci, D.S., Moreno, L., Blanco, D.: SMA based wrist exoskeleton for rehabilitation therapy. In: IROS, pp. 153–157 (2018)
26. Rahman, M., Rahman, M., Cristobal, O., Saad, M., Kenné, J., Archambault, P.: Development of a whole arm wearable robotic exoskeleton for rehabilitation and to assist upper limb movements. Robotica **33**(1), 19–39 (2015)
27. Buongiorno, D., Sotgiu, E., Leonardis, D., Marchschi, S., Solassi, M., Frisoli, A.: WRES: a novel 3 DoF wrist exoskeleton with tendon-driven differential transmission for neuro-rehabilitation and teleoperation. IEEE Robot. Autom. Lett. **3**, 2152–2159 (2018)
28. Bartlett, N.W., et al.: A soft robotic orthosis for wrist rehabilitation. J. Med. Devices **9**(3), 030918 (2015)
29. Than, T., San, A., Mynt, T.: Biokinetic study of the wrist joint. Int. J. Collab. Res. Intern. Med. Public Health **4**(5), 450–458 (2012)

Exoskeletons and Prostheses

Design and Gait Control of an Active Lower Limb Exoskeleton for Walking Assistance

Lingzhou Yu[1(✉)], Harun Leto[1], André d'Elbreil[2], and Shaoping Bai[1]

[1] Department of Materials and Production, Aalborg University, Aalborg, Denmark
liyu@mp.aau.dk

[2] Department of Robotics, École Centrale de Nantes, Nantes, France

Abstract. This paper presents an assistive lower-limb exoskeleton (ALEXO) for active walking assistance. The mechatronics design covering mechanical design, sensors selection and motor controllers are introduced. A 2-link model is built for dynamic analysis control purposes, upon which a trajectory tracking control method based on an improved computed torque control is proposed. This control method was tested with sensor data acquired from walking trials of a healthy subject, which validated the design and gait control of this exoskeleton.

Keywords: active lower-limb exoskeleton · walking gait · trajectory tracking · exoskeleton validation

1 Introduction

Lower-limb exoskeleton technology has advanced significantly for broad applications [1–8]. Most of these devices can be divided into three main lower-limb categories: industry, healthcare and military exoskeletons. Of these, assistive exoskeletons can help patients with stroke and spinal cord injuries to restore their movement abilities [6,7]. Up to date, different exoskeletons have been designed [8–13]. A few exoskeletons use hydraulic actuators, which can obtain high bandwidth, but the system stability is limited by the hydraulic fluid and the servo-valves [14]. Some exoskeletons adopt artificial pneumatic muscles, which are more flexible, but the force bandwidth of the whole system is low [15]. Most exoskeletons use electric motors, for example, the Hybrid assistive limb(HAL) exoskeleton, which can provide walking assistance for hemiplegia patients [16].

For achieving active assistance, control methods have to be developed to meet the needs of different tasks. In [17], an adaptive algorithm was proposed for a rehabilitation exoskeleton. The dynamic movement primitives(DMP) control method was applied to an exoskeleton for human power augmentation [18]. To generate a reasonable reference actuator torque for a flexible gait pattern, a central pattern generator (CPG) was utilized in [19] to produce continuous gait trajectory. A hybrid controller using CPG and admittance controller with electromyography (EMG) signals has achieved trajectory generating for both hip and knee joints [20]. In spite of these developments, control methods that are

D. Tarnita et al. (Eds.): MESROB 2023, MMS 133, pp. 127–135, 2023.
https://doi.org/10.1007/978-3-031-32446-8_14

able to achieve efficient walking assistance on active lower exoskeletons are still a major challenge.

In this paper, a design of an active lower-limb exoskeleton robot (ALEXO) is proposed for walking assistance. The exoskeleton was designed with a lightweight structure, which is suitable for users of different sizes. The sensors and control units are integrated. A computed torque control method is implemented for tracking trajectory.

The remainder of the paper is organized as follows. Section 2 introduces the concept of the exoskeleton, and Sect. 3 describes the control method. Sections 4 and 5 present the results of the simulation and the experimental results with users. The work is concluded in Sect. 6.

2 Active Lower Limb Exoskeleton Robot

2.1 The ALEXO Configuration

The concept of the ALEXO is shown in Fig. 1, which was developed on the basis of the lower-limb module of the full-body exoskeleton AXO-SUIT [21,22].

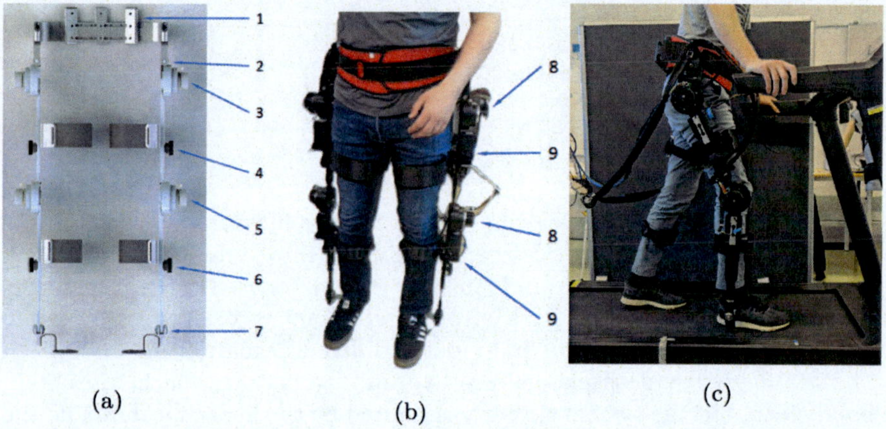

Fig. 1. Concept of ALEXO. (a) The CAD model, (b) the physical system, (c) human-exoskeleton interaction test. The system includes: 1. waist support, 2. passive adduction/abduction hip joint, 3. active flexion/extension hip joint, 4. thigh adjustment screw, 5. active flexion/extension knee joint, 6. shank adjustment screw, 7. passive plantar flexion/dorsiflexion ankle joint, 8. harmonic drive unit driven by EC60 100W brushless motors, 9. Forsentek FNG30 load sensors.

The ALEXO was designed to help individuals with walking difficulty by enhancing the lower limbs' motion in sagittal plane. The ALEXO exoskeleton has a total of 8 DOFs. The hip joint of the ALEXO has two DOFs: one active DOF in the sagittal plane to provide external active assistive torque, and a passive DOF for addiction and abduction. The knee joint has one active DOF for flexion and extension. The ankle joint is passive to accommodate dorsiflexion and plantar flexion.

The exoskeleton is adaptable to different body types and can adjust shank length, thigh length, hip width, and interchange user attachment option depending user needs. Furthermore, adjustable mechanical end-stops are present in the system to ensure user safety. The range of motion of the joint angles are shown in Table 1, which is sufficient to accommodate the lower human motion.

Table 1. Angular range of motion(ROM) and DOF of joints

Joint	DOF	Freedom Type	ROM
Hip	Flexion/Extension	Active	95°/25°
-	Adduction/Abduction	Passive	10°/15°
Knee	Flexion/Extension	Active	90°/0°
Ankle	Dorsiflexion/Plantar Flexion	Passive	20°/45°

The mechanical structures of ALEXO are made of 6061 and 7075 aluminum alloy. The light-weighted segments decrease the system's inertia. Four 3D-printed TPA cuffs attach to the thigh part and the shank part of both legs to fixate and align the human body in the exoskeleton. Each cuff consists of two curved segments, one in the front and one in the back, which is connected to an adjustable slide rail to adjust for different thigh and shank sizes. Elastic straps are used to tighten the cuffs. ALEXO is supported from the ground by two glass fiber foot attachments. Four Maxon EC60 48V 100W flat motors are selected for hip and knee joints. The motors drive integrates back-driveable harmonic gear drives with a ratio of 1:120 for the hip and 1:50 for the knee joint, respectively.

2.2 Hardware and Control Architecture

The hardware and control architecture of ALEXO are illustrated in Fig. 2. The system consists of two Teensy 4.1 micro controller boards that are serially connected to a PC. Each Teensy is connected to a leg and processes data from its hip and knee joint. In particular, each Teensy is connected to two ESCON 50/5 servo controllers, two Broadcom AEAT 6012 absolute encoders, and two HX711 load cell amplifiers. The Broadcom encoders are attached to the non-drive side of ALEXO and read the joint angle of the hip and knee directly from the pilot side of the exoskeleton.

ALEXO is operated on a hierarchical control. The high-level control is implemented on the Teensy 4.1 micro controllers. A computer connected serially to each Teensy has a user interface in which data is received and monitored in real time. By having a high-speed data serial data communication (5 ms cycle time) between the ESCON controller and sensors, the Teensy boards can compute reference trajectories and send these to the low-level ESCON 50/5 servo controller.

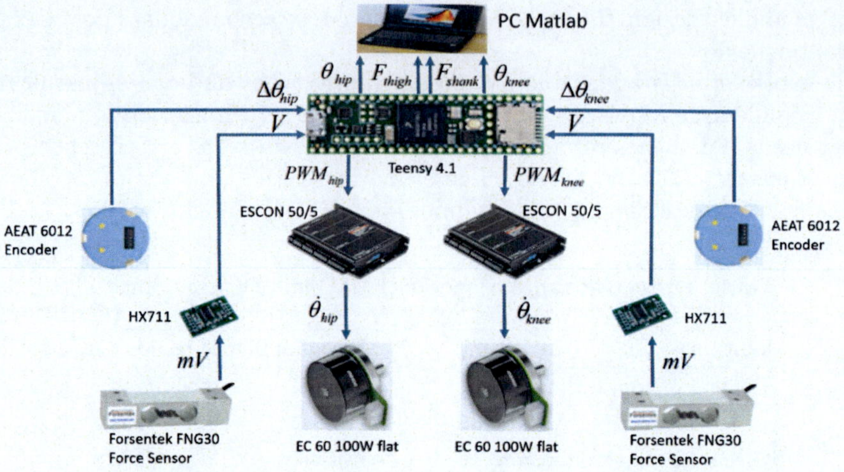

Fig. 2. The hardware and control architecture of a single leg in ALEXO

3 Trajectory Control Method

As the leg segments of the ALEXO follow the human lower limb motion with 2-DOF active, the robot movement can be described as a two-link system. Figure 3 illustrates the ALEXO exoskeleton dynamic model.

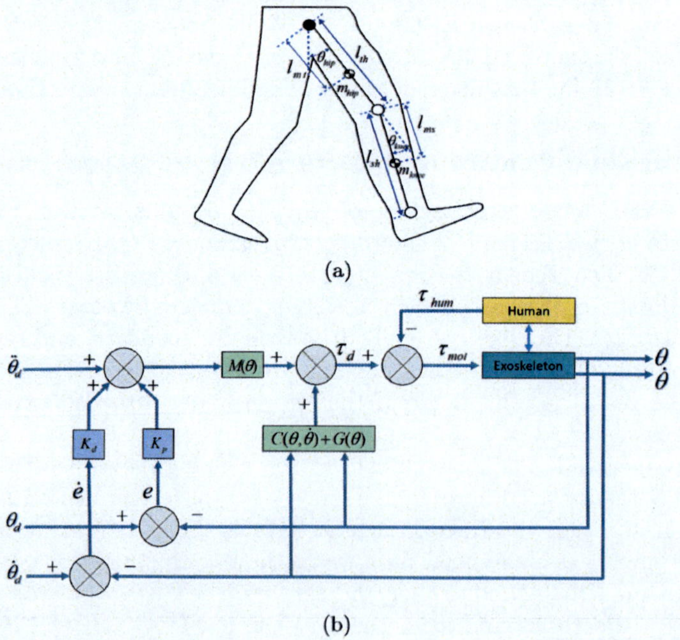

Fig. 3. (a) ALEXO exoskeleton dynamic model. (b) The control scheme of the ALEXO.

The nonlinear dynamics of the ALEXO exoskeleton interacting with the user is given as:

$$M(\theta)\ddot{\theta} + C(\dot{\theta}, \theta)\dot{\theta} + G(\theta) = \tau_{mot} + \tau_{hum} \tag{1}$$

where $M(\theta)$ is the inertial matrix, $C(\dot{\theta}, \theta)$ represents the matrix of Coriolis and centrifugal force, $G(\theta)$ donates the gravitational effect, $\theta = [\theta_{hip}\ \theta_{knee}]^T$, where θ_{hip} and θ_{knee} represent the hip joint and the knee joint of the exoskeleton respectively, τ_{mot} and τ_{hum} are torques from the exoskeleton and the human joint, respectively.

As shown in Fig. 3, a CTC trajectory control is proposed for the exoskeleton:

$$\tau_{mot} = M(\theta)(\ddot{\theta}_d + K_p e(t) + K_d \dot{e}(t)) + C(\dot{\theta}, \theta)\dot{\theta} + G(\theta) - \tau_{hum} \tag{2}$$

$$e(t) = \theta_d(t) - \theta(t) \tag{3}$$

where $\theta_d(t) = [\theta_{d,h}, \theta_{d,k}]$ represents the predefined target position of hip and knee joints; e is the difference between desired angular position and actual angle, K_p and K_d are the proportional and the derivative gains of the CTC controller.

ESCON controllers adopt velocity control. Considering the walking movement pattern, the desired velocity is written as:

$$\int_0^t \ddot{\theta}_r(t)dt = \dot{\theta}_r(t) \tag{4}$$

$\ddot{\theta}_r(t)$ are the desired acceleration, which can be described as:

$$\ddot{\theta}_r(t) = M^{-1}(\tau_{mot} - C(\dot{\theta}, \theta)\dot{\theta} - G(\theta) + \tau_{hum}) \tag{5}$$

thus eq. (4) can be described as:

$$\dot{\theta}_r(t) = \int_0^t M^{-1}(\tau_{mot} - C(\dot{\theta}, \theta)\dot{\theta} - G(\theta) + \tau_{hum})dt \tag{6}$$

4 Simulations

Simulations are conducted on MATLAB. For simulating the interaction forces, two forces, F_t and F_s that are applied on the thigh and shank, are written as:

$$F_t = 50\cos(\omega t) - 50 + f_t \tag{7a}$$

$$F_s = 40\cos(\omega t) - 40 + f_s \tag{7b}$$

where ω is set to π, f_t and f_s are random disturbance ranging from 0 to 10 N. The mass distribution of the ALEXO and the parameters of the controller gain are shown in Table 2.

The sinusoidal reference trajectories of the hip joint and the knee joint are given as:

$$\theta_h = 60\sin(\pi t - 0.194\pi) + 35 \tag{8a}$$

$$\theta_k = 45\cos(\pi t) - 45 \tag{8b}$$

The results are shown in Fig. 4. The maximum errors of trajectory tracking for the hip and knee joints are 1.50 and 2.20 °C, respectively.

Table 2. Control parameters.

	Hip	Knee
K_p	3600	6400
K_d	110	140

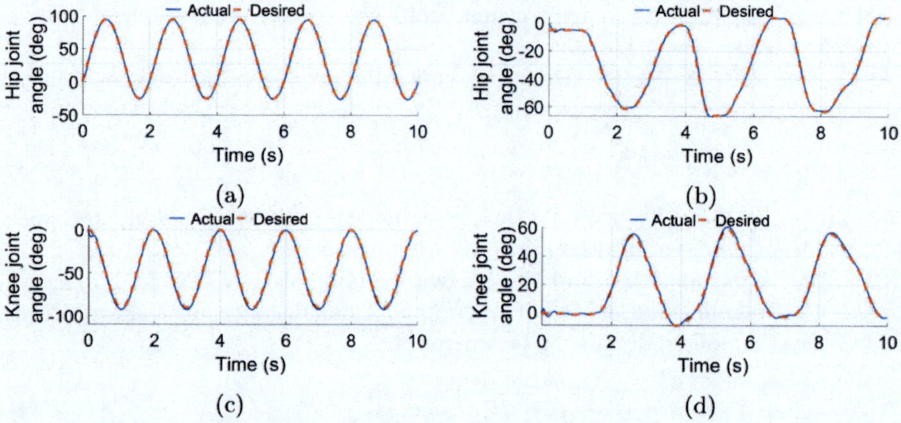

Fig. 4. Trajectory tracking simulation results: (a) hip joint with sinusoidal trajectory, (b) hip joint with real gait, (c) knee joint with sinusoidal trajectory, (d) knee joint with real gait.

5 Physical Experiments

5.1 Trajectory Tracking

The control algorithm was firstly tested on the ALEXO without users. The exoskeleton was fixed on the aluminum alloy frame, and sinusoidal trajectories were applied to the hip and the knee joints:

$$\theta_{dh} = 15\sin(\omega t),\ \theta_{dk} = 25\sin(\omega t) + 25 \tag{9}$$

The results of the sinusoidal trajectory following are shown in Fig. 5. Larger errors are shown at the beginning of the trajectory while smaller errors appear during the trajectory tracking mode, but the level of errors is generally acceptable.

A real walking gait trajectory was also used to test the performance of the trajectory tracking controller. The trajectory is obtained by putting the exoskeleton leg on the human subject and collecting joint sensor data in transparent mode. The results are shown in Fig. 5b and Fig. 5d, respectively. Although there were some errors on the knee joint, the whole exoskeleton robot had a good performance on trajectory tracking to realize walking gait.

5.2 Walking Assistance Tests

The proposed method was evaluated on walikng assistance with the ALEXO robot. Experiments were performed on a single subject with height of 179 cm and weight of 65 kg. The subject was required to walk on the treadmill wearing the ALEXO working on the trajectory tracking mode (Fig. 1c). Interaction force between the exoskeleton and the human body was collected during walking.

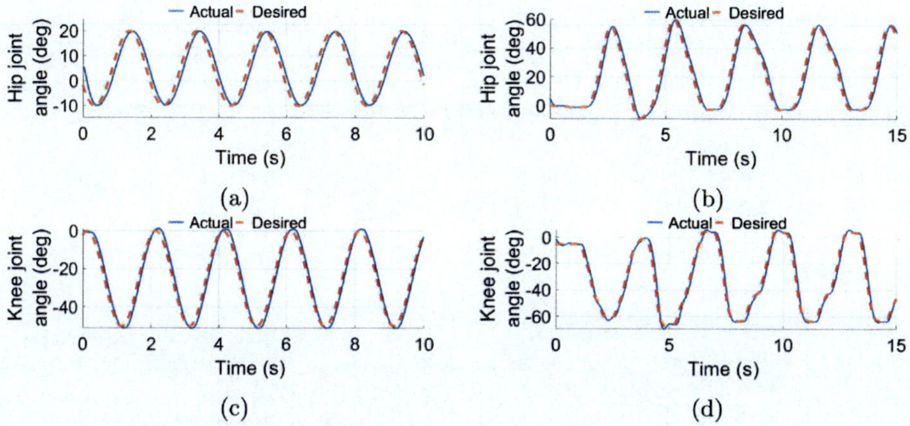

Fig. 5. Trajectory tracking results: (a) hip joint with sinusoidal trajectory, (b) hip joint with real gait, (c) knee joint with sinusoidal trajectory, (d) knee joint with real gait.

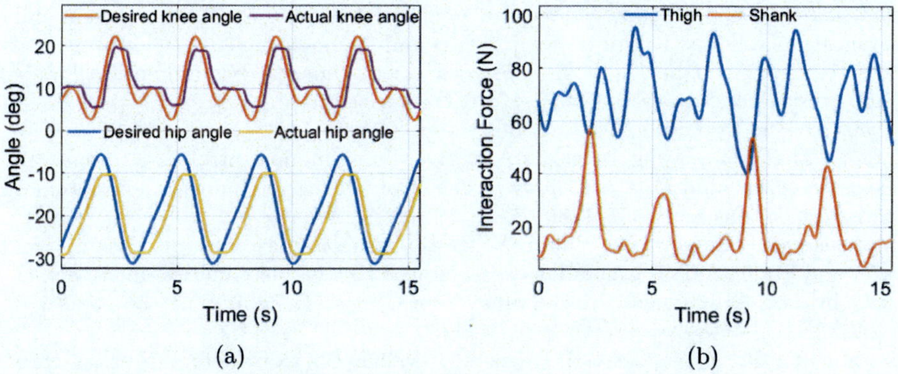

Fig. 6. Human-exoskeleton interaction test with real walking gait trajectory. (a) Angles of hip and knee joints. (b) Interaction force values of the lower limb.

As shown in Fig. 6, the exoskeleton follows the desired trajectory, while providing assistive force to the subject. Periodical force patterns can be observed during the gait cycle on the thigh and the shank segments. Maximum interaction forces of 95.83 N and 57.29 N were measured at the thigh and the shank, respectively.

6 Conclusions

This paper presents the design of an active lower limb exoskeleton (ALEXO) for walking assistance. A trajectory tracking control method is proposed, which has been simulated and tested with the physical system. Our experiments demonstrated that the ALEXO was able to provide sufficient assistance on the hip and knee joints during walking to follow a given gait.

Future work will focus on improving the control method to achieve adaptive gait control for different users. The effectiveness of the ALEXO in assisting individuals with different walking patterns will be evaluated through user studies. Furthermore, the motion primitives theory will be applied to the ALEXO, which can contribute to achieving gait control that is more robust and intelligent.

Acknowledgments. The authors acknowledge the financial support by the Frode V. Nyegaards and Wife's fund for the ALEXO project.

References

1. Nam, K.Y., Kim, H.J., Kwon, B.S., et al.: Robot-assisted gait training (Lokomat) improves walking function and activity in people with spinal cord injury: a systematic review. J. NeuroEng. Rehabil. **14**(1), 1–13 (2017)
2. Husty, M., Birlescu, I., Tucan, P., et al.: An algebraic parameterization approach for parallel robots analysis. Mech. Mach. Theory **140**, 245–257 (2019)
3. Grazi, L., Trigili, E., Proface, G., et al.: Design and experimental evaluation of a semi-passive upper-limb exoskeleton for workers with motorized tuning of assistance. IEEE Trans. Neural Syst. Rehabil. Eng. **28**(10), 2276–2285 (2020)
4. Bai, S., Virk, G.S., Sugar, T.: Wearable exoskeleton systems: design, control and application. The Institution of Engineering and Technology (2018)
5. Tu, Y., Zhu, A., Song, J., et al.: Design and experimental evaluation of a lower-limb exoskeleton for assisting workers with motorized tuning of squat heights. IEEE Trans. Neural Syst. Rehabil. Eng. **30**, 184–193 (2022)
6. Liu, J., Zhang, Y., Wang, J., et al.: Adaptive sliding mode control for a lower-limb exoskeleton rehabilitation robot. In: IEEE Conference on Industrial Electronics and Applications, pp. 1481–1486 (2018)
7. Meijneke, C., van Oort, G., Sluiter, V., et al.: Symbitron exoskeleton: design, control, and evaluation of a modular exoskeleton for incomplete and complete spinal cord injured individuals. IEEE Trans. Neural Syst. Rehabil. Eng. **09**, 330–339 (2021)
8. Patané, F., Rossi, S., Sette, F.D., et al.: WAKE-Up exoskeleton to assist children with cerebral palsy: design and preliminary evaluation in level walking. IEEE Trans. Neural Syst. Rehabil. Eng. **25**(7), 906–916 (2017)
9. Wang, X., Guo, S., Song, M., et al.: Mechanical design and experimental verification of a parallel hip exoskeleton with virtual rotation center. In: IEEE International Conference on Advanced Robotics and Mechatronics, pp. 230–235 (2021)
10. Simonsick, E.M., Newman, A.B., Visser, M., et al.: Mobility limitation in self-described well-functioning older adults: importance of endurance walk testing. J. Gerontol. Ser. A **63**(8), 841–847 (2013)

11. Zhou, X., Yu, Z., Wang, M., et al.: Design of control system for lower limb exoskeleton robot. In: International Conference on Control, Automation and Robotics, pp. 122–126 (2022)
12. Peng, X., Acosta-Sojo, Y., Wu, M., et al.: Actuation timing perception of a powered ankle exoskeleton and its associated ankle angle changes during walking. IEEE Trans. Neural Syst. Rehabil. Eng. **30**, 869–877 (2022)
13. Colins, S.H., Wiggin, M.B., Sawicki, G.S.: Reducing the energy cost of human walking using an unpowered exoskeleton. Nature. **522**(7555), 212–215 (2015)
14. Véronneau, C., Bigué, J.L., Lussier-Desbiens, A., et al.: A high-bandwidth back-drivable hydrostatic power distribution system for exoskeletons based on magnetorheological clutches. IEEE Robot. Autom. Lett. **3**(3), 2592–2599 (2018)
15. Galle, S., Malcolm, P., Collins, S.H., et al.: Reducing the metabolic cost of walking with an ankle exoskeleton: interaction between actuation timing and power. J. Neuroeng. Rehabil. **14**, 35 (2017)
16. Kawamoto, H., Kandone, H., Sakurai, T., et al.: Development of an assist controller with robot suit hal for hemiplegic patients using motion data on the unaffected side. In: International Conference of the IEEE Engineering in Medicine and Biology Society, pp. 3077-3080 (2014)
17. Zhang, A., Tu, Y., Zheng, W., et al.: Adaptive control of man-machine interaction force for lower limb exoskeleton rehabilitation robot. In: IEEE International Conference on Information and Automation, pp. 740-743 (2018)
18. Huang, R., Cheng, H., Guo, H., et al.: Hierarchical interactive learning for a human-powered augmentation lower exoskeleton. In: IEEE International Conference on Robotics and Automation, pp. 257–263 (2016)
19. Schrade, S.O., Nager, Y., Wu, A.R., et al.: Bio-inspired control of joint torque and knee stiffness in a robotic lower limb exoskeleton using a central pattern generator. In: International Conference on Rehabilitation Robotics, pp. 1387–1394 (2017)
20. Gui, K., Liu, H., Zhang, D.: A generalized framework to achieve coordinated admittance control for multi-joint lower limb robotic exoskeleton. In: International Conference on Rehabilitation Robotics, pp. 228–233 (2017)
21. Christensen, S., Rafique, S., Bai, S.: Design of a powered full-body exoskeleton for physical assistance of elderly people. Int. J. Adv. Rob. Syst. **18**(6), 1–15 (2021)
22. Bai, S., Islam, M.R., Power, V., et al.: User-centered development and performance assessment of a modular full-body exoskeleton (AXO-SUIT). Biomim. Intell. Robot. **2**(2), 100032 (2022)

Preliminary Design of a Novel ULRD Upper Limb Rehabilitation Device

Luis D. Filomeno Amador[1,2], Eduardo Castillo Castañeda[1], and Giuseppe Carbone[2(✉)]

[1] Instituto Politécnico Nacional, Queretaro, México
lfilomenoa1800@alumno.ipn.mx, ecastilloca@ipn.mx
[2] DIMEG, University of Calabria, Rende, Italy
giuseppe.carbone@unical.it

Abstract. Robotic devices are being used more frequently to support upper-limb (UL) physical therapies. The main drawback of most conventional devices is that they can only be used individually, which makes training sessions more expensive, results in low compliance, and is inaccurate for external evaluations. This paper presents a novel design for an Upper-Limb Rehabilitation Device (ULRD) based on the three key movements for an effective arm therapy session: wrist extension and flexion, radial and ulnar deviation, and pronosupination. The device's forward kinematics, inverse kinematics, and constrain analysis are presented. The previously developed NURSE device is integrated with the proposed device to gain a full system to aid with most of the UL physical therapies for performing planar rehabilitation exercises.

Keywords: Upper-limb rehabilitation · forward kinematics · inverse kinematics · anthropomorphic dimensions

1 Introduction

Repeatability and precision are important factors to consider when developing a UL rehabilitation therapy for patients who have experienced UL motor abnormalities due to various types of injuries and conditions, including those who have a restricted UL maneuver. Therefore, UL mobility restriction negatively impacts the quality of daily activities like cooking, cleaning, and doing the laundry, [1, 2]. Due to the variety of movements utilized in each session activity, the majority of patients who had any of these medical events and required arm rehabilitation were aware that the process was too extensive and complex, [3–5]. Therefore, the main problem in the majority of physiotherapy rehabilitation sessions is that more than one device is required or that an extension of a simple device is required in order to complete the scheme of maneuver rehabilitation developed by the specialist, making the rehabilitation sessions (RS) more expensive, with low compliance, and inaccurate for external evaluations, [3, 6–9].

This research project's primary goal was to analyze the forward kinematics, inverse kinematics, and constrain restrictions of an Upper Limb Rehabilitation Device (ULRD)

D. Tarnita et al. (Eds.): MESROB 2023, MMS 133, pp. 136–143, 2023.
https://doi.org/10.1007/978-3-031-32446-8_15

[10] that offers a variety of motion arrangements that include wrist flexion and extension, ulnar and radial deviation, and pronosupination of the forearm and hand. The combination of all the ULRD movements complements an RS full motion scheme.

The process involves the use of multiple rehabilitation devices creating a long-term procedure. Patients have seriously struggled to maintain regular training in the home after the session ends, so keeping this in mind, the model presented in this paper can be used in their own homes. Once the UL motion has been analyzed, the specialist assigns a specific type of exercise, but most of the time it is necessary to use more than just one exercise for a single patient [10].

2 Mechanical Design

The proposed mechanical design is based on a three-rotational-joint kinematics system (GKS), whose structure comprises the URLD prototype corresponding to hand, forearm, and elbow motion. In addition, by including the previously developed NURSE component [11], the maneuver is extended to the elbow and shoulder on a bi-dimensional framework. The ULRD CAD model is shown in Fig. 1, where: θ_1. Is used for tracking the trajectory for wrist flexion and extension; θ_2 plays the pronosupination movement; and d_2. Represents the ulnar and radial deviation joint. It is said that the mechanical structure is a passive system.

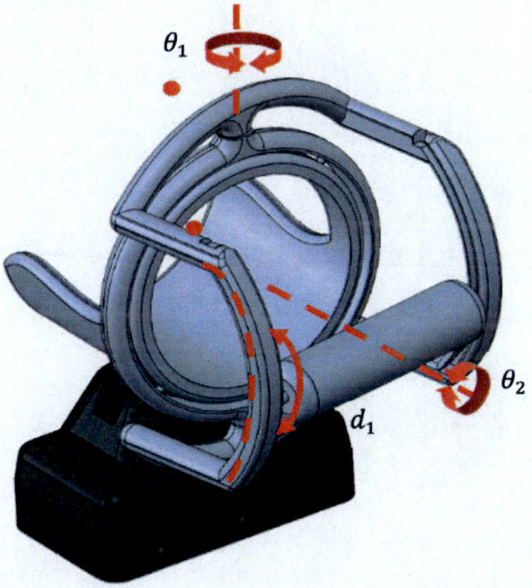

Fig. 1. The ULRD CAD model

After all the minimum requirements are established, the device can be expressed in a kinematic model, highlighting the key parameters to each joint. The main joints used on 2-D upper-limb exercises are radiocarpal flexion/extension, radiocarpal radial/ulnar deviation, and proximal/distal pronosupination.

3 Kinematic Analysis

Once all necessary minimums have been achieved, the device can be described as a kinematic model, emphasizing the crucial joint characteristics. Radiocarpal flexion/extension, radio-carpal radial/ulnar deviation, and proximal/distal pronosupination are the key joints utilized in 2-D upper-limb workouts.

3.1 Forward Kinematic Analysis

The UL analysis diagram in Fig. 2 is based on the D-H parameters presented in Table 1. The initial reference, presented by C_0 coordinate system, is moved through the d_1 and a_1 and becomes C_1 with the θ_2 DoF then this reference is displaced through the a_2 and becomes the C_2 reference position with the θ_3 DoF, and finally this reference is moved through a_3 and a_2 to develop C_3 with the a_4 distance maneuverability.

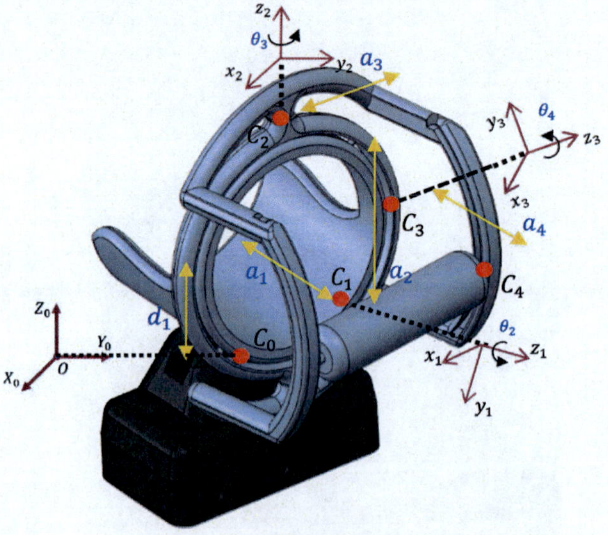

Fig. 2. IDMech study diagram

Table 1 is generated by examining Fig. 2 in the three-dimensional coordinate system and applying the D-H parameters. Which lists the four joints and the motion parameters. The five transformation matrices (2), (3), (4), (5) and (6) are obtained using Eq. 1.

$$^{0}p_4 = \prod_{i=1}^{4}\left[{}^{i-1}T_i(q_i)\right]p^4 \tag{1}$$

Table 1. ULRD D-H parameters

Joint i	α_i	a_i	d_i	θ_i
C_1	$-\frac{\pi}{2}$	a_1	d_1	θ_1
C_2	$\frac{\pi}{2}$	a_2	0	θ_2
C_3	$-\frac{\pi}{2}$	a_3	$-a_3$	θ_3
C_4	0	a_4	0	θ_4

$$^0T_1 = \begin{bmatrix} Cos(\theta_1) & 0 & -Sin(\theta_1) & a_1Cos(\theta_1) \\ Sin(\theta_1) & 0 & Cos(\theta_1) & a_1Sin(\theta_1) \\ 0 & -1 & 0 & d_1 \\ 0 & 0 & 0 & 1 \end{bmatrix} \tag{2}$$

$$^1T_2 = \begin{bmatrix} Cos(\theta_2) & 0 & Sin(\theta_2) & a_2Cos(\theta_2) \\ Sin(\theta_2) & 0 & -Cos(\theta_2) & a_2Sin(\theta_2) \\ 0 & 1 & 0 & 0 \\ 0 & 0 & 0 & 1 \end{bmatrix} \tag{3}$$

$$^2T_3 = \begin{bmatrix} Cos(\theta_3) & 0 & -Sin(\theta_3) & a_3Cos(\theta_3) \\ Sin(\theta_3) & 0 & Cos(\theta_3) & a_3Sin(\theta_3) \\ 0 & -1 & 0 & 0 \\ 0 & 0 & 0 & 1 \end{bmatrix} \tag{4}$$

$$^3T_4 = \begin{bmatrix} Cos(\theta_4) & -Sin(\theta_4) & 0 & a_4Cos(\theta_4) \\ Sin(\theta_4) & Cos(\theta_4) & 0 & a_4Sin(\theta_4) \\ 0 & 0 & 1 & 0 \\ 0 & 0 & 0 & 1 \end{bmatrix} \tag{5}$$

$$^0T_4 = \begin{bmatrix} U_x & V_x & W_x & q_x \\ U_y & V_y & W_y & q_y \\ U_z & V_z & W_z & q_z \\ 0 & 0 & 0 & 1 \end{bmatrix} \tag{6}$$

where

$$U_x = -C\theta_4(S\theta_1S\theta_3 - C\theta_1C\theta_2C\theta_3) - C\theta_1S\theta_2S\theta_4$$
$$U_y = C\theta_4(C\theta_1S\theta_3 + C\theta_2C\theta_3S\theta_1) - S\theta_1S\theta_2S\theta_4$$
$$U_z = -C\theta_2S\theta_4 - C\theta_3C\theta_4S\theta_2$$
$$V_x = S\theta_4(S\theta_1S\theta_3 - C\theta_1C\theta_2C\theta_3) - C\theta_1C\theta_4S\theta_2$$
$$V_y = -S\theta_4(C\theta_1S\theta_3 + C\theta_2C\theta_3S\theta_1) - C\theta_4S\theta_1S\theta_2$$
$$V_z = C\theta_3S\theta_2S\theta_4 - C\theta_2C\theta_4$$
$$W_x = -C\theta_3S\theta_1 - C\theta_1C\theta_2S\theta_3$$

$$W_y = C\theta_1 C\theta_3 - C\theta_2 S\theta_1 S\theta_3$$
$$W_z = S\theta_2 S\theta_3$$
$$q_x = a_1 C\theta_1 + a_2 C\theta_1 C\theta_2 - a_2 C\theta_1 S\theta_2 - a_3 S\theta_1 S\theta_3 + a_3 C\theta_1 C\theta_2 C\theta_3$$
$$q_y = a_1 S\theta_1 + a_2 C\theta_2 S\theta_1 + a_3 C\theta_1 S\theta_3 - a_2 S\theta_1 S\theta_2 + a_3 C\theta_2 C\theta_3 S\theta_1$$
$$q_z = a_1 - a_2(C\theta_2 + S\theta_2) - a_3 C\theta_3 S\theta_2$$

3.2 Inverse Kinematic Analysis

In real life, each theta value is not available but the end-effector location is well known [4], therefore Eqs. (2–6) can be used to determine the position of the end effector knowing the value of each joint $(\theta_1, \theta_2, \theta_3, \theta_4)$. The algebraic method (AM) is used to solve Eq. 6 and compute the joint angles from a desired trajectory. The main constraint to make the AM applied to the IKA analysis easier is, $\theta_1 = 0$. This condition was established by the NURSE system examination that has already been studied.

1. In first place, Eq. 7 is computing using ${}^1T_4$

$$ {}^1T_4 = \left({}^0T_1\right)^{-1} {}^0T_4 \tag{7}$$

2. Now, θ_3 is calculated using q_z from Eq. 6, giving Eq. 8.

$$\theta_3 = \sin^{-1}\left(\frac{q_y}{a_3}\right) \tag{8}$$

3. Once θ_3 is computed, θ_2 can be solved using W_y and W_z from Eq. 6 getting Eq. 9:

$$W_z^2 + W_y^2 = \sin\theta_2^2 \sin\theta_3^2 + \cos\theta_3^2$$

$$\sin\theta_2^2 = \frac{W_z^2 + W_y^2 - \cos\theta_3^2}{\sin\theta_3^2}$$

$$\theta_2 = \sin^{-1}\left(\frac{W_z^2 + W_y^2 - \cos\theta_3^2}{\sin\theta_3^2}\right) \tag{9}$$

with $\theta_3 \neq 0$

4. Calculating θ_4, it is essential to use U_x and U_z from Eq. 6, getting:

$$\begin{aligned} U_x &= \cos\theta_2 \cos\theta_3 \cos\theta_4 - \sin\theta_2 \sin\theta_4 \\ -U_z &= \cos\theta_3 \cos\theta_4 \sin\theta_2 + \cos\theta_2 \sin\theta_4 \end{aligned} \tag{10}$$

$$\boldsymbol{A}\overrightarrow{x} = \boldsymbol{b}$$

$$\boldsymbol{A} = \begin{bmatrix} \cos\theta_2 \cos\theta_3 & -\sin\theta_2 \\ \cos\theta_3 \sin\theta_2 & \cos\theta_2 \end{bmatrix}, \overrightarrow{x} = \begin{bmatrix} \cos\theta_4 \\ \sin\theta_4 \end{bmatrix}, \boldsymbol{b} = \begin{bmatrix} U_x \\ -U_z \end{bmatrix}$$

$$\theta_4 = \tan^{-1}\left(-\frac{U_x \sin\theta_2 + U_z \cos\theta_2}{U_x \frac{\cos\theta_2}{\cos\theta_3} - U_z \frac{\sin\theta_2}{\cos\theta_3}}\right) \tag{11}$$

3.3 Constraint Analysis

Using the relationship between Fig. 2 and Eqs. 8, 9, and 11, it is possible to derive the velocity and acceleration components after computing the, θ_2, θ_3, and θ_4. Values corresponding to the joint angles defined as follows:

$$^0\dot{T}_n = \begin{bmatrix} \dot{R}_n & \dot{V}_n \\ 0 & 1 \end{bmatrix} = \sum_{i=1}^{n} \begin{bmatrix} \dot{\theta}_i Z_{i-1} & -\dot{\theta}_i Z_{i-1} P_{i-1} + d_i Z_{i-1} \\ 0 & 1 \end{bmatrix}$$

Equation 12 offers the Jacobian formulation of the kinematical analysis, assuming that all the links are homogenous with a relatively small cross-section position center of mass is given by, P_{i-1}. The Jacobian matrix brings the relation between joint and end-effector variables [12], in this way.

$$\dot{x} = J\dot{q} \tag{12}$$

$$\dot{x} = \begin{bmatrix} \sum_{i=1}^{n} [\dot{\theta}_i (Z_{i-1} x^{i-1} P_n) + Z_{i-1} \dot{d}_i] \\ \sum_{i=1}^{n} [\dot{\theta}_i Z_{i-1}] \end{bmatrix}$$

where

$$Z_{i-1} = {}^0R_{i-1} \begin{bmatrix} 0 & 0 & 1 \end{bmatrix}^T$$

$$^{i-1}r_i = \begin{bmatrix} a_i \cos\theta_i & a_i \sin\theta_i & d_i \end{bmatrix}^T$$

$$^{i-1}P_n = {}^0R_{i-1}{}^{i-1}r_i$$

$$J(:, i) = \begin{bmatrix} Z_{i-1} x^{i-1} P_n \\ Z_{i-1} \end{bmatrix} \tag{13}$$

It is possible to determine the limit constraints, as can be shown in Fig. 4, where the type of deracination and the constrained level is presented based on the type of movement. Figure 3 displays the fusion prototype using the NURSE appliance [13] and the ULRD.

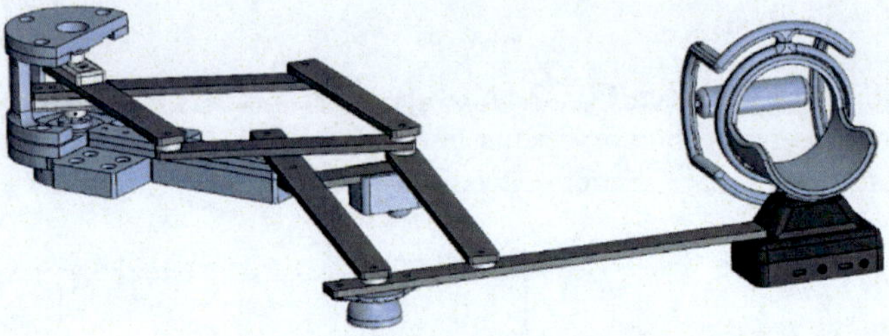

Fig. 3. ND and ULRD fusion

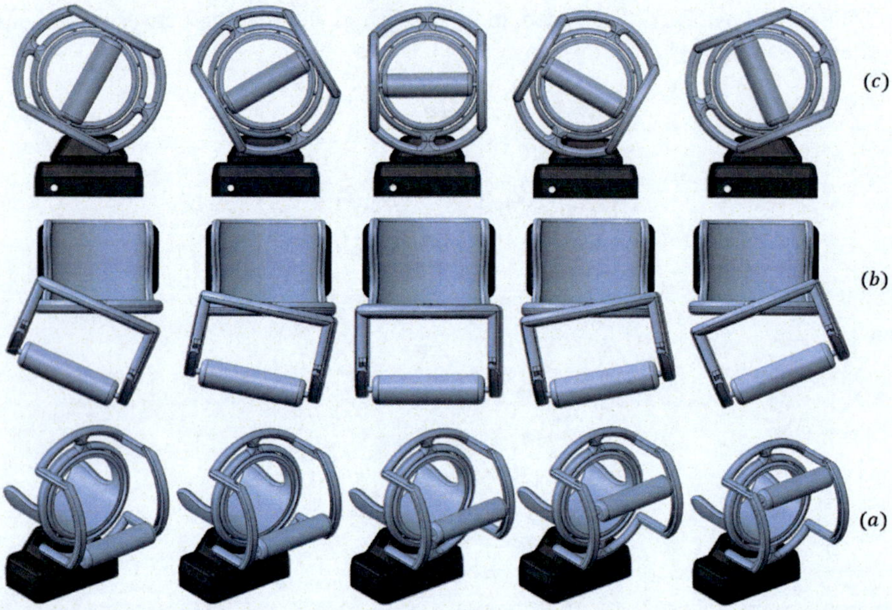

Fig. 4. ULRD wrist extension and flexion (a), radial and ulnar deviation (b), and pronosupination (c), movements animation

4 Conclusions

The main activity in recovery operations and mobility health nowadays is upper-limb physiotherapy, but this process can be extremely difficult, imprecise, and unmeasurable utilizing a variety of technologies. We propose a solution to overcome these limitations with a cost-oriented design solution. The proposed design solution is studied in terms of direct and inverse kinematics analysis by considering the main requirements and constraints of the wrist extension and flexion, radial and ulnar deviation, and arm pronosupination). This calculation enables the full incorporation of a six DoF system tracking the majority of training sessions rehabilitation tasks.

Acknowledgements. This paper has been partially funded by the PNRR Next Generation EU "AGE-IT" - CUP H23C22000870006.

References

1. Bos, R.A., et al.: A structured overview of trends and technologies used in dynamic hand orthoses. J. Neuroeng. Rehabil. **13**, 62 (2016)
2. Hatem, S.M., et al.: Rehabilitation of motor function after stroke: a multiple systematic reviews focused on techniques to stimulate upper extremity recovery. Front. Hum. Neurosci. **10**, 442 (2016)
3. Brewer, B.R., McDowell, S.K., Worthen-Chaudhari, L.C.: Poststroke upper extremity rehabilitation: a review of robotic systems and clinical results. Top Stroke Rehabil. **14**(6), 22–44 (2014)
4. Zariffa, J., et al.: Feasibility and efficacy of upper limb robotic rehabilitation in a subacute cervical spinal cord injury population. Spinal Cord **50**, 220–226 (2011)
5. Veerbeek, J.M., et al.: What is the evidence for physical therapy poststroke a systematic review and meta-analysis. PLoS ONE **9**, Article no. e87987 (2014)
6. Cafolla, D., Russo, M., Carbone, G.: CUBE, a cable-driven device for limb rehabilitation. J. Bionic Eng. **16**(3), 492–502 (2019)
7. Carbone, G., Gherman, B., Ulinici, I., Vaida, C., Pisla, D.: Design issues for an inherently safe robotic rehabilitation device. In: Ferraresi, C., Quaglia, G. (eds.) RAAD 2017. MMS, vol. 49, pp. 1025–1032. Springer, Cham (2018). https://doi.org/10.1007/978-3-319-61276-8_110
8. Tucan, P., et al.: Fuzzy logic-based risk assessment of a parallel robot for elbow and wrist rehabilitation. Int. J. Environ. Res. Public Health **17**, 654 (2020)
9. Vaida, C., et al.: Systematic design of a parallel robotic system for lower limb rehabilitation. IEEE Access **8**, 34522–34537 (2020)
10. Amador, L.D.F., Castañeda, E.C., Carbone, G.: A novel design for an upper-limb rehabilitation assisting device. In: Niola, V., Gasparetto, A., Quaglia, G., Carbone, G. (eds.) IFToMM Italy 2022. Mechanisms and Machine Science, vol. 122, pp. 514–522. Springer, Cham (2022). https://doi.org/10.1007/978-3-031-10776-4_59
11. Chaparro-Rico, B., Cafolla, D., Ceccarelli, M., Castillo-Castañeda, E.: NURSE-2 DoF device for arm motion guidance: kinematic, dynamic, and FEM analysis. Appl. Sci., 2139 (2020)
12. Spong, M.W., Vidyasagar, M.: Robot Dynamics and Control. Wiley, Hoboken (1984)
13. Contreras-Calderón, M.G., Castillo-Castañeda, E.: PRSX: an end-effector for pronation and supination adaptable to arm rehabilitation devices. In: Zeghloul, S., Laribi, M., Sandoval Arevalo, J. (eds.) RAAD 2020. Mechanisms and Machine Science, vol. 84, pp. 149–158. Springer, Cham (2020). https://doi.org/10.1007/978-3-030-48989-2_17

Development of a Passive Ankle-Foot Exoskeleton for Variable Force Resistance Training

Avinash S Pramod[1](✉), Poongavanam Palani[1], Santhakumar Mohan[2], and Asokan Thondiyath[1]

[1] Indian Institute of Technology Madras, Chennai, India
avinashspramod@gmail.com
[2] Indian Institute of Technology Palakkad, Palakkad, India

Abstract. Patients with muscle atrophy undergo rehabilitation exercises by applying resistive force and obstructing foot movement to strengthen their muscles and engage with their neuromuscular system. This can be successfully accomplished without the intervention of a physiotherapist through the use of passive wearable ankle-foot exoskeleton. The existing devices in the market cannot offer bidirectional and variable resistance rehabilitation. This paper proposes the design and development of a passive ankle rehabilitation exoskeleton for bidirectional resistance training with variable stiffness element for ankle torque variation. The conceptual design of the exoskeleton with a variable stiffness element made of Grade 5 Titanium alloy (Ti6Al4V) has been presented along with its kinematic and static analysis. The fabricated prototype of the device was validated using surface electromyogram (sEMG), and the observation clearly depicted improvement in the signal energy during plantar flexion and dorsiflexion.

Keywords: Passive wearable ankle-foot exoskeleton · variable stiffness · bidirectional resistance · surface electromyography

1 Introduction

The human ankle is a synovial joint equivalent to a hinge joint, which forms at the joining point of the shank and the foot, between the distal tibia, distal fibula, and talus bones. The ankle joint has a critical role in human gait and other day-to-day activities. The foot movements are possible due to specific muscles such as the tibialis anterior, extensor hallucis longus, and extensor digitorum longus facilitate the dorsiflexion motion of the foot. The gastrocnemius, plantaris, soleus, and fibularis longus facilitate plantar flexion of the foot [1]. Ankle motion range varies based on age, gender, and disability; for a large number of the population, the range of motion in the sagittal plane is limited to 10–20° of dorsiflexion motion and 40–55° of plantar flexion [2]. Chronic musculoskeletal ankle disorders such as muscle atrophy can affect the strength of muscles, which can lead to changes in the range of motion, affecting the ability of an individual to carry out day-to-day activities [3]. The non-surgical techniques such as stretching and physiotherapy

D. Tarnita et al. (Eds.): MESROB 2023, MMS 133, pp. 144–151, 2023.
https://doi.org/10.1007/978-3-031-32446-8_16

including resistance exercise, using passive rehabilitation devices, are effective and have shown better and long-lasting results compared to an invasive surgical method [4]. The portability and weight of an exoskeleton depends on the type of actuation mechanism that is used in it. If the wearable robot is heavier, it may negatively affect the rehabilitation process and cause muscle fatigue [5]. Most of the existing passive devices use helical springs, torsional springs or lightweight pneumatic actuated muscle (PAM) as the energy-storing module for the purpose of resistance rehabilitation [6, 7]. These mechanical elements cannot provide bidirectional resistance unless they are used in pairs. The major drawback of these devices is that the stiffness cannot be varied without changing these elastic elements. In order to facilitate variable resistive force training for the patient, the stiffness of the element must be changed. From the available literature, it is found that the existing passive ankle rehabilitation devices cannot provide bidirectional resistance during the dorsiflexion and plantar flexion motion using a single elastic element. Also, they fail to provide variable resistance for different levels of resistance training for the patients, which can contribute to the gradual increase in muscle strength and neuromuscular recovery. On considering these drawbacks in the existing wearable passive rehabilitation devices, a simple and lightweight wearable ankle rehabilitation device must be developed to be used by patients for ankle rehabilitation at home without professional assistance.

This paper focuses on developing a novel, low-cost, one-degree-of-freedom, wearable passive ankle-foot exoskeleton (PAFE) to perform in-home ankle resistive training at different resistive loads without professional assistance. In the following sections, the concept selection, and design of the exoskeleton based on the kinematic and static analysis are briefly discussed. The device is then validated by conducting a performance test using sEMG as a physiological indicator.

2 Proposed System Design

The design of the wearable PAFE is carried out by considering the major functional design requirements. These are: (1) It should provide bidirectional resistance for carrying out plantar flexion/dorsiflexion resistance training exercise, (2) The user should be able to carry out the exercise at different resistive forces in a seated position, (3) The mechanism used in the device should not interfere with the free movement of the foot and should be able to trace the motion of the foot about the ankle joint without any self-collision, and (4) The device should be adjustable to foot size variations and should be easily wearable. Based on these requirements, four conceptual models are proposed, as shown in Fig. 1. The design I has two helical springs attached to the tethers to provide bidirectional resistance. One end of each tether is attached to the footrest, and the other is attached to the shank attachment wound through a tensioner. The helical springs are used to provide bidirectional resistance, and the tensioner is used to vary the stiffness of the spring. In design II, a torsional spring is used for bidirectional resistance. The spring is attached to two rotation adjustment knobs by means of a Prismatic-Revolute joint. In design III, two rubber strips are attached to the shank attachment, and by varying the clamp length of the rubber strip, the resistance force can be varied. Design IV makes use of a four-bar mechanism and a single curved spring connected to the diagonal joints of the mechanism to provide bidirectional resistance. The resistance is varied by varying the stiffness of the spring by changing the position of the clamp along the length of the spring. The best possible design is chosen based on Pugh's selection matrix [8]. The selection is based on the performance criteria such as ease of handling, ease of use, portability, ease of manufacturing, ease of resistance adjustability, the capability of offering variable resistance, bidirectional resistance, and dexterity in range of motion (ROM). From the four conceptual designs, design IV is selected as the final design based on the above selection process. A CAD model and the kinematic diagram of the PAFE based on design IV is shown in Fig. 2. The footrest, where the foot will be placed is the crank; the shank is the fixed link which will be attached to the human leg and tightened using the elastic velcro band. The variable stiffness element is attached to the ankle joint and the joint between the rocker link and coupler link. The variable stiffness is achieved by varying the clamp length along the spring of Grade 5 Titanium alloy (Ti6Al4V). The sizing of the links has been carried out based on the kinematic and static analysis of the mechanism.

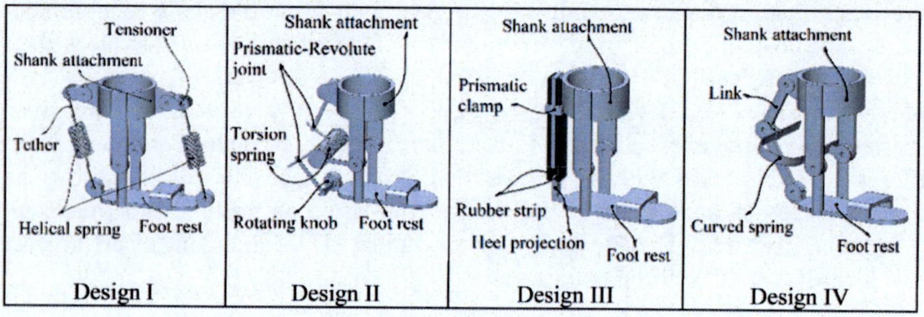

Fig. 1. Conceptual designs

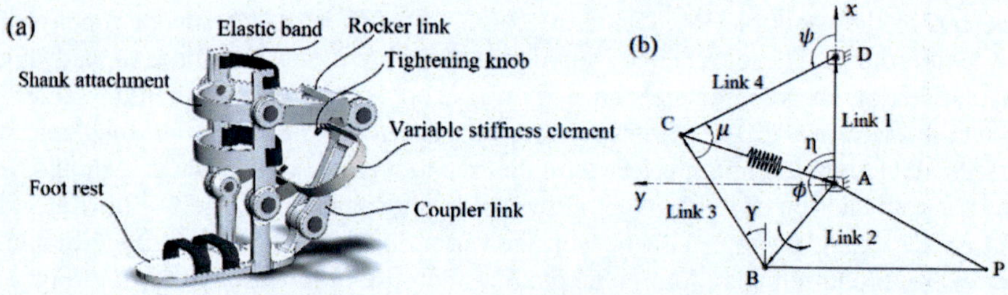

Fig. 2. (a) CAD model of passive ankle resistive training rehabilitation device with variable stiffness element (b) Kinematic diagram of the 4-Bar ankle mechanism

3 Kinematic Analysis

The kinematic modeling and analysis of the proposed mechanism are carried out to obtain appropriate sizing of the links. Figure 2(b) shows the kinematic diagram of the four-bar mechanism with the spring, where AD, ABP, BC, and CD are link 1, link 2, link 3, and link 4 having revolute joints respectively. The angles ϕ, Υ, ψ, and η represent the angle made by a crank, coupler, rocker, and the spring with the x-axis, respectively. The transmission angle between the coupler and rocker link is represented by μ. The four-bar mechanism has a single degree of freedom which is used to assist the dorsiflexion/ plantar flexion motion of the human ankle. The three positions of the mechanism P_1, P_2andP_3 during dorsiflexion, rest, and plantar flexion of the foot, respectively, are represented in Fig. 3(a). The link 1, link 2, link 3 and link 4 are represented as $\vec{R}_1$, $\vec{R}_2$, $\vec{R}_3$and$\vec{R}_4$ with corresponding link lengths given as r_1, r_2, r_3 and r_4 respectively. Link 2 is taken as the input link considering the foot to be attached to it while the link 4 is taken as the output link. The input and output angles during dorsiflexion, rest, and plantar flexion position are represented by ϕ_1, ϕ_2, ϕ_3 and ψ_1, ψ_2, ψ_3 respectively. The dimensions $r_1 = 0.150$ m and $r_2 = 0.128$ m are geometrically calculated using anthropometric foot dimensions for a particular group of people with a maximum body height of 1.750 m, ankle joint height from heel within 0.100 m, and foot length within 0.260 m, and the distance from the heel to the ankle joint is within 0.080 m [9]. The length of the shank attachment is such that it will not affect the relaxation and contraction of the anterior tibialis muscle. This makes it easy to mount the wearable PAFE onto the tibia without restricting muscle mobility and change in volume. The dimensions of the coupler and the rocker link are determined analytically from the equation of transmission angle.

$$r_1^2 + r_2^2 - r_3^2 - r_4^2 + 2r_3r_4\cos\mu - 2r_1r_2\cos\phi_1 = 0 \tag{1}$$

The maximum and minimum value of transmission angle μ is obtained by taking,

$$\frac{d\mu}{d\phi} = \frac{r_1r_2\sin\phi_1}{r_3r_4\sin\mu} = 0 \tag{2}$$

Since the link lengths r_1 and r_2 are not zero, the maximum and minimum transmission angles occur when $\phi_1 = 180°$ and $\phi_1 = 0°$respectively. To ensure that the mechanism can provide maximum torque transmission to the output link, it is synthesized within the transmission angle limit of $\mu = 90°$ at which the torque transmission is maximum. The transmission angle μ is considered for the dimensional synthesis of the mechanism as the variable stiffness element is directly connected to the output link of the mechanism. Solving Eq. (1) at $\phi_1 = 161.34°$ and $\mu = 90°$, the dimensions of the coupler and the output link are obtained as $r_3 = 0.184$ m and $r_4 = 0.203$ m respectively. This mechanism is synthesized at $\phi_1 = 161.34°$, to maintain the transmission angle within $\mu = 90°$ throughout the motion of the foot during plantar flexion. The output angles corresponding to the input angles of the mechanism are calculated using Freudenstein's equation [10] as

$$\cos(\phi - \psi) = K_1 + K_2\cos\psi + K_3\cos\phi \tag{3}$$

where,

$$K_1 = \frac{r_1^2+r_2^2+r_4^2-r_3^2}{2r_2r_4};\ K_2 = \frac{r_1}{r_2};\ K_3 = \frac{-r_1}{r_4}$$

Three positions of the mechanism are simulated and it is observed that the transmission angle is within the desired limit of $90° \geq \mu > 45°$. Therefore, the mechanism is free of any toggle positions and provides maximum torque transmission within the required ROM. The synthesized mechanism satisfies Grashoff's law and is a type one crank-rocker mechanism. The thickness of each link is determined from static force analysis of the mechanism, which is discussed in the following section.

4 Static Analysis

Static analysis of the exoskeleton is carried out to calculate the cross-sectional dimension of the links to withstand the stress due to axial loading and bending moment during the resistive rehabilitation process using the exoskeleton. The forces and moments acting on the links are calculated considering the whole system is in static equilibrium, as shown in Fig. 3(b). The forces acting on each link are calculated from the force-momentum equilibrium equations. The peak ankle joint resistive torque of a healthy human during passive plantar flexion motion is up to 15 Nm, and during dorsiflexion is up to 5 Nm [11]. Hence, a maximum torque of 15 Nm is applied on the second link, for which the spring exerts maximum resistance at the two extreme configurations of the mechanism within the range of human foot motion. Solving the equations, it is identified that link 3 experienced the maximum amount of axial and bending load of 211 N and 3.6 Nm respectively. The maximum axial load acting on the spring is 215 N. Based on these loads the thickness of the links and the spring dimensions are determined.

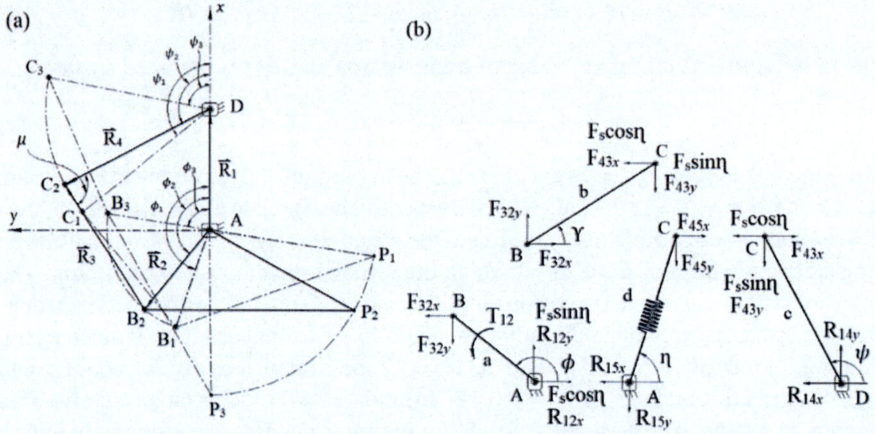

Fig. 3. (a) Path traced by the 4-Bar ankle mechanism during dorsiflexion, rest, and plantar flexion position (b) Free body diagram of the four-bar mechanism with a diagonal elastic element in static equilibrium, where F_S is the spring force which can be either compressive or tensile in nature based on the direction of motion.

5 Experimental Results

5.1 Finite Element Analysis of the Coupler

The thickness of the coupler is determined from Finite element analysis (FEA) of the PAFE carried out using Solidworks 2019 software. The material used for the part is polylactic acid (PLA). An axial load of 211 N and a bending moment of 3.6 Nm is applied at the nodes of one hinge joint, and the nodes are fixed on the other hinge joint. The link thickness is selected based on different trials of the static stress simulation at an assumed safety factor of 27 for a 27% infill of PLA. The maximum stress generated within the link is 2.262 MPa which is less than the maximum yield strength of the material, which is 60 MPa. The maximum deflection is observed to be 3.554×10^{-04} m which is negligible. Hence, selected dimensions are safe and the optimum thickness of the coupler is 0.020 m.

5.2 Experimental Verification of the Variable Stiffness Spring

The spring attached between joint A and C of the mechanism as in Fig. 2(b) is designed and tested for a maximum required stiffness of 2826 N/m, to provide resistance in the motion. The designed spring is a curved strip of Ti6Al4V which weighs about 0.13 kg, having 2.5×10^{-03} m thickness, width of 0.020 m, and a length of 0.600 m, which is cold rolled to get the desired shape. The stiffness of the element is varied by changing the distance of the clamp along the length of the strip from its tip. FEA results are verified by experimentation on the Ti alloy spring. Different stiffness provided by the spring along its length at different distances from its tip are measured using the setup shown in Fig. 4(a). The FEA and experimental results in Fig. 4(b) show the same trend of stiffness variation throughout the strip length. The developed spring can provide a resistance between 2.2 kg to 20.3 kg for the required application without failure.

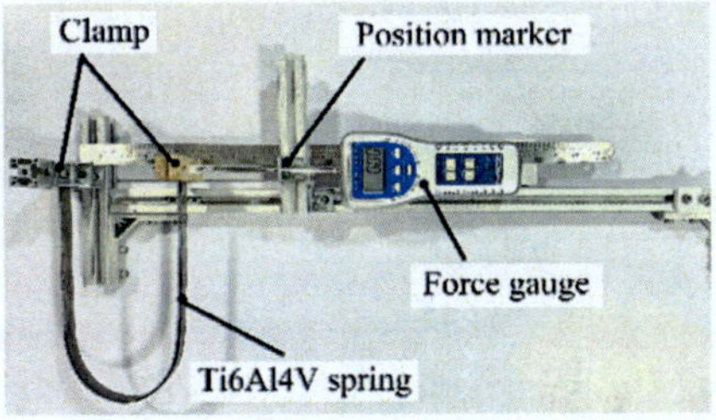

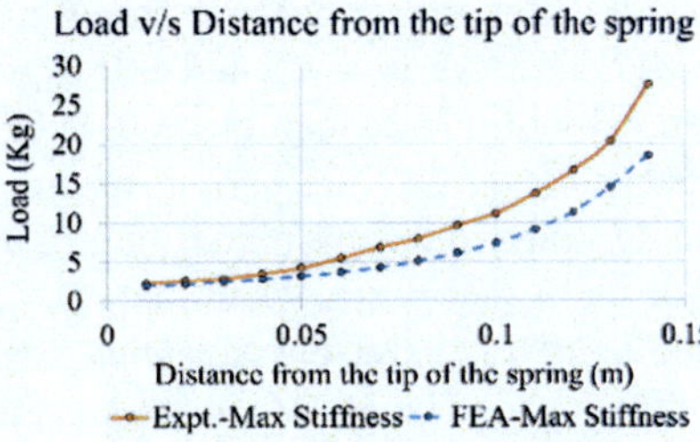

Fig. 4. (a) Experimental setup (b) Maximum experimental and FEA stiffness

5.3 Performance Test of the PAFE

Indirect muscle force measurement can be performed by measuring the electrical activity of the muscle when using the PAFE. Plantar flexion (PF) is predominantly controlled by the Gastrocnemius (GM) muscle, whereas dorsiflexion (DF) is controlled by the Tibialis Anterior (TA) muscle. The contribution of GM and TA during DF and PF respectively is analyzed in this validation study. Four sets of tasks are performed with the sEMG sensor band (8-channel EMG armband, Mindrove Kft, EU) worn around the muscle belly of the GM muscle and at the same time covering the TA muscle as seen in Fig. 5(a). The protocol followed is seen in Fig. 5(b) and adheres to the Declaration of Helsinki. A healthy volunteer performed PF and DF under T1, T2, T3 and T4 epochs for 40 s each with rest periods in-between to avoid muscle fatigue.

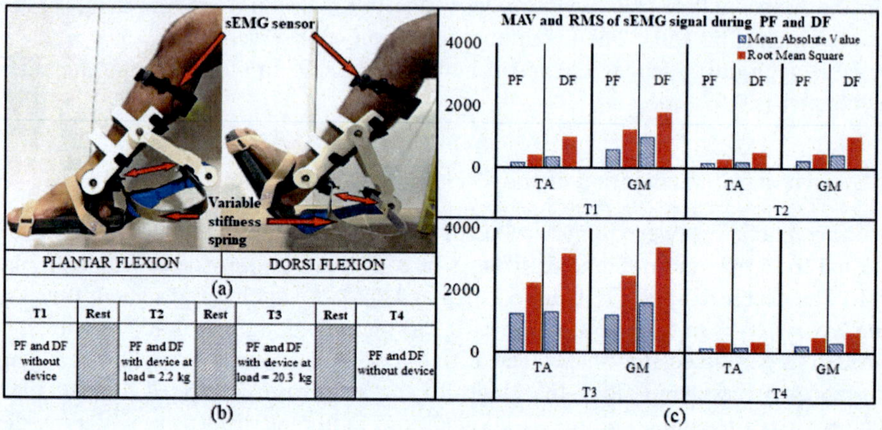

Fig. 5. (a) Device validation setup depicting the variable stiffness spring changes during PF and DF (b) Protocol to evaluate device performance (c) MAV and RMS value of sEMG signal acquired from TA and GM muscle during PF and DF movements

Mean absolute value (MAV) and Root mean square (RMS) have been utilized frequently in the literature to describe the sEMG signals as two significant temporal domain properties [12]. MAV is computed as the average of the summation of the absolute value of the signal while RMS can be calculated as the square root of the average power of the signal in the given time period. From Fig. 5(c), it can be seen that the RMS value of TA and GM muscles are higher before using the resistive training device in T1. The energy of the signal peaks when maximum load is applied at T3 than during minimal load training in T2. After the resistance exercise sessions, in T4 the RMS value is considerably reduced. The MAV value also shows a similar trend. During PF in T4, RMS reduces by 24% for TA and by 60% for GM muscle while MAV reduces by 26% for TA and 62% for GM.

Similarly, during DF in T4, RMS reduces by 66% for TA and by 63% for GM while MAV reduces by 53% for TA and 68% for GM muscle. From the observations, it is clear that the PAFE can provide intended resistance training results over the TA and GM muscles.

6 Conclusion

The PAFE with a variable stiffness element presented in this paper is a simple four-bar mechanism with a diagonally attached variable stiffness element. The proposed design is lighter in weight and of low cost which makes it easy to carry and affordable for the average population. The mechanism is designed to mimic the human foot trajectory during plantar flexion and dorsiflexion movement. The exoskeleton facilitates the user with weak muscles to carry out bidirectional resistance training exercises for plantar flexion/ dorsiflexion motion of the foot at variable resistive forces. The outcomes from the validation experiment showed good improvement in the energy level of the plantar flexor and dorsi flexor muscles.

The prototype can be further developed by modifying the footrest into a footwear attachment for better foot grip. It can be made automatic or semi-automatic by incorporating actuators and force sensors, which can be used to control the stiffness based on the user feedback and training requirements.

Acknowledgement. The authors would like to thank the Indian Institute of Technology, Madras and Indian Institute of Technology Palakkad Technology IHub Foundation (IPTIF) for providing the lab and resources to conduct the research.

References

1. Enderle, J., Bronzino, J. (eds.): Introduction to Biomedical Engineering. Academic Press, Cambridge (2012)
2. Engsberg, J.R., Grimstom, S.K., Hanley, D.A.: Differences in ankle joint complex range of motion as a function of age. Foot Ankle **14**(4), 215–222 (1993)
3. Hiller, C.E., et al.: Prevalence and impact of chronic musculoskeletal ankle disorders in the community. Arch. Phys. Med. Rehabil. **93**(10), 1801–1807 (2012)
4. Zhang, M., Davies, T.C., Xie, S.: Effectiveness of robot-assisted therapy on ankle rehabilitation–a systematic review. J. Neuroeng. Rehabil. **10**(1), 1–16 (2013)
5. Yu, H., et al.: Mechanical design of a portable knee-ankle-foot robot. In: IEEE International Conference on Robotics and Automation, pp. 2183–2188. IEEE (2013)
6. Wang, X., Guo, S., Qu, B., Song, M., Qu, H.: Design of a passive gait-based ankle-foot exoskeleton with self-adaptive capability. Chin. J. Mech. Eng. **33**(1), 1–11 (2020)
7. Alvarez-Perez, M.G., Garcia-Murillo, M.A., Cervantes-Sánchez, J.J.: Robot-assisted ankle rehabilitation: a review. Disabil. Rehabil. Assist. Technol. **15**(4), 394–408 (2020)
8. Guler, K., Petrisor, D.M.: A Pugh Matrix based product development model for increased small design team efficiency. Cogent Eng. **8**(1), 1923383 (2021)
9. Suga, T., et al.: Calcaneus height is a key morphological factor of sprint performance in sprinters. Sci. Rep. **10**(1), 1–10 (2020)
10. Freudenstein, F.: Design of Four-Link Mechanisms. Columbia University (1954)
11. Mizuno, S., Sonoda, S., Takeda, K., Maeshima, S.: Measurement of resistive plantar flexion torque of the ankle during passive stretch in healthy subjects and patients with poststroke hemiplegia. J. Stroke Cerebrovasc. Dis. **25**(4), 946–953 (2016)
12. Noor, A., et al.: Decoding of ankle joint movements in stroke patients using surface electromyography. Sensors **21**(5), 1575 (2021)

Design and Performance Analysis of Ankle Joint Exoskeleton

Zhetenbayev Nursultan[1,2](✉), Marco Ceccarelli[3], and Gani Balbayev[4]

[1] Satbayev University, Almaty, Kazakhstan
n.zhetenbayev@gmail.com
[2] Almaty University of Power Engineering and Telecommunications, Almaty, Kazakhstan
[3] LARM2 Laboratory of Robot Mechatronics, University of Rome Tor Vergata, Rome, Italy
marco.ceccarelli@uniroma2.it
[4] Eurasian National University, Nur-Sultan, Kazakhstan

Abstract. This paper presents the design and modeling of an ankle exoskeleton for a human rehabilitation system. The proposed, low-cost new exoskeleton is designed to perform the basic tasks of human motion with low-cost and easy-to-use functions. The correct kinematic and static model of the proposed exoskeleton is developed and deployed in the Solidworks environment. An appropriate 3D CAD model is developed, and the entire exoskeleton of the leg is modelled and simulated in the SolidWorks Motion environment. The results of the simulation show that the proposed system is technically achievable.

Keywords: Medical Devices · Biomechanics · Motion Assisting Devices · Ankle Exoskeleton · Design

1 Introduction

Recently, the exoskeletons of the lower extremities have become a very interesting research topic because they run parallel to the leg of a wearer. Exoskeletons can perform functions such as walking assist, heavy lifting and physiotherapy support for patients who are unable to walk again. However, portable power supplies, light actuators and high-performance transmissions are some of the most important factors that need further improvement [1]. As for exoskeletons specially designed to restore the human motor system, they can be divided into two main categories: one category consists of exoskeletons that serve as robotic systems in an assist mode to restore gait patterns in people with partial mobility; the other category is represented by exoskeletons specially designed to help the elderly in performing everyday tasks. Exoskeletons in the first category have been specifically designed for those suffering from neuromotor disorders or stroke as in research works [2, 3]. However, exoskeletons [4, 5] have been specially developed for the implementation of programs for the temporary restoration of human walking, intended for people who have undergone orthopedic surgery. In both categories, there are four-wheel drive exoskeletons [6] for all lower limb joints of an individual in rehabilitation programs. Considering the exoskeletons used in temporary recovery programs

D. Tarnita et al. (Eds.): MESROB 2023, MMS 133, pp. 152–159, 2023.
https://doi.org/10.1007/978-3-031-32446-8_17

[7], they can activate individual joints of the patient's motor system (one joint, a pair of joints or a group of joints of the lower extremities of a person is activated). Furthermore, they are characterized by personalized therapy protocols that allow you to restore a joint, namely one that has been involved in surgery. Most existing exoskeletons have several design requirements, such as comfort during rehabilitation programs, complex actuation, principles of low or high cost, usability, and practical interfaces [8].

Almaty Ankle Exo is featured in this article as a lightweight robot to carry to support, ankle movement with an architecture controlled by electric linear actuators. In addition, numerical simulations are included to test the suitability of the Almaty Ankle Exo for the entire range of ankle joint mobility to characterize the performance of this new design in terms of range of motion, drive tension, ankle joint load and engine power.

2 Motion Requirements from Ankle Biomechanics

However, studies have shown that ROM may vary with age and gender. Ankle movements mainly happen about talocrural and subtalar joints. Talocrural joint is formed by talus, tibia, and fibula bones. Top of the talus fits inside the socket formed by the tibia and fibula. This joint is mechanically like a mortise and tenon joint providing plantarflexion-dorsiflexion. Bottom of the talus locates on the calcaneus forming subtalar joint that allows eversion-inversion and abduction-adduction of the ankle. Thus, joint complex supports triplane motions. Collection of muscles is responsible for generating the motions of foot segment during ambulation. The tibialis anterior, extensor digitorum longus, extensor hallucis longus and fibularis tertius muscles with tendons dorsiflexes the foot. The gastrocnemius, soleus, planters, fibularis longus, fibularis brevis, tibialis posterior, flexor digitorum longus and flexor hallucis longus muscles with tendons plantar flexes the foot. Fibularis longus, Fibularis brevis, Fibularis treats muscles, and their tendons perform the eversion. Tibialis anterior and tibialis posterior muscles along with related tendons performs the inversion of the ankle (Fig. 1).

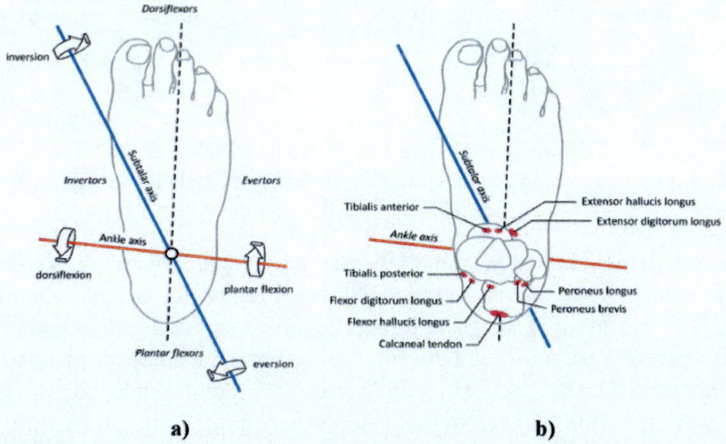

Fig. 1. a) Rotation directions b) Structure of ankle joint

According to biomechanics studies, synovial hinge joints at ankle plays a crucial role in supporting motions of the human lower extremity. The fitting of the exoskeleton at the ankle is more difficult than hip and knee, due to the strict requirements of smaller space as well as anatomical complexity introduced by talocrural and subtalar joints. The anatomical axes of talocrural and subtalar joints are placed in an oblique sensory that cause foot to move across all three planes allowing pronation and supination to occur during walking. Hence, constraining motions to a single plane can lead to abnormal joint movements, poor muscle recruitment and increasing overall energetic cost. Ground irregularities, body weight and walking speed directly affect the mechanical stiffness assumed by the ankle and foot. Hence, the exoskeleton should adjust the system resistance to account for the variable stiffness of the biological counterpart during walking, running, etc. If stiffness not properly adjusted, it may even lead to loss of stability or even injury of the joint. The motion ranges in humans are ±20 deg for dorsiflexion, ±50 deg for plantar flexion; ±10 deg for abduction, and ± 12 deg for inversion.

3 Design of a Wearable Device for Ankle Motion Assistance

The design of the (Almaty Ankle Exo) a wearable device for helping with the movement of the ankle joint, Fig. 2. The above-mentioned problems are solved by indicating the directions of movement and the scheme of the system with an electric linear drive, which is also equipped with appropriate sensors (S) for monitoring and control purposes.

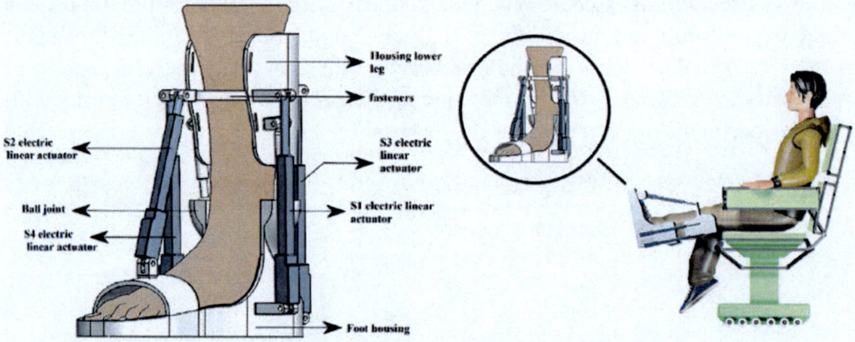

Fig. 2. Conceptual design of the Almaty Ankle Exo with main components [7]

The use of the device can range from motion control when performing exercises and increasing the volume of the ankle joint to movement assistance during rehabilitation and physiotherapy treatment of the ankle joint. The movement of the ankle joint relative to the shin (the part of a person's leg between the knee and the ankle) is planned by the relative movement of the foot platform, which may even include shoes for wearing the system, relative to the shin. a platform that can be shaped like a ring to be worn on the shin. The motors (M) increase or decrease the drive length to guide this relative motion by means of a mechanical structure consisting of a pulley and a servo motor. The control system can use information from sensors (S), which can be either on board the device or worn by the patient. These sensors may include accelerometers and IMUS that allow gait analysis. Sensors (S) can be used not only to control the operation of the device, but also to monitor the condition of the ankle, for example, to measure temperature, muscle reaction and blood pressure, as required in the device application. In Fig. 2 shows the design of a mechanical solution in CAD, emphasizing the lightness and compactness of the conceptual design, providing portability and user-orientation. The power supply can also be integrated into a foot platform, a shin platform, or a box next to the device.

Advantages of the proposed exoskeleton with 4 electric linear actuators:

Lightweight: Using electric linear drives instead of motors reduces the weight of the exoskeleton, making it more comfortable and comfortable to wear for a long time.

Simple Design: Compared to other exoskeleton designs, the design with 4 electric linear actuators is relatively simple, which reduces the complexity of the control system and increases the reliability of the system.

Low Cost: The cost of an exoskeleton with 4 electric linear drives is usually lower than that of other designs, which makes it more affordable for a wider population.

Increased Range of Motion: The design with 4 electric linear actuators provides a greater range of motion in the joints, which may be important for certain applications such as rehabilitation.

4 Procedure of Design

The degree of freedom (DOF) of an ankle exoskeleton refers to the number of independent directions in which it can move. Generally, ankle exoskeletons are designed to provide one DOF, corresponding to plantarflexion and dorsiflexion movements.

The spatial mechanism of the ankle exoskeleton involves a combination of rigid and flexible components that work together to achieve the desired range of motion. The mechanism typically includes a footplate that attaches to the wearer's foot and a rigid frame that attaches to the lower leg. The footplate is connected to the frame by a hinge joint that allows for rotation in the sagittal plane, corresponding to plantarflexion and dorsiflexion movements (Fig. 3).

According to the Somov – Malyshev formula, the number of degrees W of freedom of the mechanism for a spatial kinematic structure is determined as follows:

$$W = 6 \cdot (n - 1) - 5 \cdot p_5 = 6 \cdot 8(-)1 - 5 \cdot 9 = 3$$

The application of this formula is possible if no additional conditions are imposed on the movements of the links that make up the mechanism (the axes of all rotational pairs were parallel, intersected at one point, etc.). These additional requirements change the nature of the movements of the mechanism and, accordingly, change the form of its structural formula.

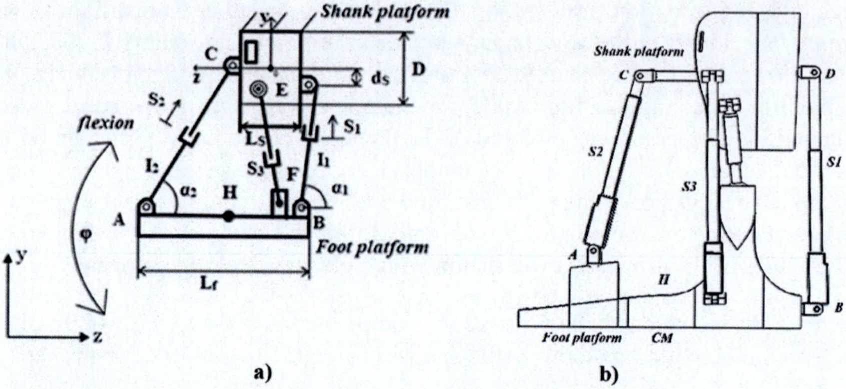

a) b)

Fig. 3. The proposed Ankle Exoskeleton: a) kinematic design with parameters; b) CAD design.

In a spherical mechanism, all three kinematic chains impose the same connections, and the axes of all pairs intersect at one point. In the proposed design there are three power screws and three kinematic mutual screws. These are the zero parameter screws. To determine the number of degrees of freedom, we apply the Dobrowolski formula:

$$W = 3 \cdot (n - 1) - 2 \cdot p_5 - p_4 = 3 \cdot (8 - 1) - 2 \cdot 9 = 3$$

If the last rotational pairs are replaced by spherical ones, then in this case each chain imposes one bond. The number of degrees of freedom is determined by the Somov-Malyshev formula:

$$W = 6 \cdot (n - 1) - 5 \cdot p_5 - 4 \cdot p_4 - 3 \cdot p_3 = 6 \cdot (8 - 1) - 5 \cdot 6 - 3 \cdot 3 = 3$$

5 Performance Analysis

A 3D modeling and simulation calculations were performed in a virtual environment using the Solidworks Simulation software, and the Motion Simulation package. Using Solidworks Simulation an electric linear actuator input is given, which generates movement of the ankle joint. Figure 4B shows simulated Abduction and Abduction obtained using Solidworks Simulation. Adduction the range of motion in this movement will be up 22.0 deg to 36 deg, while the Simulation will bend to 15 deg. The range of motion in Abduction is from 15.4 deg to 25.9 deg, and in Simulation, binding is up to 10 deg.

A 3D modeling and simulation calculations were performed in a virtual environment using the Solidworks Simulation software, and the Motion simulation supplement. Using Solidworks Simulation an electric linear actuator input is given, which generates movement of the ankle joint. Figure 4A shows the movement of the dorsal flexion plantar flexion ankle in a normal position. Figure 4 shows snapshot of simulated assisted motions using Solidworks Simulation. The dorsal flexion is given with a range of motion up to 20°, while the Simulation in Fig. 4A will bend to 15°. The range of motion in plantar flexion is from 40 to 50°, and in Simulation, bending is up to 20°.

Figure 6 shows driving force by the linear actuators: F1 is force of the linear actuator in front side of the leg, F2 is the force of the linear actuator in back side of the leg, respectively. The computing results of the forces F1 and F2 reach 0.8 N.

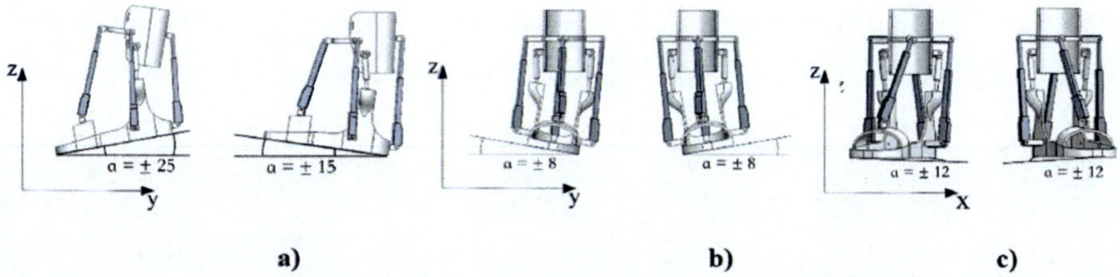

Fig. 4. Snapshot of simulated assisted motions in a) dorsiflexion – plantarflexion; b) abduction – adduction; c) inversion – eversion.

Figure 5A shows components of linear displacement of the platform. From the plot, the motions from all directions are with peaks of maximum values 100 deg/s^2. Represented for X – component and less than 85 deg/s^2 for another components.

Figure 5B shows components of linear displacement of the linear actuators. From the plot, the motions from all directions are with peaks of maximum values 30 deg/s^2. Represented for Y – component and less than 25 deg/s^2 for another components.

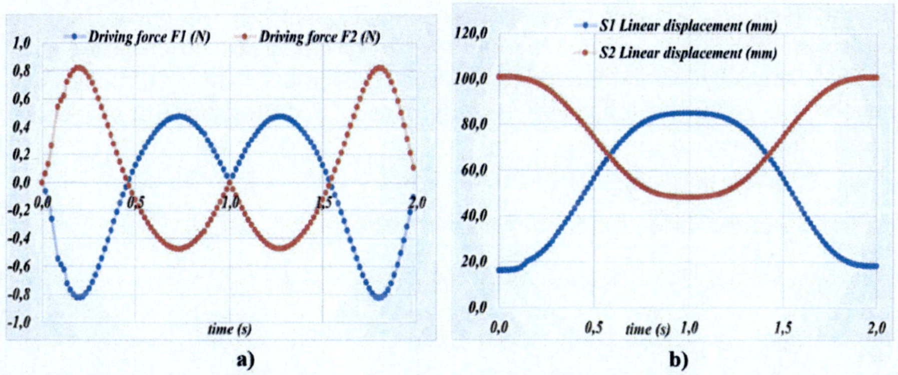

Fig. 5. Simulation results for the motion in Fig. 4A by linear actuators in terms of a) driving force; b) actuators' movement.

Translational motion relative to the angle is shown in Fig. 4 B. The highest conversion value of 37 N is near the top position, the bottom position is 28 N. Translational motion is a motion in which all points of a moving body move uniformly along the same line or in the same direction. If an exoskeleton makes a translational movement, then its orientation relative to a fixed point does not change. With this type of motion, all points of the body have velocities and accelerations that are the same in magnitude and direction at each moment of time. All points describe the same trajectories. By this we mean that

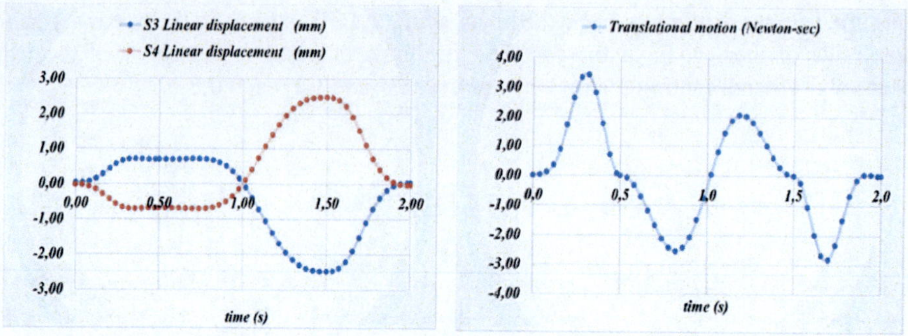

a) b)

Fig. 6. Simulation results for the motion in Fig. 4 B by linear actuators in terms of: a) driving force; b) actuators movement.

the trajectories would coincide if they were located one above the other. Basically, the orientation of the body remains fixed relative to the fixed axis.

When the drive moves or moves from one point to another, it is a movement in which all the points of the moving body move uniformly in one line or direction. If the exoskeleton body moves forward, its orientation relative to the fixed point does not change.

Angular movements are produced by changing the angle between the bones of a joint. The angular movement is shown in Fig. 7A 2 s 45 N seconds.

Figure 7 B shows the computed results in of components of Center of gravity position of the platform. The movements of this point along Z axis are equal to 30 mm. The Center of gravity in this study shows the stability of the equilibrium positions of bodies and continuous media under the influence of gravity, namely: in the resistance of materials – when using the Vereshchagin rule.

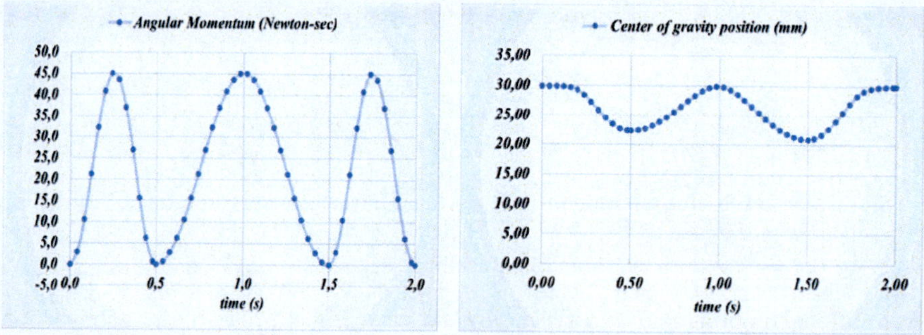

a) b)

Fig. 7. Simulation results for the motion in Fig. 4 C by linear actuators in terms of: a) driving force; b) actuators movement.

The center of gravity (COG) of the human body is a hypothetical point around which the force of gravity appears to act. It is point at which the combined mass of the body appears to be concentrated. However, since humans do not remain fixed in the anatomical position, the exact location of the center of gravity changes constantly with each new position of the body and limbs. Human body proportions will also affect the location of COG.

6 Conclusion

To restore the patient's ability to move, the proposed exoskeleton is intended for external use for moving the lower part of the body, as well as for lifting the weight of the victim. The proposed ankle exoskeleton is made from lightweight, low-cost components. The design is finalized and validated by means of simulation analysis with performance characterization. A prototype with three degrees of rotational freedom around a virtual stationary center is developed for intensive and repetitive leg recovery exercises. Each joint is equipped with a motor and a specific mechanism, a four-position mechanism for linear training and wrist joints. This increases the speed and effectiveness of the model, the results of which are examined in terms of performance characteristics. The prototype is assembled to pilot the new concept, and future work will provide a practical description.

Acknowledgement. This research has been funded by the Ministry of Science and Higher Education of the Republic of Kazakhstan, Grant № AP13268857.

References

1. Na, L., Lei, Y., Hua, Q., Jian, W., Sen, M., Yanbei, L.: Design and simulation analysis of an improved lower limb exoskeleton. J. Vibroeng. **16**(7) (2014)
2. Bortole, M., et al.: The H2 robotic exoskeleton for gait rehabilitation after stroke: early findings from a clinical study. J. Neuroeng. Rehabil. **12**, 1–14 (2015)
3. Federici, S., Meloni, F., Bracalenti, M., de Filippis, M.L.: The effectiveness of powered, active lower limb exoskeletons in neurorehabilitation: a systematic review. J. Neuro Rehabil. **37**, 321–340 (2015)
4. Dumitru, N., Copilusi, C., Geonea, I., Tarnita, D., Dumitrache, I.: Dynamic analysis of an exoskeleton new ankle joint mechanism. In: Flores, P., Viadero, F. (eds.) New Trends in Mechanism and Machine Science. MMS, vol. 24, pp. 709–717. Springer, Cham (2015). https://doi.org/10.1007/978-3-319-09411-3_75
5. Geonea, I.D., Margine, A., Dumitru, N., Copiluşi, C.: Design and simulation of a mechanism for human leg motion assistance. In: Advanced Materials Research, vol. 1036, pp. 811–816. Trans Tech Publications Ltd., Bäch, Switzerland (2014)
6. Galle, S., Malcolm, P., Derave, W., De Clercq, D.: Adaptation to walking with an exoskeleton that assists ankle extension. Gait Posture **38**, 495–499 (2013)
7. Zhetenbayev, N., Balbayev, G., Iliev, T., Bakhtiyar, B.: Exoskeleton for the ankle joint design and control system. In: 2022 International Conference on Communications, Information, Electronic and Energy Systems (CIEES 2022), 24–26 November 2022, Veliko Tarnovo, Bulgaria (2022)
8. Copilusi, C., Dumitru, S., Geonea, I., Ciurezu, L.G., Dumitru, N.: Design Approaches of an Exoskeleton for Human Neuromotor Rehabilitation. Appl. Sci. 2022, 12(8), 3952; https://doi.org/10.3390/app12083952

A Leg Exoskeleton Mechanism for Human Walking Assistance

Cristian Copilusi[1](✉), Marco Ceccarelli[2], Sorin Dumitru[1], Alexandru Margine[1], and Ionut Geonea[1]

[1] University of Craiova, 200512 Craiova, Romania
cristian.copilusi@edu.ucv.ro
[2] University of Rome Tor Vergata, Rome. Lazio, Italy

Abstract. This research addresses attention to a conceptual mechanism design for a leg exoskeleton used in human walking assistance. The proposed mechanism is designed as based on three classical mechanisms, namely Chebyshev, pantograph mechanism and Stephenson III six-bar mechanism. The research core was focused on the extended actuation for the human ankle joint based on functional and structural analyses. Thus, a leg exoskeleton mechanism was identified, that is characterized by low-cost features and motion ability for human walking assistance.

Keywords: Biomechanics · Human Locomotion · Exoskeletons · Leg Mechanisms · Ankle Joint Design

1 Introduction

Nowadays several humanoid robots, walking machines, and rehabilitation exoskeletons types are designed as based on theoretical analyses, modelling, simulations, and experimental experiences, for solving clinical health tasks. These solutions are designed by having a starting point from analyses of human motions especially developed for walking activities.

By analyzing significant biped walking system designs [1–8] it can be noted two major categories, namely complex exoskeletons that are characterized by a large number of actuators like [2, 3, 7] and simple ones that are characterized by a limited number of actuators like the ones reported in [5, 6, 8].

Most of those solutions have actuation at the level of hip and knee joints like [5, 6] and the ankle joint is substituted by an elastic element that compensate this motion.

Thus, this research was focused on human ankle joint motion during walking when implemented on some leg exoskeletons that are designed with different mechanisms, and combinations of them.

This research has a starting point represented by a leg exoskeleton characterized by three types of mechanisms namely pantograph, Chebyshev and a cam mechanism as presented in [9–11]. This leg exoskeleton conceptual design was analysed several times, and even a prototype was tested in [11]. But the inserted cam mechanism for ankle

D. Tarnita et al. (Eds.): MESROB 2023, MMS 133, pp. 160–167, 2023.
https://doi.org/10.1007/978-3-031-32446-8_18

joint actuation presents some major disadvantages like wear, imprecise motions during overloads, the backlash between the cam follower and the cam body, so that they can lead to improper motions during walking activity phases.

Thus, this work represents continuity for identifying optimal solutions in the case of a leg exoskeleton design based on low-cost and easy-operation features criteria.

This paper is organized as follows. The first section is dedicated for presenting the motivation for elaborating a new conceptual leg exoskeleton by considering the walking machines existing solutions as a starting point for a new exoskeleton design. In the second section are presented characteristics of human walking activity with proper attention on the human ankle joint. This is discussed through an experimental analysis with the aid of motion analysis equipment. Based on the existent solutions especially designed for walking machines combination of pantograph, Chebyshev, cam mechanism, and Stephenson III six bar mechanism are studied from a structural viewpoint in the third section. Thus by considering these structural schemes for obtaining a low-cost leg exoskeleton solution with a single actuator, it is designed a proper leg exoskeleton that is presented and analysed from functional and structural viewpoints in the fourth section of this research.

2 Experimental Evaluation of Human Ankle Joint

For the experimental evaluation of the human ankle joint, two main interest parameters are analyzed, namely ankle trajectory and ankle angular variation. This was possible only through experimental analysis, by using special video-analysis equipment.

University of Craiova – Faculty of Mechanics use this type of equipment that is CONTEMPLAS [12]. This experimental analysis aimed to create a database with motion laws developed by 30 human subjects during walking. From this database, it was retained data from a single human subject, respectively a female with known anthropometrical data with an age of 30 years, as in the example in Fig. 1.

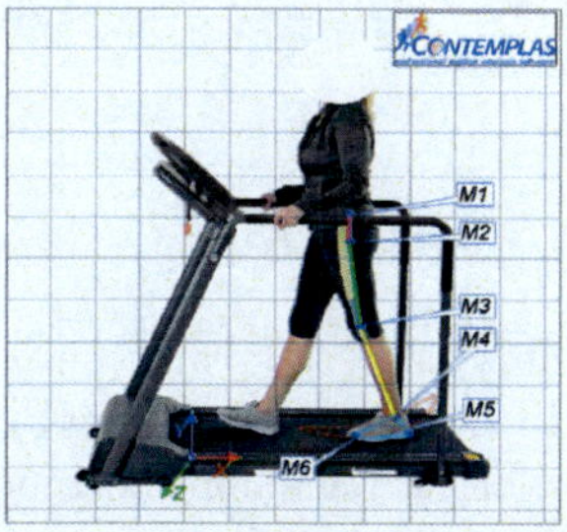

Fig. 1. Example by using CONTEMPLAS with markers

The analysis procedure consists of monitoring the position of the markers that are attached on each joint centre as it can be seen in Fig. 1 where it shows the markers location and the ankle experimental trajectory during experimental tests. The labels represented in Fig. 1 correspond to the following notation: M1 – pelvis mass centre; M2 – hip joint; M3 – knee joint; M4 – ankle joint; M5 – heel extreme point; M6 – distal phalanges.

It was recorded the experimental test for a complete gait on a treadmill, with the use of two high-speed cameras characterized by 350 frames/second. First camera was placed on the lateral side and the second was mounted in front. Thus, the results interest was represented by the first camera recordings, while the second monitors additional data about passive movements of the analysed joints. The interested results are shown in Fig. 2, and these represents constraints for the design of the parametrized exoskeleton by using the combination of the specified mechanism.

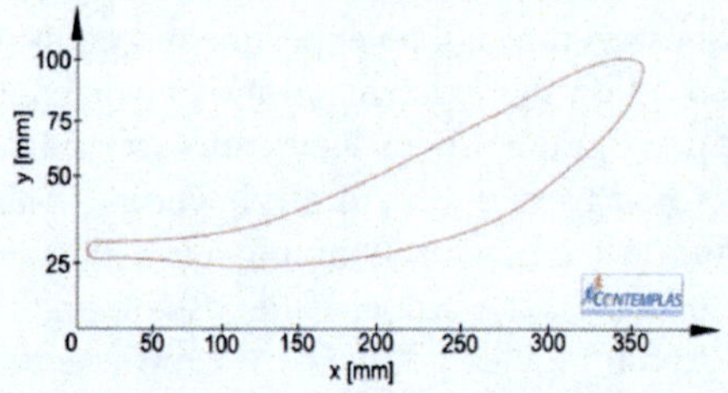

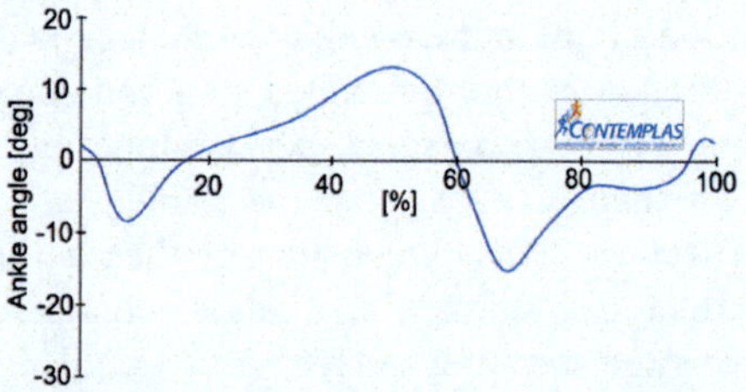

Fig. 2. An example of experimental analysis of walking by using CONTEMPLAS with results on: a) trajectory on ankle joint; b) angle variation of ankle joint

From Fig. 2-a) it can be observed that the trajectory is represented in X-Y coordinate system and on Y – axis records a displacement of 101.456 mm and in X- axis it was developed a displacement of 365.209 mm. In the case of human ankle joint angular variation reported in Fig. 2-b), it can be remarked an angular variation from −18.67° to 18.45°, respectively angular amplitude of 37.12° during walking. The obtained results reported through graphs from Figs. 2 and 3 correspond with the ones existent in data literature from [13]. For the human ankle joint functional recovery, there are a few medical recovery devices that have an extension to this joint only for plantar/dorsal flexion of this. In the case of persons with injuries this motion has angular amplitude with limitations.

3 Ankle Joint Actuation Mechanisms

This research represents a continuity in mechanism types especially adapted for motion extension at the ankle joint level from the exoskeletons structure. The basic criteria in developing and designing exoskeletons for human locomotion rehabilitation purposes were simplicity, low-cost, user-friendly interface, and a minimum number of actuators – preferably one actuator. Thus in previous research presented in [9–11] there were conceived exoskeleton leg types by combining a pantograph and Chebyshev mechanisms for efficient reproduction of human walking. The obtained mechanism addresses only the hip and knee joints. Furthermore, the research was extended to mechanisms for ankle joint actuation as it was presented in [9], respectively a cam mechanism with a proper profile. This mechanism has 4 links, 7 revolute joints, and one cam mechanism. By having in sight this mechanism, a prototype was elaborated and experimental tests were done. During these tests, it appears some specific cam mechanism disadvantages and for this reason, it was conceived another mechanism solution based on Stephenson III six-bar mechanism [14, 15]. Figure 3 it is shown a structural scheme of this mechanism type, where it can be remarked the ovoid trajectory developed by the final link, which can be imposed on a new leg exoskeleton structure.

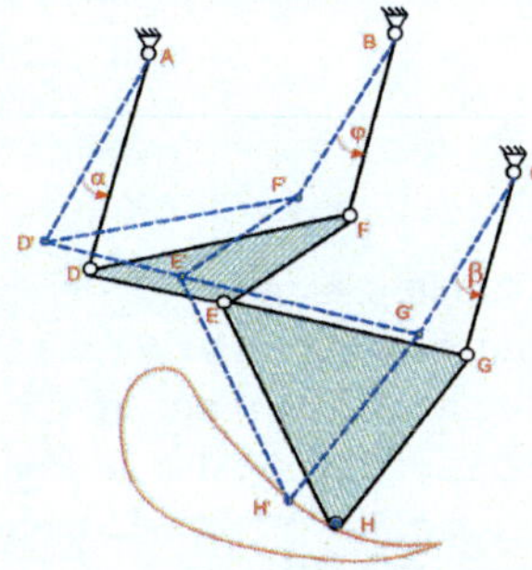

Fig. 3. Stephenson III six-bar mechanism general structural scheme for the proposed ankle joint mechanisms [15]

In order to eliminate the cam mechanism disadvantages, the main target was to modify and adapt the Stephenson III six-bar mechanism onto the pantograph and Chebyshev mechanism combination. Thus it was conceived a novel leg exoskeleton and the crossing phases are shown in Fig. 4.

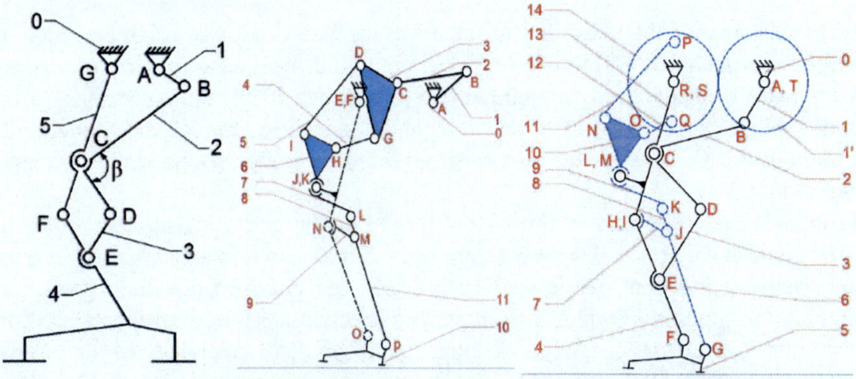

Fig. 4. Low-cost exoskeleton structural schemes: a) mechanism with pantograph and Chebyshev; b) the modified Stephenson III six-bar mechanism for actuating the ankle joint; c) mechanism with the pantograph, Chebyshev and a modified Stephenson III six-bar.

The structural parameters for the presented solutions in Fig. 4 are listed in Table 1 whose characterization is given through the range of mobility.

In Fig. 4-a) it is presented the base structural scheme for actuating a leg exoskeleton for hip and knee joints.

Table 1. Leg exoskeleton structural comparison based on Fig. 4

Mechanism	*Number of links*	*Number of joints*	*DoF*	*Range of mobility*
Figure 4 a)	5	7	1 DoF = 7 joints	1
Figure 4 b)	11	16	1 DoF = 16 joints	1
Figure 4 c)	14	20	1 DoF = 20 joints 2DoF = 1 Gear mechanism	1

The presented solution in Fig. 4-b) represents the obtained solution for implementing Stephenson III six-bar mechanism for actuating only the ankle joint.

At first look, the leg exoskeleton structural scheme from Fig. 4-c) seems to be a complex one due to a large number of links. Also in Fig. 4-c) it can be identified a gear mechanism for a parallel motion of the modified Stephenson III mechanism which actuates the ankle joint (links marked with dotted lines). As mention, it can be observed that the drive gear (1') is fixed with the drive link (1).

The advantage of the solution from Fig. 4-c) is that it can have a precise motion for a complete gait for three main actuated joints, namely: hip (R), knee (I), and ankle (F). Also, this linkage can be a parametrized one for other research or it can be designed with adjustable links.

4 A Leg Exoskeleton Concept and Functional Evaluations

In order to demonstrate the feasibility of the novel leg exoskeleton solution presented in Fig. 4-c), it was designed a 3D model in a parametrized form according to the anthropometrical data from the analyzed human subject shown in Fig. 1. According to the structural scheme from Fig. 4-c) it was designed a simplified model and numerically processed with MSC Adams/AdamsView program. The model of one leg exoskeleton is shown in Fig. 5.

In Fig. 6 it can be remarked the virtual model of the entire exoskeleton with the major remark that the left and right legs are mirrored as position and orientation from the main frame (equivalent pelvic segment). It can be remarked that both gear pairs for actuating the modified Stephenson III six-bar mechanism for ankle actuation. This have, for both exoskeleton legs, 28 links connected through 40 revolute joints and 2 gear mechanisms defined in MSC Adams environment. According to the Fig. 5, the link sizes in millimeters are the following: $l_1 = 35$; $l_2 = 215$; $l_3 = 225$; $l_4 = 260$; $l_5 = 320$; $l_6 = 335$; $l_7 = 120$; $l_8 = 40$; $l_9 = 400$; $l_{10} = 250$; $l_{11} = 20$; $l_{12} = 120x103x60$; $l_{13} = 80$; $l_{14} = 55$; $l_{15} = 15$.

As regards the actuation, it was considered a drive link l_1, with a complete rotation which corresponds to a complete gait cycle. Other parameters can be processed like connection forces, after applying a body force on foot equivalent to element l_7. This can be done and it can be the object for other case studies in this research which will generate analysis in processed in a dynamic mode.

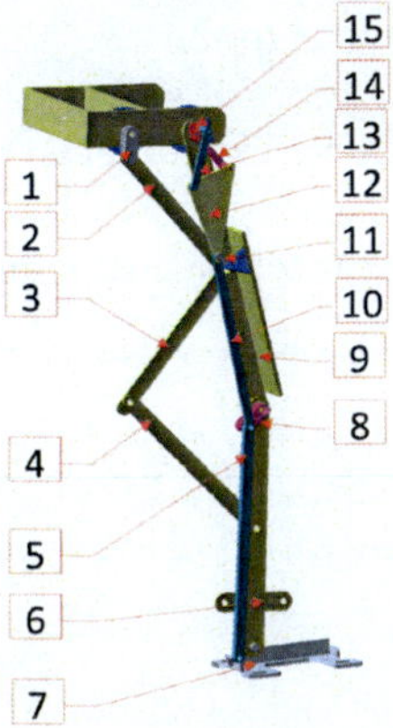

Fig. 5. A leg simplified model

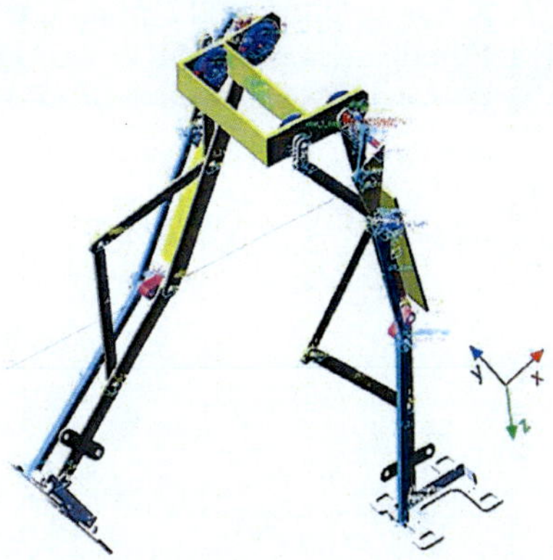

Fig. 6. The parametrized exoskeleton imported in MSC Adams

This model was simulated from kinematic viewpoints to obtain the foot trajectory and also the ankle joint motion law for one desired exoskeleton leg. For this, it was considered a complete gait, which was performed in a time of 1.25 s almost equal to the real-time developed during human gait experimental analysis. The ground contact was neglected. During virtual simulation, there were obtained some snapshots of the simplified model, which is reported in Fig. 7, where it can be observed the marker trajectory from the right ankle joint.

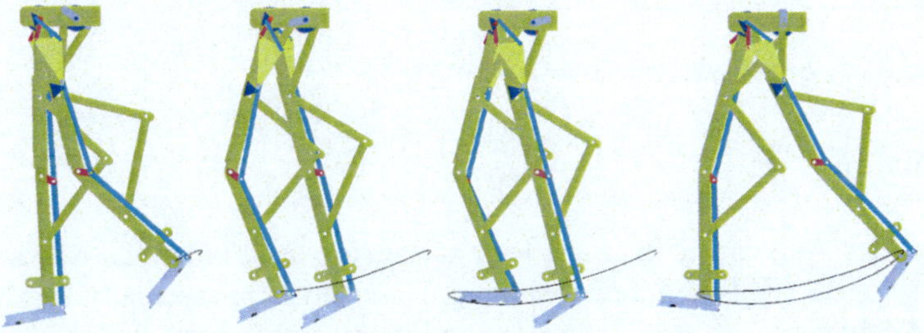

Fig. 7. Snapshots during virtual simulations of the simplified model of the proposed exoskeleton

During this virtual simulation, performed from a kinematic viewpoint, the main results were focused on the leg exoskeleton ankle joint behavior. These results were represented through diagrams that characterize the ankle joint planar trajectory and ankle joint angular variation for a complete gait. These results are shown through graphs reported in Figs. 8 and 9.

In Fig. 8 it can be remarked the ankle joint angular variation which develops an angular amplitude of 35.25° (this was calculated between 67.41° and 102.66°). Also, this variation has a similar path like the one reported in Fig. 2.

Regarding the ankle joint trajectory, this was obtained in an X-Y coordinate system as it can be observed in Fig. 9, where it can be found displacement on x-axis of 349.092

mm and on y-axis of almost 112 mm. The trajectory is similar to the one plotted in Fig. 2. In fact there are some small errors due to the position errors of global reference system in MSC Adams/Adams View and the one considered from experimental tests of a human subject during walking for a complete gait.

Thus, the obtained main results allow continuing with this mechanism combination due to the precise motion of the ankle joint exoskeleton.

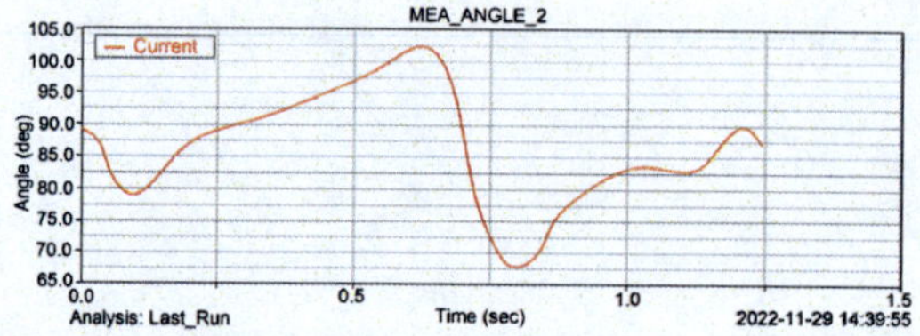

Fig. 8. Equivalent ankle joint angular variation [degrees] vs. time [seconds]

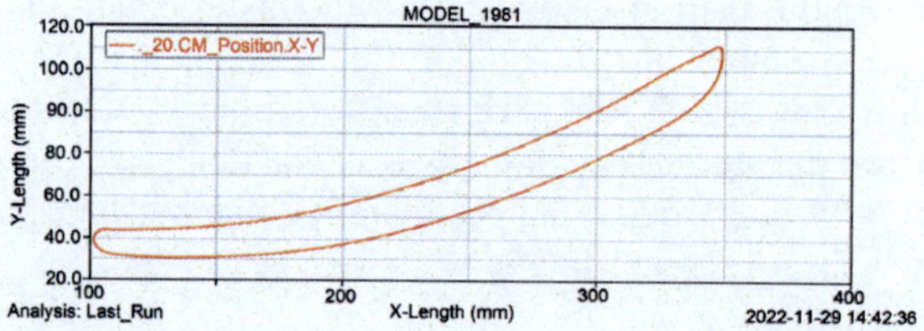

Fig. 9. Trajectory developed in x-y system coordinates developed by an ankle center marker [millimeters]

5 Conclusions

A conceptual design is presented for a leg exoskeleton used in human walking assistance. By having in sight the human walking characteristics, especially for the ankle joint, a leg mechanism has been elaborated and its kinematic structure can be used in wearable exoskeletons structures for walking rehabilitation purposes. The proposed leg mechanism can be parametrized and it can be designed with adjustable size devices. A final solution is proposed and evaluated with capabilities for motion of hip, knee and ankle articulations. Moreover, ankle joint motion is obtained by combining three classical mechanisms. The leg exoskeleton conceptual design was evaluated through virtual simulations based on structural and functional considerations.

Acknowledgment. This work was supported by a grant of the Ministry of Research, Innovation and Digitization, CCCDI – UEFISCDI, project number PN-III-P2–2.1-PED-2021–1917, within PNCDI III.

References

1. Ganguly, A., Sanz-Merodio, D., Puyuelo, G.: Wearable pediatric gait exoskeleton- a feasibility study. In: IEEE/RSJ International Conference on Intelligent Robots and Systems (IROS), pp. 4667–4672. Spain (2018)
2. Lerner, Z., Damiano, D., Bulea, T.: A lower-extremity exoskeleton improves knee extension in children with crouch gait from cerebral palsy. Sci. Transl. Med. **23**(9)(404), 10 (2017)
3. Shepherd, M., Rouse, E.: Design and validation of a torque-controllable knee exoskeleton for sit-to-stand assistance. In: IEEE/ASME Trans Mechatron. **22**(4), 1695–1704 (2017)
4. Eilenberg, M.F., Geyer, H., Herr, H.: Control of a powered ankle-foot prosthesis based on a neuromuscular model. IEEE Trans. Neural Syst. Rehabil. Eng. **18**(2), 164–173 (2010)
5. Liang, C., Ceccarelli, M., Takeda, Y.: Operation analysis of a one-DOF pantograph leg mechanisms. In: Proceedings of the RAAD '08. In: 17th International Workshop on Robotics in Alpe-Adria-Danube Region September 15–17, pp. 1–10 (2008)
6. Li, T., Ceccarelli, M.: An experimental characterization of a rickshaw prototype. Int. J. Mech. Control **12**(2), 29–48 (2012)
7. Copilusi, C., Dumitru, S., Geonea, I., Colici, F., Dumitru, N.: Design and numerical characterization of a new leg exoskeleton for human neuromotor rehabilitation. Acta Tech. Napocensis. Series Appl. Math. Mech. Eng. **64**(1) (2021)
8. Tavolieri C., Ottaviano E., Ceccarelli M.: Analysis and design of a 1-DOF Leg for walking machines. In: Proceedings of RAAD'06, 15th International Workshop on Robotics in Alpe-Adria-Danube Region, Balantonfured, CD Proceedings, pp. 63-71 (2006)
9. Copilusi, C., Ceccarelli, M., Carbone, G., Margine, A.: Mechanism of a leg exoskeleton for walking rehabilitation purposes. In: Petuya, V., Pinto, C., Lovasz, EC. (eds) New Advances in Mechanisms, Transmissions and Applications. Mechanisms and Machine Science, vol. 17. Springer, Dordrecht. (2014). https://doi.org/10.1007/978-94-007-7485-8_14
10. Copilusi C., Ceccarelli M., and Carbone G.: Design and Numerical Characterization of a New Leg Exoskeleton for Motion Assistance, pp. 1–16. Robotica Cambridge University Press (2014)
11. Copilusi, C., Ceccarelli, M., Dumitru, N., Carbone, G.: Design and simulation of a leg exoskeleton linkage for a human rehabilitation system. In: Visa, I. (eds.) The 11th IFToMM International Symposium on Science of Mechanisms and Machines. Mechanisms and Machine Science, vol. 18. Springer, Cham. (2014). https://doi.org/10.1007/978-3-319-01845-4_12
12. CONTEMPLAS Motion Analysis Equipment user manual (2010)
13. Williams M., Biomechanics of Human Motion. Saunders Co. Philadelphia & London (1996)
14. Batayneh, W., et al.: Biomimetic design of a single DOF Stephenson III leg mechanism. Mech. Eng. Res. **3**(2), 43 (2013)
15. Plecnik, M., McCarthy, J.M.: Kinematic synthesis of Stephenson III six-bar function generators. Mech. Mach. Theory **97**,112–126 (2015)

Dynamic Analysis and Structural Optimization of a New Exoskeleton Prototype for Lower Limb Rehabilitation

Ionut Geonea(✉), Cristian Copilusi, Alexandru Margine, Sorin Dumitru, Adrian Rosca, and Daniela Tarnita

Faculty of Mechanics, University of Craiova, 200512 Craiova, Romania
ionut.geonea@edu.ucv.ro

Abstract. This paper presents a new exoskeleton robot solution for assisting human walking. As a novel feature of the present research work, a new solution for the design of a mechanism for the legs of an exoskeleton robot is proposed. A virtual prototype is made, based on which the proposed exoskeleton robot solution is analysed kinematically and dynamically. Following this analysis, it is found that the proposed solution achieves motion laws in the hip and knee joints similar to those obtained in normal human walking. The kinematic elements of the exoskeleton are conceived with a design that ensures manufacturability by rapid prototyping technique, easy assembly as well as structural strength. For this purpose, a structural optimization study will be carried out with the finite element method to obtain the best design solution.

Keywords: exoskeleton robot · dynamic analysis · structural optimization · mechanism design

1 Introduction

Robotics for rehabilitation treatment is an emerging field that is expected to grow as a solution for rehabilitation automation [1]. Robotic rehabilitation can: replace the physical training effort of a therapist, allowing for more intense repetitive movements and providing therapy at a reasonable cost; and quantitatively assess the level of motor recovery by measuring force and movement trajectories [2, 3]. The issues addressed in this paper are related to the kinematic and dynamic analysis of exoskeleton robotic systems intended for the rehabilitation of people with locomotor disabilities. This category of mobile robotic systems has undergone two directions of development: the development of open kinematic chains with motors placed in the system joints, and the development of closed kinematic chains with a single drive motor [4–6]. In the last decade, several robotic lower limb rehabilitation systems have been developed to restore mobility to affected limbs. These systems can be grouped according to the rehabilitation principle and they follow: treadmill systems with patient suspension system; underfoot plate-based gait systems; ground-based gait systems, stationary systems, chair-based systems, ankle rehabilitation systems [7–11]. Studies on the experimental determination of the

D. Tarnita et al. (Eds.): MESROB 2023, MMS 133, pp. 168–178, 2023.
https://doi.org/10.1007/978-3-031-32446-8_19

laws of motion performed in normal human gait are presented in [12, 13]. As a novelty, we found from the literature study, that systems with a dual functional role have been developed, as a gait trolley and as an exoskeleton for assisting upright position and gait [14]. Aspects of 3D printing technologies are detailed in [15].

The paper is structured in four parts. After the introductory part, the kinematic solution of a new mechanism that is used as the leg of an exoskeleton is presented. This robotic system is virtually modelled and analyzed kinematically and dynamically. For the physical realization of the robotic system, a structurally optimized solution of the shape of the component elements is proposed.

2 The Proposed Structural Solution

Both solutions of exoskeleton robot leg mechanisms are driven by a single motor, i.e. they have a single degree of freedom, placed in kinematic joint A. The proposed solution to design the exoskeleton leg mechanism is based on a previously developed one shown in Fig. 1a [16]. It can be seen from Fig. 1b, that the new solution is simplified, having only 7 kinematic links in the structure, compared to 9 links as the first solution has. In addition, the new design is simplified in terms of the drive kinematic chain, having in its structure only crank 1 and connecting rod 2. The foot mechanism has a quadrilateral (CDFH) and a pantograph (GJIF) kinematic chain structure. The E and G joints model the hip and knee joint, similar to the human foot structure.

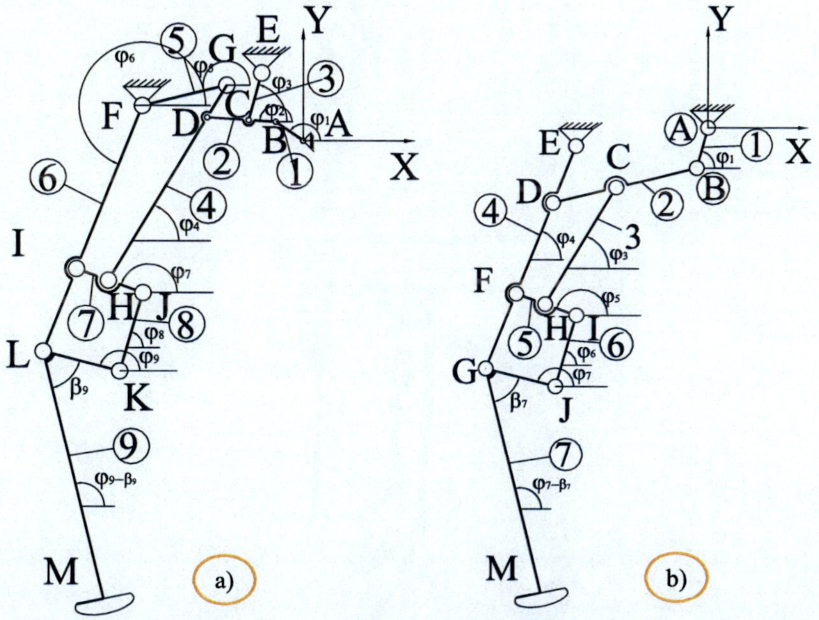

Fig. 1. Previous structural solution and newly developed solution for the exoskeleton leg mechanism.

Among the advantages of the new structural solution, we can highlight the following: - the drive part is placed further back than the kinematic chain of the foot, in this way being a more ergonomic solution, easier to wear by humans; - the angle variation laws of the hip and knee joints have amplitudes very close to those of the human, for normal gait; -the stride length is greater than in the previous solution.

For kinematic and dynamic modelling, the prototype in Fig. 2a is made. In the first stage of making the virtual model we designed the kinematic elements as bars. This solution is not suitable for the realization of a real model, because it does not allow to mount the bearings in the joints. In order to optimize the design solution, it is necessary to design the elements of the mechanism as shown in Fig. 2b, where the ends must be fork-shaped to allow mounting the bearings on a shaft. The manufacturing of the exoskeleton will be based on the prototype in Fig. 2b, where the elements have been made with a design that allows the mounting of axles with bearings, and ensures the correct transmission of connecting forces in the kinematic joints.

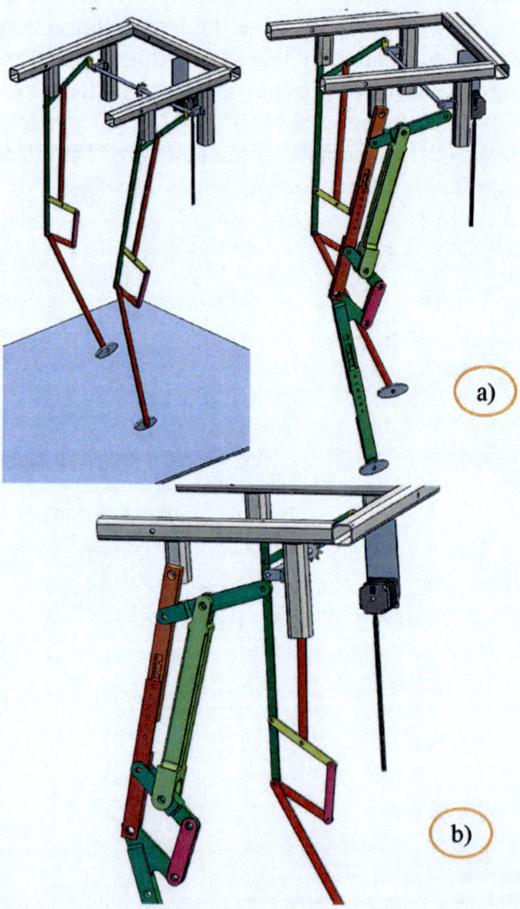

Fig. 2. Design of the constructive solution of the exoskeleton robot.

The kinematic modelling of the exoskeleton's leg mechanism is carried out in a first phase in the situation where it operates with the upper frame fixed to the base. In this situation the angles in the foot joints (hip and knee) and the shape of the trajectory made by the sole (M-point) are of interest. They are shown in Fig. 3.

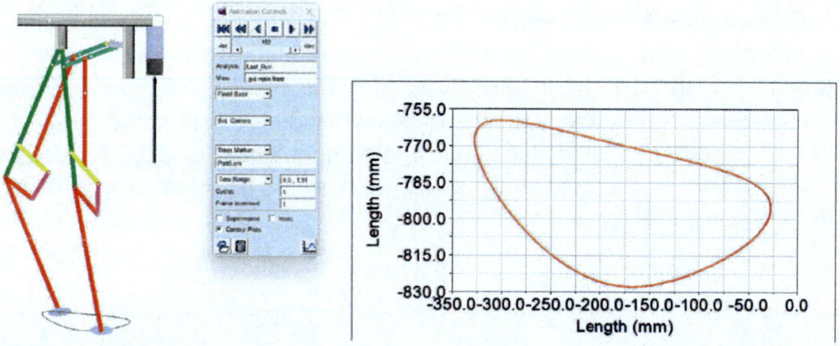

Fig. 3. The path performed by point M, corresponding to the ankle joint, calculated in ADAMS.

The laws of variation of the angles in the hip and knee joints of the exoskeleton (E and G joints, according to the kinematic scheme) are shown in Fig. 4. According to these plots the angle variation in the knee joint is between -21.066° and 19.049°, i.e. it has an amplitude of 40.115°. The angle in the hip joint has a variation between −12.64° and 20.814°, i.e. it has an amplitude of 33.454°. These angles are comparable to those made by humans during normal walking [12].

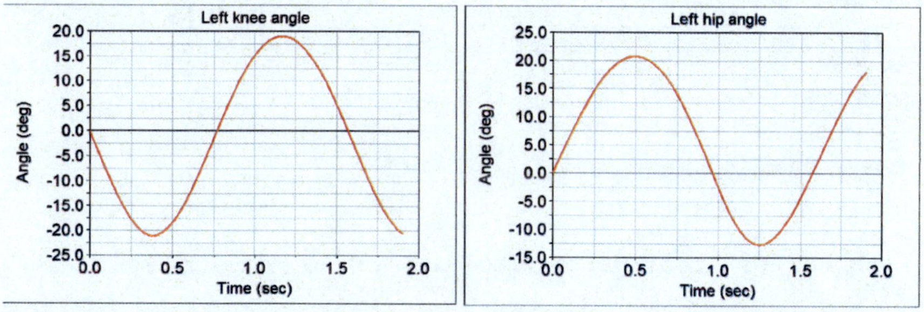

Fig. 4. Laws of variation of angles in the hip and knee joints of the exoskeleton leg.

For the second phase of the study, we performed dynamic modelling of the exoskeleton robot, in the situation where it performs the activity of walking on the ground, and takes the full weight of the attached patient. The trajectory described by a point located on the exoskeleton sole, obtained by numerical simulation in ADAMS is depicted in Fig. 5. In Fig. 5b, the laws of variation of the coordinates of point M, which belongs to element 7 of the left foot, are shown. It can be seen that the robot steps in the opposite direction of the X-axis, and performs in 10 s a displacement over a distance of 3250 mm.

Also, at this stage of dynamic analysis we obtained the laws of variation of the connection forces in the kinematic joins of the robot leg mechanism. Thus in Fig. 6, the laws of variation of the connection forces in the exoskeleton knee joint are shown. The Y-axis is the vertical axis, and as can be seen the connection force component has the highest value along this axis. The peaks recorded with positive values, come due to the shock, produced by the impact between the exoskeleton sole and the ground, which are considered rigid solids. In the operation of the exoskeleton, this does not happen because the exoskeleton sole will be provided with a deformable rubber support.

Figure 7. Shows the connection forces in the hip joint obtained in the case of exoskeleton ground walking. Again, the components of the bending forces show jumps at heel contact with the ground. These shocks reach maximum values of 2200 N. Unlike the knee, in this joint, the maximum value is along the X-axis. The value recorded when the foot is in contact with the ground reaches 650 N.

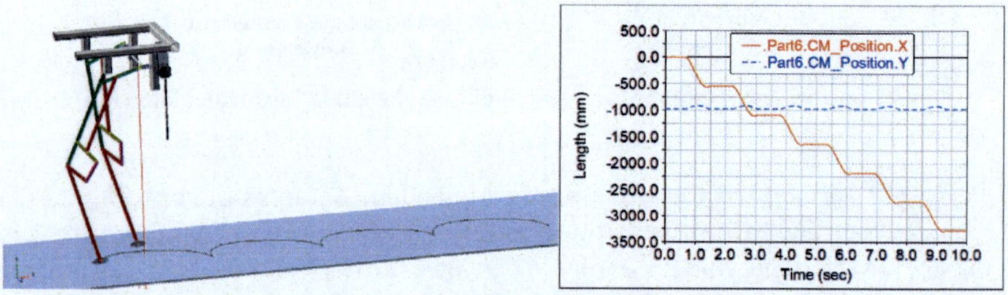

Fig. 5. The trajectory computed during the exoskeleton gait simulation a), and b) the laws of variation of the coordinates of point M, attached to the sole of the exoskeleton foot.

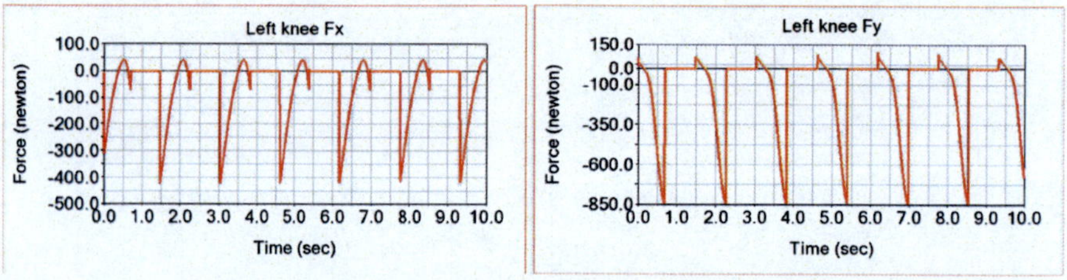

Fig. 6. Laws of variation of connection forces in the exoskeleton knee joint.

From the analysis of the graphs shown in Fig. 6 and 7 we can conclude as follows. For both the knee and hip joint, the Y-axis is oriented upwards. The presence of the ABCD kinematic drive chain, changes the distribution of reactions in the F joint, corresponding to the hip joint. Thus, a pronounced increase for a short period of time of the connection force component upon the X (horizontal) axis is observed. This increase occurs when the left leg touches the ground and the drive element is in a vertical position.

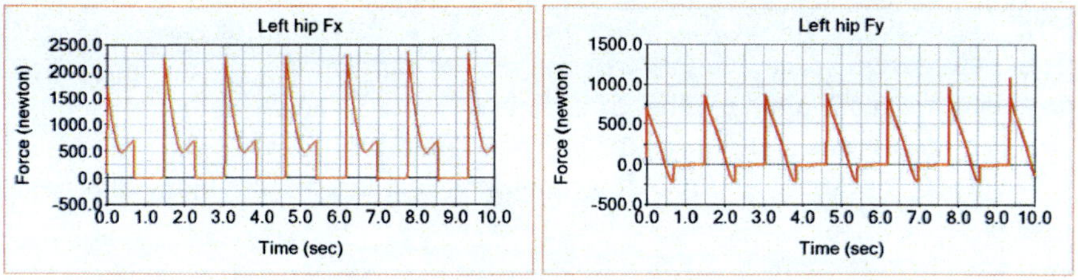

Fig. 7. Laws of variation of connection forces in the exoskeleton hip joint.

3 Structural Optimization of Robot Kinematic Elements

Optimization can be defined as the process of maximizing or minimizing a desired objective function with the satisfaction of constraints [17]. Mechanical structures are often analysed with the finite element method, which is a widely used technique for structural analysis. Finite element analysis is used to analyze the dynamic response, and to analyze mechanical strains and stresses in structures that are subjected to loads and boundary conditions. From a mathematical point of view optimization can be considered as a numerical computation technique to analyze problems governed by partial derivative equations, which describe the behavior of the system under study.

The optimization problem based on the finite element method can generally be expressed as:

Minimize $f(x, U)$
Subject to $g_i(x, U) \leq 0$, i = 1,...m
and $h_j(x, U) = 0$ j = 1,...m

where U is the vector of nodal displacements (n dof x 1), for which the field of displacements u (x, y, z) is determined. The relationship between U and x is governed by the equilibrium differential equations:

$$K(x)U = F(x)$$

where K is the quadratic stiffness matrix (n dof x n dof) and F is the vector of loads (n dof x 1).

Depending on the type of design variables **x** finite element-based optimization may be classified as parameter or size, shape and topology optimization. In parameter or size optimization the objective function f is typically the weight of the structure, and g_i are the constraints reflecting limits on stress and displacement. The design variable set x can take various forms.

In our case, we propose to structurally optimize the link 2 of the robot, which has the geometrical shape shown in Fig. 8. As design parameters, we have the thickness of the stiffening wall in the middle, as well as the two radii of the connection. The objective function is to reduce the mass of the element (minimization), and the constraint is to maintain an equivalent mechanical stress not exceeding a certain value. The limits of variation of the extrusion height are specified in the range 10.8...13.2 mm. Similarly, the ranges of variation are specified for the radii of the connection, between 2.7...3.3 mm.

Design of experiments (DOE) can be defined as a procedure for choosing a set of samples in the design space, with the general goal of maximizing the amount of information gained from a limited number of samples. Figure 9 shows the input parameters and their variation limits and Fig. 10 the objective function. These limits have been set to obtain a possible design solution. After running the algorithm, we obtained the results shown in Fig. 11.

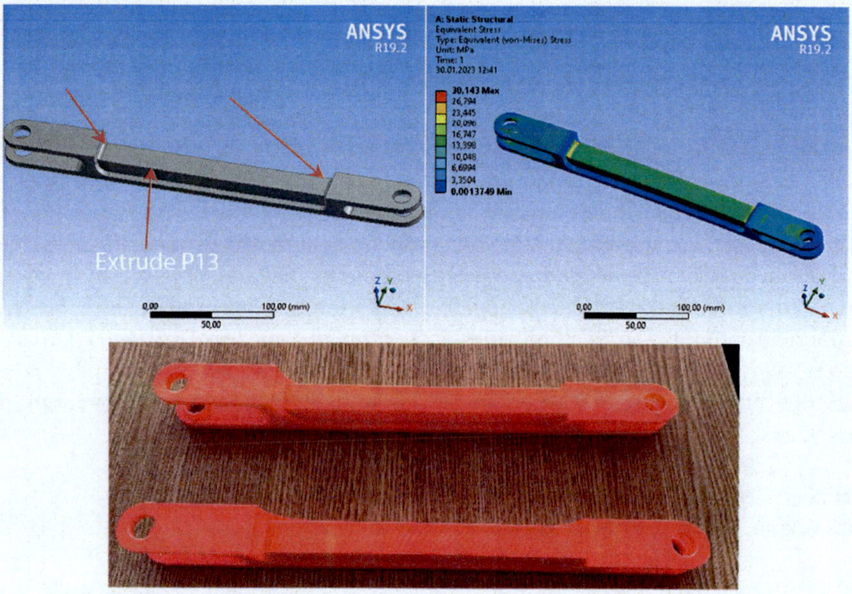

Fig. 8. Defined design parameters and equivalent stress distribution according to the von Mises method as well as 3D printed elements.

	A	B	C	D
1	⊟ Input Parameters			
2	Name	Lower Bound	Upper Bound	
3	P11 - FBlend8.FD1 (mm)	2,7	3,3	
4	P12 - FBlend10.FD1 (mm)	2,7	3,3	
5	P13 - Extrude8.FD1 (mm)	10,8	13,2	
6	⊟ Parameter Relationships			
7	Name	Left Expression	Operator	Right Expression
*	New Parameter Relationship	New Expression	<=	New Expression

Fig. 9. Optimization input parameters.

	A	B	C	D	E	F	G
1	Name	Parameter	Objective		Constraint		
2			Type	Target	Type	Lower Bound	Upper Bound
3	Minimize P6	P6 - Solid Mass	Minimize		No Constraint		
4	P7 <= 33 MPa	P7 - Equivalent Stress Maximum Maximum Value Over Time	No Objective		Values <= Upper Bound		33
*		Select a Parameter					

Fig. 10. Specify the objective function and the optimization constraint.

Table of Outline A2: Design Points of Design of Experiments

	A	B	C	D	E	F	G	H
1	Name	P11 - FBlend8.FD1 (mm)	P12 - FBlend10.FD1 (mm)	P13 - Extrude8.FD1 (mm)	P5 - Total Deformation Maximum (mm)	P6 - Solid Mass (kg)	P7 - Equivalent Stress Maximum Maximum Value Over Time (MPa)	P8 - Equivalent Elastic Strain Maximum (mm mm^-1)
2	1 DP 2	3	3	12	0,57741	0,35311	30,143	0,00042996
3	2	2,7	3	12	0,57783	0,35309	32,611	0,00045948
4	3	3,3	3	12	0,57695	0,35313	29,824	0,00042212
5	4	3	2,7	12	0,57788	0,35309	31,317	0,00044295
6	5	3	3,3	12	0,57691	0,35313	29,047	0,00041104
7	6	3	3	10,8	0,77085	0,34014	35,815	0,00050455
8	7	3	3	13,2	0,43889	0,36604	26,485	0,00037429
9	8	2,7561	2,7561	11,024	0,73055	0,34254	37,626	0,00053253
10	9	3,2439	2,7561	11,024	0,7295	0,34257	37,534	0,00053043
11	10	2,7561	3,2439	11,024	0,72951	0,34257	33,137	0,00047858
12	11	3,2439	3,2439	11,024	0,72851	0,3426	32,682	0,00046227
13	12	2,7561	2,7561	12,976	0,46176	0,3636	30,394	0,00043083
14	13	3,2439	2,7561	12,976	0,4615	0,36362	30,318	0,00042985
15	14	2,7561	3,2439	12,976	0,4611	0,36364	26,646	0,00037666
16	15	3,2439	3,2439	12,976	0,46088	0,36365	26,498	0,00037436

Fig. 11. Design point of design of experiments.

Figure 12 shows the response surfaces for the output parameter P6 -Solid Mass, as a function of the input parameters: P11 and P12- Radius of connection, P13-Extrude feature.

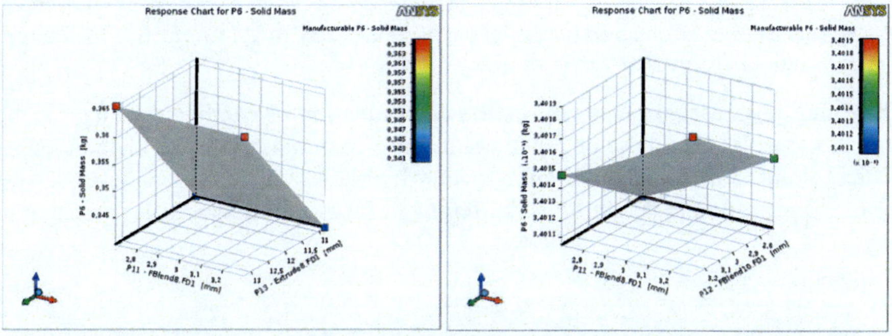

Fig. 12. Response surface obtained for the output parameter P6 -Solid Mass.

Figure 13 shows the response surfaces for the output parameter P7 - Equivalent Stress Maximum, as a function of the input parameters: P11and P12 - Radius of Connection, P13-Extrude feature.

Figure 14 shows the response surfaces for the output parameter P5 -Total Deformation maximum, as a function of the input parameters: P11and P12- radius of connection, P13-Extrude feature.

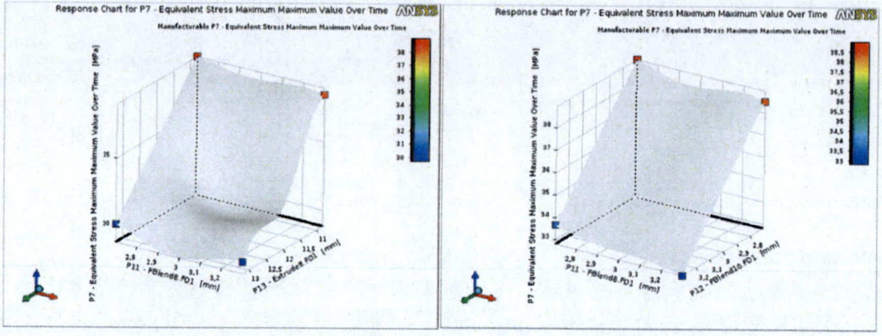

Fig. 13. Response surface obtained for the output parameter P7 -Equivalent Stress Maximum.

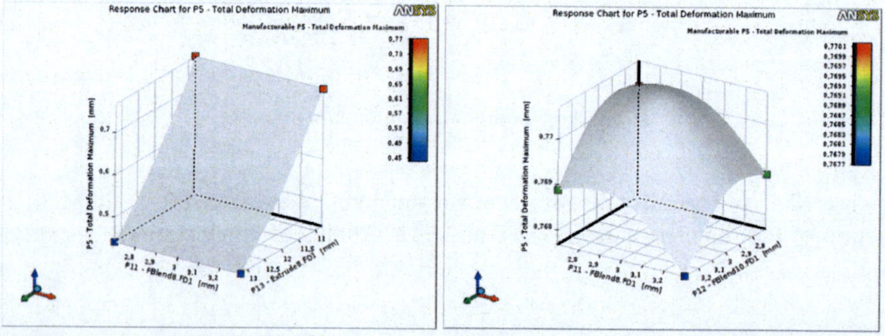

Fig. 14. Response surface obtained for the output parameter P5- Total Deformation Maximum.

Obtaining response surfaces, allows the determination of candidate points for the optimal design solution. These obtained points are 3 in number. Among them the most convenient point is the candidate Point 1, for which the radii of the connection have values of 3.3 mm and the height of the stiffening portion is 10.8 mm, as is presented in Fig. 15.

	A	B	C	D	E	F
1–2	Reference	Name	P11 - FBlend8.FD1 (mm)	P12 - FBlend10.FD1 (mm)	P13 - Extrude8.FD1 (mm)	P5 - Total Deformation Maximum (mm)
3	○	Candidate Point 1	3,3	3,3	10,8	0,76767
4	○	Candidate Point 2	2,7	2,7	13,2	0,44078
5	●	Candidate Point 3	3,3	3,3	13,2	0,43968
*		New Custom Candidate Point	2,7	2,7	10,8	

Fig. 15. Candidate points obtained as the optimal solution.

4 Conclusions

In this paper we have presented a new constructive solution for the leg mechanism of an exoskeleton intended for locomotor assistance of people with disabilities. The constructive solution is characterized by the fact that it is simple, having in its structure 7 kinematic elements and is driven by a single motor. This solution is analysed from a kinematic and dynamic point of view using the ADAMS software, which allows the study of mobile multibody systems. The motion laws from the hip and knee joints of the exoskeleton leg are obtained. For the dimensioning of the exoskeleton elements, the dynamic simulation of the exoskeleton robot and the connection forces from the kinematic joints are obtained. These forces are required for structural analysis with the finite element method. As a way to execute the elements, the rapid prototyping technique of the optimized design shape is proposed. To obtain the optimal design, we used ANSYS software. The optimization involved reducing the mass of the elements, and reducing the mechanical stress concentrators. As future research direction we aim to realize the physical prototype of the exoskeleton robot.

References

1. Shi, D., Zhang, W., Zhang, W., Ding, X.: A review on lower limb rehabilitation exoskeleton robots. Chin. J. Mech. Eng. **32**(1), 1–11 (2019)
2. Chaichaowarat, R., Prakthong, S., Thitipankul, S.: Transformable wheelchair-exoskeleton hybrid robot for assisting human locomotion. Robotics **12**(1), 16 (2023)
3. Hu, B., Liu, F., Cheng, K., Chen, W., Shan, X., Yu, H.: Stiffness optimal modulation of a variable stiffness energy storage hip exoskeleton and experiments on its assistance effect. IEEE Trans. Neural Syst. Rehabil. Eng. (2023)
4. Carbone, G., Laribi, M.A.: Recent trends on innovative robot designs and approaches. Appl. Sci. **13**(3), 1388 (2023)
5. Rodrigues-Carvalho, C., et al.: Benchmarking the effects on human–exoskeleton interaction of trajectory, admittance and EMG-triggered exoskeleton movement control. Sensors, **23**(2), 791 (2023)
6. Jayaraman, C., et al.: Modular hip exoskeleton improves walking function and reduces sedentary time in community-dwelling older adults. J. Neuroeng. Rehabil. **19**(1), 1–12 (2022)
7. Arcos-Legarda, J., Torres, D., Velez, F., Rodríguez, H., Parra, A., Gutiérrez, Á.: Mechatronics design of a gait-assistance exoskeleton for therapy of children with duchenne muscular dystrophy. Appl. Sci. **13**(2), 839 (2023)
8. Veneman, J.F., Kruidhof, R., Hekman, E.E., Ekkelenkamp, R., Van Asseldonk, E.H., Van Der Kooij, H.: Design and evaluation of the LOPES exoskeleton robot for interactive gait rehabilitation. IEEE Trans. Neural Syst. Rehabil. Eng. **15**(3), 379–386 (2007)
9. Huo, W., Mohammed, S., Moreno, J.C., Amirat, Y.: Lower limb wearable robots for assistance and rehabilitation: a state of the art. IEEE Syst. J. **10**(3), 1068–1081 (2014)
10. Zhou, J., Yang, S., Xue, Q.: Lower limb rehabilitation exoskeleton robot: a review. Adv. Mech. Eng. **13**(4), 16878140211011862 (2021)
11. Lee, H., Ferguson, P.W., Rosen, J.: Lower limb exoskeleton systems—overview. Wearable Robot. 207–229 (2020)
12. Tarnita, D., Marghitu, D.: Nonlinear dynamics of normal and osteoarthritic human knee. Proc. Rom. Acad. **18**(4), 353–360 (2017)
13. Tarniţă, D., Geonea, I., Petcu, A., Tarniţă, D. N.: Experimental characterization of human walking on stairs applied to humanoid dynamics. In: Rodić, A., Borangiu, T. (eds.) Advances in Robot Design and Intelligent Control: Proceedings of the 25th Conference on Robotics in Alpe-Adria-Danube Region (RAAD16), pp. 293–301. Springer International Publishing (2017). https://doi.org/10.1007/978-3-319-49058-8_32

14. Geonea, I.D., Tarnita, D.: Design and evaluation of a new exoskeleton for gait rehabilitation. Mech. Sci. **8**(2), 307–321 (2017)
15. Tarnita, D., Berceanu, C., Tarnita, C.: The three-dimensional printing–a modern technology used for biomedical prototypes. Mater. Plastice **47**(3), 328–334 (2010)
16. Geonea, I., Ceccarelli, M., Carbone, G.: Design and analysis of an exoskeleton for people with motor disabilities. In: Proceedings of the 14th IFToMM World Congress, pp. 33–40 (2015)
17. Husty, M., Birlescu, I., Tucan, P., Vaida, C., Pisla, D.: An algebraic parameterization approach for parallel robots analysis. Mech. Mach. Theory **140**, 245–257 (2019)

Developments in the Design of an Ankle Rehabilitation Platform

Ioan Doroftei(✉) and Cristina-Magda Cazacu

"Gheorghe Asachi" Technical University of Iasi, Bvd. D. Mangeron, 43, 700050 Iasi, Romania
idorofte@mail.tuiasi.ro

Abstract. Because the ankle joint is intensively used in a person's daily activities, it can often suffer injuries. In addition to the doctor's intervention and to the use of medicines, therapy sessions to recover its movements are mandatory. For doing that, in addition to the classic ankle recovery devices, numerous robotic recovery platforms have been proposed in recent years. To ensure a qualitative recuperation of the ankle joint movement, the rehabilitation devices should ensure coincidence between the center of the ankle joint and the intersection point of the rotation axes for the sole supporting plate. To counter drawbacks of their previous designs of a rehabilitation platform, the authors will propose an improved design in this paper. For this new design, direct and inverse kinematic problems results are shown. In addition, the simulation of the 3D virtual rehabilitation platform will be performed.

Keywords: ankle joint · rehabilitation platform · improved design

1 Introduction

The ankle joint fulfils a very important role in a person's daily activity, either just to allow him/her to move, or to allow him/her to perform various movements in sports activities. Because this joint is highly stressed during the day, injuries can occur, due to accidents, due to making a wrong movement or due to its overuse. When the ankle joint is injured, in addition to the use of medicines, subsequent recovering sessions are necessary in order to completely solve the problem.

Beside the classic devices, such as elastic bands and foam rollers, used for the recovery of the ankle joint, rehabilitation robotic platforms have been designed and built in recent years [1–3]. Among the advantages of these platforms, it can be mentioned that the therapist can follow, simultaneously, the recovery sessions for several patients. At the same time, the recovery sessions can also take place in the absence of the therapist, at home.

There are two main categories of robotic rehabilitation devices. The first one is related to wearable devices, which can be robotic orthoses [4] and exoskeletons [5], used to correct the gait of patients and to improv the performance of the ankle joint during walking. The second category includes robotic platforms, which are intended only to improve the performance of the ankle joint [6]. Devices from this second category have

D. Tarnita et al. (Eds.): MESROB 2023, MMS 133, pp. 179–187, 2023.
https://doi.org/10.1007/978-3-031-32446-8_20

a fixed platform and a movable footplate, and can have a single [7] or more degrees of freedom [8].

To allow patients to have access to such rehabilitation platforms, these devices must be user-friendly and, also, they must have a low price in order to be rented. In this paper, developments in the design of such rehabilitation platform and, also, simulation results will be presented.

2 Developments on the Rehabilitation Platform Design

2.1 Previous Designs

Based on the ankle joint movements (Fig. 1), [1], few solution designs of ankle rehabilitation devices with two degrees of freedom (d.o.f.) have been proposed and discussed previously. Some of these designs are using the Scotch-Yoke mechanism as the device structure and some others are based on the spatial four-bar mechanism (SF-BM). All of them have been proposed to recover the dorsiflexion/plantar flexion and inversion / eversion movements. In this paper, we will refer to the second category of designs.

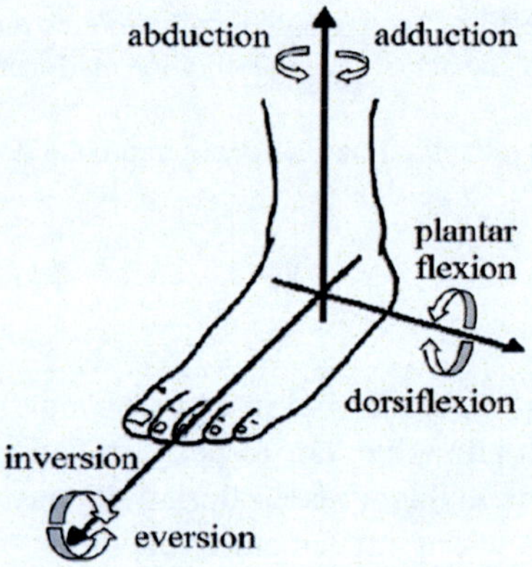

Fig. 1. Ankle joint movements [3].

To avoid ankle joint movements during the rehabilitation, it is recommended that both rotational axes of the plate supporting the sole (PSS) should be coincident with the ankle joint axes. This was the case for the design shown in Fig. 2.

Unfortunately, numerical simulation and also CAD simulation demonstrated that this constructive solution does not cover the range of the mentioned ankle joint movements. For this reason, this constructive solution has been abandoned after simulations.

The second design based on the kinematics of SF-BM has the superior surface of the PSS coincident with the plane containing both its rotational axes (Fig. 3). As consequence, the ankle joint axes are in a plane placed over the PSS rotational axes.

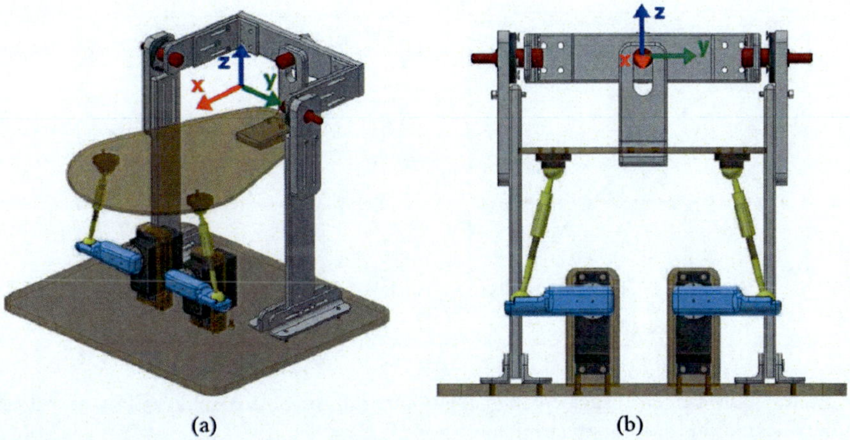

Fig. 2. Ankle rehabilitation platform (ARP) design with rotational axes of the PSS coincident with the ankle joint axes: a) isometric view; b) front view.

It means that the ankle joint will suffer some displacements along all the three axes of the reference frame placed in the middle of the ankle joint (Fig. 4). These displacements could affect the quality of the ankle joint recovering process and could also produce a discomfort to the patient during recovering sessions if the shank is fixed.

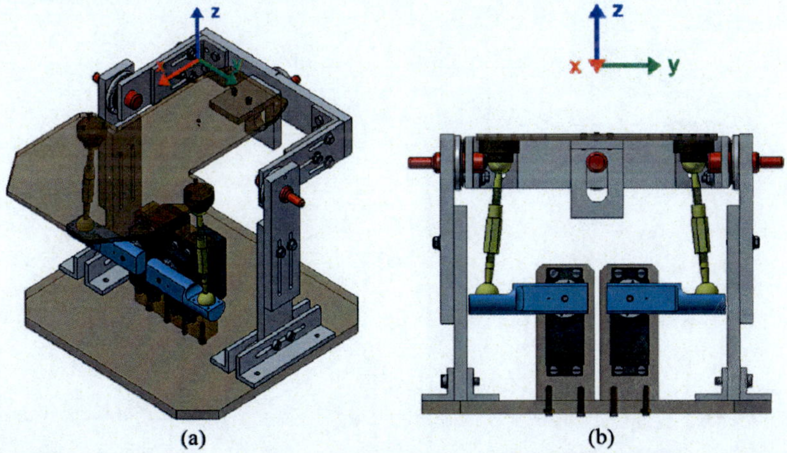

Fig. 3. ARP design with ankle joint axes over the plane containing the rotational axes of the PSS: a) isometric view; b) front view [3].

Despite these inconveniences, the previously studied and realized robotic platform demonstrated, during practical tests on a patient, that it can successfully contribute to the recovery of ankle joint movements [3].

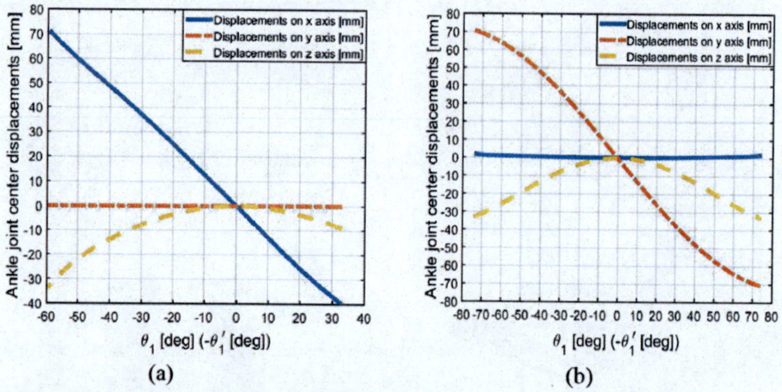

Fig. 4. Ankle joint center displacements along the reference system axes: a) for plantar flexion/dorsiflexion; b) for inversion/eversion.

2.2 New Design

To eliminate the shortcomings mentioned above, a third improved constructive solution is proposed. The kinematics of this design is shown in Fig. 5.

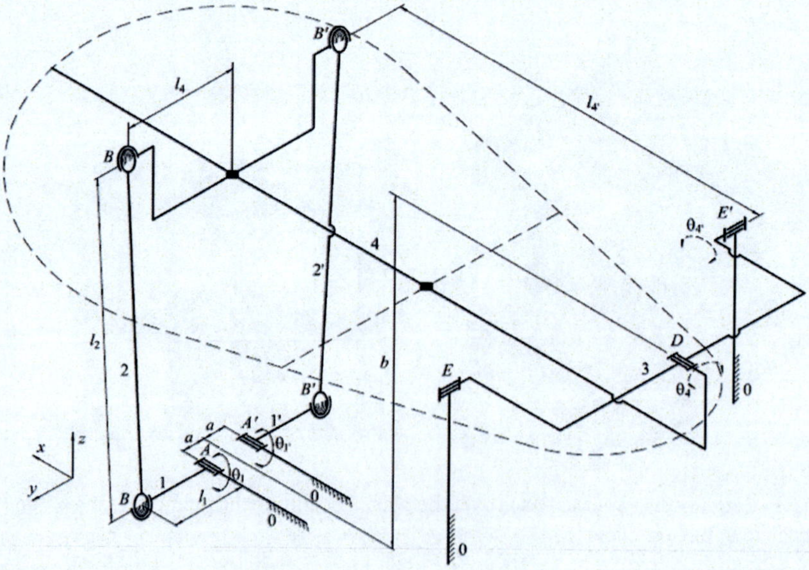

Fig. 5. Kinematics of the rehabilitation platform with optimized constructive solution.

Based on this kinematics, a new constructive solution of the platform has been designed, with rotational axes of the PSS coincident with the ankle joint axes (Fig. 6).

To recover the inversion/eversion movement of the ankle joint, the link 3 in Fig. 5 is considered fixed (see Fig. 7). For this movement, both driving links (1 and 1') are rotating in the same direction, with the same angle, $\theta_1 = \theta_{1'}$. Solving the direct kinematics problem for this movement, we will get:

$$\theta_4 = 2\text{atan}\left(\frac{-B_1 \pm \sqrt{A_1^2 + B_1^2 - C_1^2}}{C_1 - A_1}\right), \tag{1}$$

where

$$\begin{cases} A_1 = -2l_4(a + l_1 \cos\theta_1) \\ B_1 = 2l_4(b - l_1 \sin\theta_1) \\ C_1 = 2l_1(a\cos\theta_1 - b\sin\theta_1) + l_1^2 - l_2^2 + l_4^2 + a^2 + b^2 \end{cases} \tag{2}$$

Inverse kinematics problem leads to:

$$\theta_1 = \theta_{1'} = 2atan\left(\frac{-B_2 \pm \sqrt{A_2^2 + B_2^2 - C_2^2}}{C_2 - A_2}\right), \tag{3}$$

where

$$\begin{cases} A_2 = 2l_1(a - l_4 \cos\theta_4) \\ B_2 = -2l_1(b + l_4 \sin\theta_4) \\ C_2 = 2l_4(b\sin\theta_4 - a\cos\theta_4) + l_1^2 - l_2^2 + l_4^2 + a^2 + b^2 \end{cases} \tag{4}$$

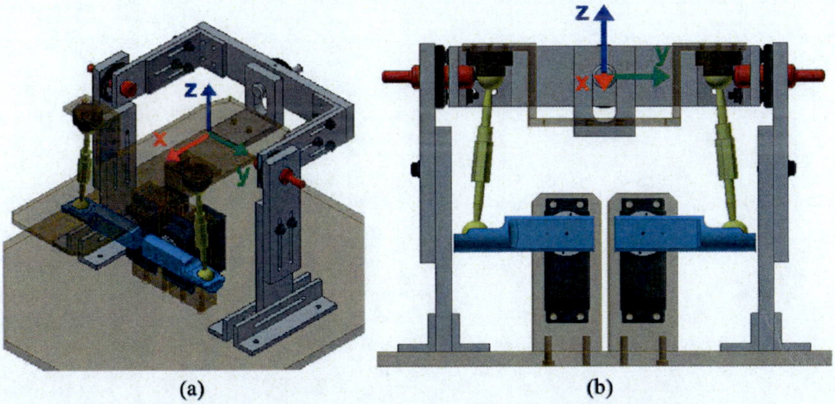

Fig. 6. ARP with optimized design: a) isometric view; b) front view.

The plantar flexion/dorsiflexion movement is produced considering that the links 3 and 4 are connected together (the joint D does not work for this movement), Fig. 8. In this case, the driving links 1 and 1’ are rotating in opposite direction, with the same angle, $\theta_1 = -\theta_{1'}$. The direct kinematics problem for this movement leads to:

$$\theta_{4'} = 2\mathrm{atan}\left(\frac{-B_3 \pm \sqrt{A_3^2 + B_3^2 - C_3^2}}{C_3 - A_3}\right), \tag{5}$$

where

$$\begin{cases} A_3 = -2l_{4'}^2 \\ B_3 = -2l_{4'}(l_2 - l_1 \sin\theta_1) \\ C_3 = 2l_1[(a - l_4)\cos\theta_1 - b\sin\theta_1] + l_1^2 - l_2^2 + l_4^2 + a^2 + b^2 + 2l_{4'}^2 - 2al_4 \end{cases} \tag{6}$$

Solving the inverse kinematics, we will get:

$$\theta_1 = -\theta_{1'} = 2\mathrm{atan}\left(\frac{-B_4 \pm \sqrt{A_4^2 + B_4^2 - C_4^2}}{C_4 - A_4}\right), \tag{7}$$

where

$$\begin{cases} A_4 = 2l_1(a - l_4) \\ B_4 = 2l_1(l_{4'}\sin\theta_{4'} - b) \\ C_4 = -2l_{4'}(l_2\sin\theta_{4'} + l_{4'}\cos\theta_{4'}) + l_1^2 - l_2^2 + l_4^2 + a^2 + b^2 + 2l_{4'}^2 - 2al_4 \end{cases} \tag{8}$$

After a mechanism dimensional synthesis, considering the extreme positions of the driven link 4 for both recovered movements, a numerical simulation and also a CAD simulation have been realized. The results are presented in Figs. 7 and 8, where θ_4 is the angular stroke of the PSS for inversion/eversion movement and $\theta_{4'}$ for plantar flexion/dorsiflexion movement.

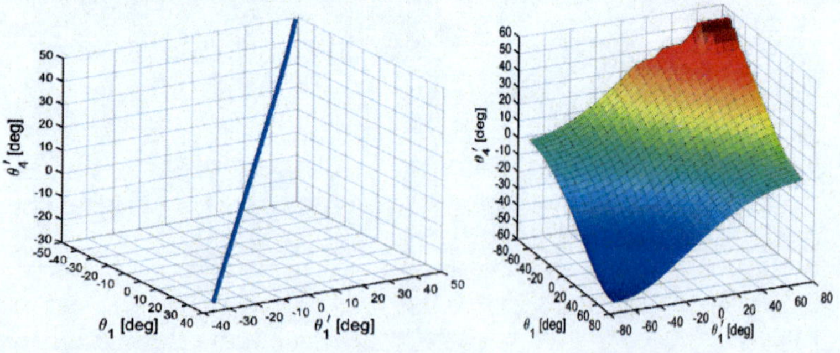

(a) (b)

Fig. 7. Simulation results for plantar flexion/dorsiflexion movement: a) for the actual plantar flexion / dorsiflexion movement; b) the limits of the driving links angular positions ensure the two rehabilitation movements.

In Fig. 9 changes of driving and driven links angular positions over time are presented.

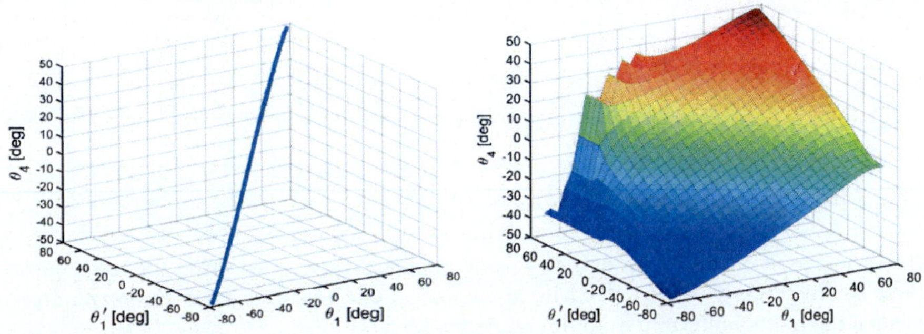

Fig. 8. Simulation results for inversion/eversion movement: a) for the actual inversion/eversion movement; b) the limits of the driving links angular positions ensure the two rehabilitation movements.

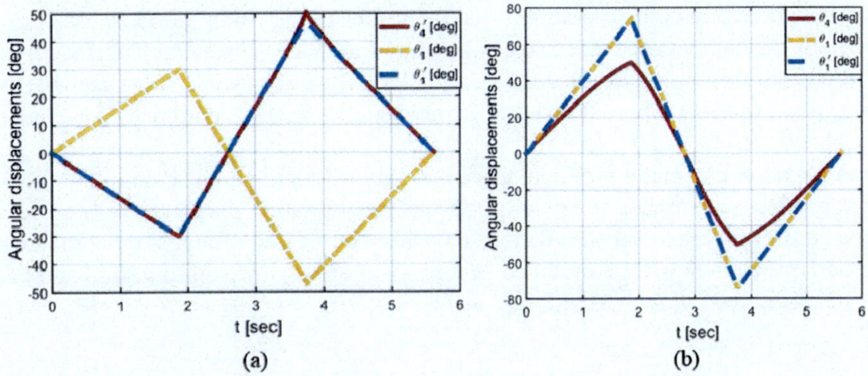

Fig. 9. Angular displacement of the driving and driven links, over time: a) for plantar flexion/dorsiflexion; b) for inversion/eversion.

Comparing the results of numerical simulation with the results of the simulation for the 3D virtual rehabilitation platform, we may see that they are identical (Fig. 10).

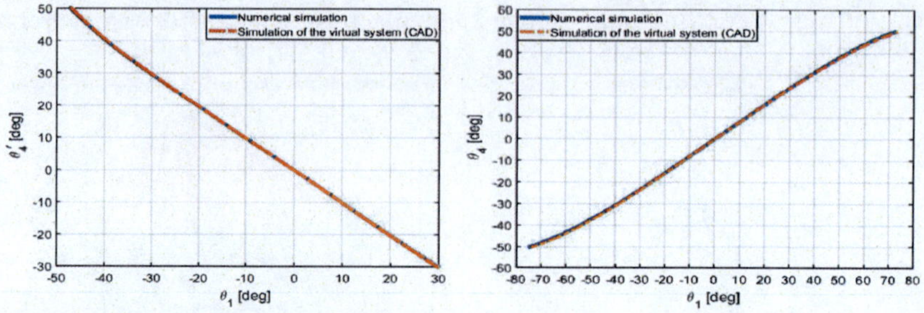

(a) (b)

Fig. 10. Comparison of the results obtained from numerical simulation, using the equations of the inverse kinematics problem, and from the simulation of the 3D virtual rehabilitation platform: a) for plantar flexion/dorsiflexion; b) for inversion/eversion.

3 Conclusion

To ensure a qualitative recuperation of the ankle joint movement, the rehabilitation devices should ensure coincidence between the center of the ankle joint and the intersection point of the rotation axes for the sole supporting plate. The authors of this paper have been developed previous rehabilitation platforms, which present some drawbacks from this point of view. These drawbacks have been previously mentioned. To counter these problems, in this paper an improved design has been proposed. For this new design, direct and inverse kinematic problems have been solved and numerical simulation has been done. Also, the simulation of the 3D virtual rehabilitation platform has been performed and the results of both simulations have been compared. The real rehabilitation device built previously will be modified according to the new proposed design and the testing results will be presented in future work.

References

1. Payedimarri, A.B., Ratti, M., Rescinito, R., Vanhaecht, K., Panella, M.: Effectiveness of platform-based robot-assisted rehabilitation for musculoskeletal or neurologic injuries: a systematic review. Bioengineering **9**(4), 129 (2022)
2. Gherman, B., Birlescu, I., Plitea, N., Carbone, G., Tarnita, D., Pisla, D.: On the singularity-free workspace of a parallel robot for lower-limb rehabilitation. Proc. Roman. Acad. **20**(4), 383–391 (2019)
3. Doroftei, I., Racu, C. M., Baudoin, Y.: Development of a robotic platform for ankle joint rehabilitation. Acta Technica Napocensis-Series Appl. Math. Mech. Eng. **64**(1-S2), 301–310 (2021)
4. Park, Y.L., Chen, B.R., Pérez-Arancibia, N.O.: Design and control of a bio-inspired soft wearable robotic device for ankle-foot rehabilitation. Bioinspir. Biomim. **9**, 016007 (2014)
5. Roy, A., Krebs, H., Williams, D.: Robot-aided neurorehabilitation: a novel robot for ankle rehabilitation. IEEE Trans. Neural. Syst. Rehabil. Eng. **25**, 569–582 (2009)
6. Mohammed, S., Amirat, Y., Rifai, H.: Lower-limb movement assistance through wearable robots: State of the art and challenges. Adv. Robot. **26**, 1–22 (2012)

7. Zhang, L.Q., Chung, G., Bai, Z.: Intelligent stretching of ankle joints with contracture/spasticity. IEEE Trans. Neural. Syst. Rehabil. Eng. **10**, 149–157 (2002)
8. Saglia, J.A., Tsagarakis, N.G., Dai, J.S.: Control strategies for patient-assisted training using the ankle rehabilitation robot (ARBOT). IEEE/ASME Trans. Mechatron. **18**, 1799–1808 (2013)

Effect of a Passive Shoulder Support Exoskeleton on Fatigue During Working with Arms over Shoulder Level

Annina Brunner[1(✉)], Rachel van Sluijs[2], Volker Bartenbach[2], Dario Bee[2], Melanie Kos[2], Lijin Aryananda[2], and Olivier Lambercy[1]

[1] ETH Zurich, Zurich, Switzerland
relab.publications@hest.ethz.ch
[2] Auxivo AG, Zurich, Switzerland
https://relab.ethz.ch/

Abstract. Work-related musculoskeletal disorders have a high prevalence across industries and are a leading cause for days away from work. Exoskeletons can assist their users during physically demanding tasks to reduce the workload and the prevalence of work-related musculoskeletal disorders. This paper explores the physiological effect of a novel passive shoulder exoskeleton on the development of fatigue during overhead work.

A sample of 32 healthy participants performed a two-minute isometric task simulating tool handling above shoulder level with and without the exoskeleton. Muscular activation and fatigue in the arm, shoulder, neck and back muscles were recorded using surface electromyography. Cardiac cost was measured using optical heart rate tracking at the wrist.

The exoskeleton significantly reduced muscle activity in shoulder, neck and back muscles up to 32% ($p<0.01$) and reduced the rate of fatiguing up to 45% ($p<0.01$) in the $\text{Deltoid}_{anterior}$. The cardiac cost while performing the task with the exoskeleton was 16% ($p<0.05$) less than without the exoskeleton.

Using the proposed passive shoulder support exoskeleton substantially reduced the muscular load and perceived effort as well as the cardiovascular load. This suggests users can perform overhead tool-handling tasks for longer periods of time while feeling less tired. It also might positively influence the development of injuries.

Keywords: muscle fatigue · muscle activity · occupational exoskeletons · preventive technology · textile spring

1 Introduction

Work-related musculoskeletal disorders (WRMSD) are disorders affecting the muscles, tendons, cartilage, and nerves that often develop gradually and are caused by overuse during physically demanding work. It has been shown that prolonged overhead work, defined as work with hands and arms on or above shoulder height, lead to biomechanical strains in the shoulder joint resulting in

D. Tarnita et al. (Eds.): MESROB 2023, MMS 133, pp. 188–197, 2023.
https://doi.org/10.1007/978-3-031-32446-8_21

shoulder-related WRMSD. Risk factors for developing WRMSD include non-neutral postures, heavy load lifting and repetitive work [1]. The "European Agency for Safety and Health at Work" reported that 41% of the working population suffered from muscular pain in the shoulders, neck and upper limbs [11]. The median days away from work for nonfatal occupational injuries and illnesses of the shoulder are 23 days, hence nearly a month per year [2,10]. The sickness absence and expenses for treatment further result in high disorder associated costs [11].

Measures to reduce the prevalence of WRMSD include ergonomic optimization of the workplace, integration of worker rotations, ergonomic training and introduction of periodic rest phases. Implementing these preventive measures is important but unlikely to solve the problem as long as risk factors are still present. An emerging solution is to provide physical support through the use of exoskeletons, i.e. wearable devices that support work-specific movements [14]. Several such systems to support the shoulder have been developed in academia and industry and are being validated, evaluated and tested in the field [4]. Considering the trade-off between the amount of support, comfort of use and cost, most of the existing shoulder exoskeletons are passive, using gas springs, metal springs or flexible beams to support the user [4].

While production workers in the automotive manufacturing industry report reduction of fatigue as an important requirement for an overhead support system [8], only a few studies evaluated the physiological effect of exoskeletons on endurance and fatigue [13,17,18]. When wearing two different passive systems the endurance time (time until discomfort) of a static task increased up to 56% [17,18]. Furthermore, positive effects of a passive system on perceived effort and fatigue related changes in muscle activity amplitude and frequency were reported [13].

In this study, we evaluate the workload reduction of a novel shoulder support exoskeleton during static overhead work. Like the study by Lee et al. [13] shoulder fatigue using perceived effort was assessed, as well as objective changes in muscle activity while following exoskeleton benchmarking guidelines for occupational exoskeletons [4]. We hypothesized that the use of the passive exoskeleton will (1) result in reductions in muscle activity, which will (2) delay the onset of muscle fatigue and reduce perceived exertion, as well as (3) reduce the cardiac cost of working in overhead position.

2 Methods

2.1 Participants

Thirty-two healthy volunteers (15 female) of working age (20 to 65 years, Mean: 26.7y, SD: 10.2y) were included, without any history of upper limb musculoskeletal disorders. Participant height ranged from 160 cm to 194 cm (Mean: 174 cm, SD: 8.8 cm) and weight ranged between 43.8 kg and 98.1 kg (Mean: 72.1 kg, SD: 13.5 kg).

2.2 Passive Shoulder Support Exoskeleton

In this study, a prototype of the Auxivo AG DeltaSuit was used (Fig. 1(a)). The DeltaSuit is a shoulder support exoskeleton that consists of a vest to attach to the wearer's upper body, an exoskeleton mechanism generating a supporting shoulder flexion torque using textile springs, and cuffs that attach to the arms above the elbow. The weight of the device is around 2 kg. The prototype was available in two sizes: S-M and L-XL. In our sample, 26 participants wore the S-M and 6 the L-XL version. The user can choose from two levels of support: level 1 provides 5.2 Nm of support, and level 2 provides 6.6 Nm.

A key difference between existing exoskeletons and the DeltaSuit is the attachment to the torso through a vest without any additional attachments at the hip. This design choice allows a significant reduction in device size and simplifies usability as it removes the need for back length adjustment and allows for unconstrained movements when bending forward. It comes at a potential risk that the ability to support the users shoulder is reduced as the attachment to the torso only might be less robust. It also bears the risk that the load on the back of the user might be increased during work as it is not directly supported but rather loaded with the exoskeletons weight.

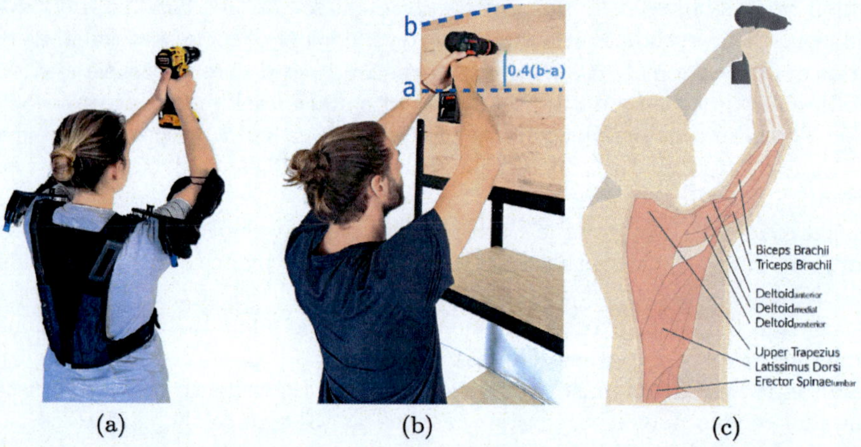

Fig. 1. (a) Illustration of the exoskeleton prototype used in this experiment. The exoskeleton attaches to the torso and upper arm of the user and force is applied around the shoulder joint using a textile spring. (b) Participants held a load of 1.8 kg at an overhead working height defined as $a + 0.4(b - a)$ with [a] hand height with the shoulder and elbow flexed at 90° and [b] upper arm in full extension [4,16]. (c) Surface electromyography sensors were placed on the arm, shoulder, neck and back muscles.

2.3 Protocol

Participants were instrumented with surface electromyography (EMG) electrodes (Trigno and Avanti, Delsys Europe, UK) and an optical heart rate tracker

(Polar Ignite 2, Polar Global, USA). On the dominant hand side, muscle activity on the following neck, arm, shoulder and back muscles was recorded: Upper Trapezius (UT), Biceps Brachii (BB), Triceps Brachii (TB), $\text{Deltoid}_{anterior}$ (AD), Deltoid_{medial} (MD), $\text{Deltoid}_{posterior}$ (PD), Erector Spinae_{lumbar}(ES) and Latissimus Dorsi (LD) (Fig. 1(c)). Normalization values were obtained by performing isometric maximal voluntary contractions (MVC) (highest of two attempts). Baseline heart rate was recorded while participants were sitting idle for 60 s. Participants were then instructed on exoskeleton use and performed a series of dynamic and static tasks with the exoskeleton prior to the reported fatigue task.

In this study, two conditions were compared: a baseline condition without the exoskeleton (OFF) and an active condition with high support (EXO). The order of the conditions was randomized.

To reliably assess fatigue an isometric task was chosen. Participants were instructed to hold a drill weighing 1.8 kg (representative for a powered drill or plastering trowel and recommended for standardized testing [4]) for 120 s (Fig. 1(b)). The tool was held at an overhead working height defined as $a + 0.4(b - a)$ with (a) hand height with the shoulder and elbow flexed at 90° and (b) hand height with the upper arm in full extension [4,16] (Fig. 1(b)). A standardized break of 15 min between the task conditions (OFF and EXO) was provided.

Participants rated their perceived exertion, discomfort and constrain on a scale from 0 to 10 after each condition. No exertion was rated as 0, and maximal effort as 10. After both conditions were completed the Quebec User Evaluation of Satisfaction with assistive Technology (QUEST) was filled out [6].

The protocol was approved by the university ethics committee (2022-N-132).

2.4 Data Processing and Statistics

For each muscle, the EMG signals were filtered using a bidirectional 4th order Butterworth bandpass filter (Fc: 10 Hz and 500 Hz), and two infinite impulse response notch filters (296 Hz and 370 Hz) with Q factor 20 to remove noise at these frequencies observed in the spectral plots. The root mean square (RMS) of the muscle activity over the entire duration of the task was calculated. Furthermore, the median frequency (MDF) of the signal was calculated every second [12]. When muscles fatigue a shift in the recruitment of type 2 to type 1 muscle fibers takes place, which lowers the EMG median frequency. This change in MDF over time can be quantified using linear regression [12,13]. Here the slope of the linear regression analysis is reported with the y-intercept of the regression indicating the initial MDF (value at $t = 0$). The slope of the linear regression fit is reported in % of initial MDF per second.

Logistic regression of the heart rate during each entire task was computed. The cardiac cost was calculated as the median of the regression line during the last 10 s of the task minus the median baseline heart rate.

Data visualization and statistical testing were performed using Matlab 2019b (MathWorks, USA). Paired sample t-tests were used to compare OFF and EXO conditions for the continuous data (RMS, MDF slope and cardiac cost). Wilcoxon signed-rank tests were used for the discrete questionnaire data.

3 Results

3.1 Effect on Muscle Activity

Medial and anterior shoulder muscle activity was significantly lower when wearing the exoskeleton ($p_{Deltoid,anterior}$ <0.001, $p_{Deltoid,medial}$<0.001), see Fig. 2 and Table 1. The reduction was 25.2% of baseline activity in the Deltoid_{medial} and 21.9% in the $\text{Deltoid}_{anterior}$. The exoskeleton also significantly reduced lower back muscle activity ($p_{ErectorSpinae,lumbar}$<0.01). The activity in the Erector Spinae at lumbar level was 12.1% lower while wearing the exoskeleton compared to the baseline condition, where the Latissimus Dorsi activity was 8.4% lower, although this change was not significant. With the support of the exoskeleton, a 26.8% reduction in neck muscle activity was observed ($p_{Trapezius}$<0.001).

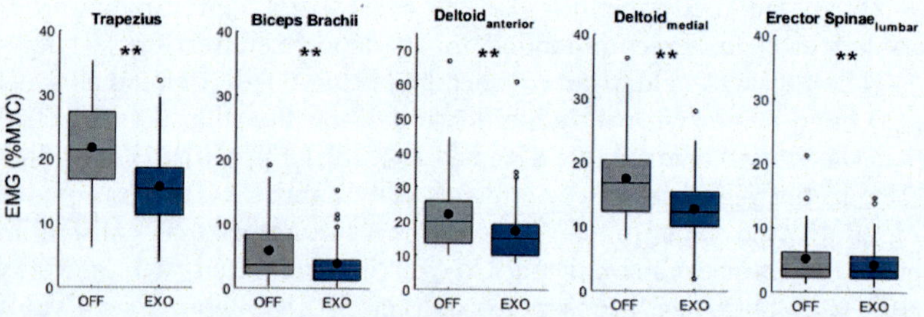

Fig. 2. Change in EMG(%MVC) RMS amplitude as percent of maximal voluntary contraction between the OFF (grey) and EXO (blue) condition for the five most relevant muscles. The data are displayed as box plots, with a dot representing the mean value. Paired t-test statistics were performed, *: p<0.05, **: p<0.01. (Color figure online)

Table 1. Table with mean and standard deviations (M(SD)) of the RMS muscle activity during the off condition, the exo condition and the % change, the number of participants included in each analysis (n) and the p-value of the paired t-test.

	RMS_{off} (%MVC)	RMS_{exo} (%MVC)	Δ off-exo (%off)	n	t-test p-value
Trapezius	21.7 (7.2)	15.7(7.3)	26.8(19.9)	30	<0.001
Biceps Brachii	5.9 (5.0)	3.9 (3.6)	31.8(18.9)	32	<0.001
Triceps Brachii	5.9 (3.5)	5.6 (3.0)	2.8 (24.5)	32	n.s
$\text{Deltoid}_{anterior}$	22.1 (11.3)	17.2(10.5)	21.9(19.9)	32	<0.001
Deltoid_{medial}	17.5 (6.3)	12.8(5.5)	25.2(27.6)	31	<0.001
$\text{Deltoid}_{posterior}$	14.3 (9.7)	10.8(7.5)	21.2(22.5)	32	<0.001
$\text{Erector Spinae}_{lumbar}$	5.2 (4.3)	4.3 (3.2)	12.1(22.5)	31	<0.01
Latissimus Dorsi	19.6 (13.9)	17.8(12.6)	8.4 (19.9)	32	n.s

[a]RMS values >100%MVC were excluded from analysis in pairwise fashion.

3.2 Objective and Perceived Fatigue

All participants were able to complete the task in both conditions. An example of the development of fatigue in the $Deltoid_{anterior}$ of one participant can be seen in Fig. 3(a). In some muscles and participants, little fatigue was observed, making the regression fit unreliable, these slope values were excluded from further analysis. This was considered the case if the residual sum of squares per second was larger than the initial MDF. The number of included data points is reported (Table 2). The change in MDF slope from baseline to exo condition in the $Deltoid_{anterior}$ was -0.03%$MDF_{initial}$/s (45% reduction, $p_{Deltoid,anterior} < 0.01$), suggesting that fatigue developed more slowly in this muscle. A significant change in slope was also observed in the Biceps Brachii ($p_{BicepsBrachii} < 0.01$) where the slope changed from -0.10%$MDF_{initial}$/s without the exoskeleton to -0.04%$MDF_{initial}$/s with the exoskeleton (59% reduction) and at the neck with a change from -0.04 to -0.01%$MDF_{initial}$/s (75% reduction, $p_{Trapezius} < 0.05$). Further, the exoskeleton prevented the development of fatigue in the back muscles, although no significant change was observed, see Fig. 3(d).

Besides objective fatigue, wearing the exoskeleton significantly reduced perceived exertion by 1.3 points ($p < 0.01$), reducing the rating from hard (M: 6.4, SD: 1.4) to somewhat hard with the exoskeleton (M: 5.2, SD: 1.9), see Fig. 3(b).

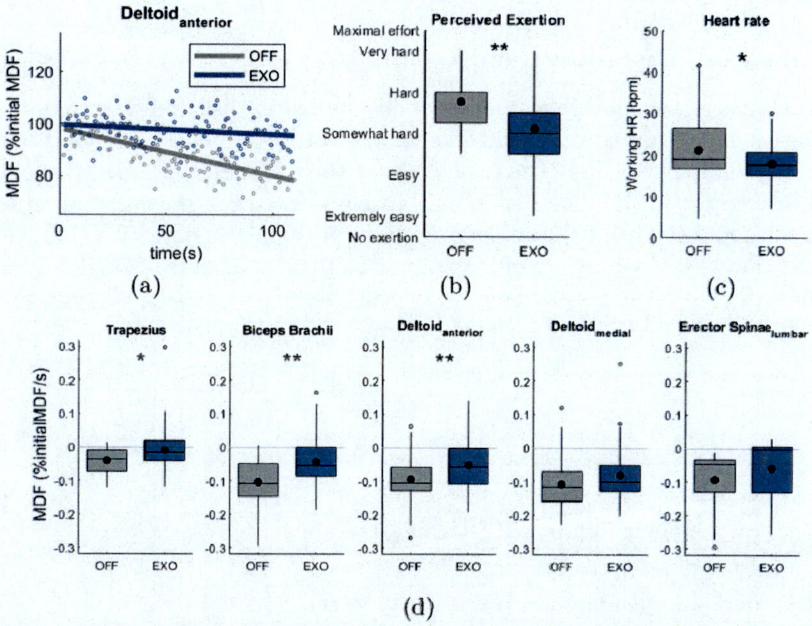

Fig. 3. (a) Example of the change in median frequency (MDF) during the task in the OFF (grey) and EXO (blue) condition. (b) Ratings of perceived exertion. (c) Cardiac cost (heart rate - resting heart rate). (d) The slope of the EMG median frequency. Data is displayed as box plots, with a dot representing the mean value. Paired t-test (MDF, heart rate) and Wilcoxon signed-rank (exertion) statistics were performed, *: $p < 0.05$, **: $p < 0.01$. (Color figure online)

Table 2. Table with changes in fatigue for the relevant muscles and stats

	$slope_{off}$ (%$MDF_{initial}$/s)	$slope_{exo}$ (%$MDF_{initial}$/s)	Δoff-exo (%$MDF_{initial}$/s)	n	t-test p-value
Trapezius	−0.04(0.04)	−0.01(0.07)	−0.01 (0.07)	32	<0.05
Biceps Brachii	−0.10(0.08)	−0.04(0.08)	−0.04 (0.10)	28	<0.01
Triceps Brachii	−0.09(0.08)	−0.09(0.08)	−0.01 (0.08)	22	n.s
$Deltoid_{anterior}$	−0.09(0.07)	−0.05(0.07)	−0.03 (0.08)	29	<0.01
$Deltoid_{medial}$	−0.11(0.08)	−0.08(0.09)	−0.02 (0.12)	27	n.s
$Deltoid_{posterior}$	−0.10(0.06)	−0.06(0.09)	−0.05 (0.10)	32	<0.05
Erector $Spinae_{lumbar}$	−0.09(0.11)	−0.06(0.11)	−0.04 (0.09)	6	n.s
Latissimus Dorsi	−0.08(0.08)	0.01 (0.13)	0.01 (0.07)	25	n.s

3.3 Cardiac Cost

Due to missing data, the heart rate analysis is based on 25 datasets. The average cardiac cost was 21.3 bpm (SD: 8.8 bpm) during off condition and 18 bpm (SD: 5.1 bpm) while wearing the exoskeleton (Fig. 3(c)). The exoskeleton significantly reduced cardiac cost during the 2 min task by 16% ($p<0.05$).

3.4 Constrain, Discomfort and Usability

Participants perceived the highest levels of discomfort in the shoulders (moderate discomfort: 3.9/10), upper arm (mild discomfort: 3.1/10) and neck (minor discomfort: 1.3/10) while performing the task without the exoskeleton. Exoskeleton use reduced discomfort in the shoulder to mild discomfort (2.6/10), in the upper arm to minor discomfort (1.9/10) and solving discomfort in the neck (0.3/10). Constrain was rated by the participants as minor to little constrain (M:2.6, SD: 2.2)

Table 3. Quebec User Evaluation of Satisfaction with Assistive Technology.

	QUEST score		
	MD	*Q1*	*Q3*
dimensions (size, height, length, width)	4	4	4
weight	5	4	5
ease of adjusting (fixing, fastening)	4	3	5
sense of safety and security	5	4	5
durability (endurance, resistance to wear)	5	4	5
ease of use	5	4	5
comfort	4	3	4
effectiveness (extent to which needs are met)	4	3	5
device subscale score	**4.3**	**4**	**4.4**

[a]Satisfaction on a scale from 1 (not satisfied at all) to 5 (very satisfied).

when the task was performed with the exoskeleton. On a scale from 1 (not satisfied at all) to 5 (very satisfied), participants reported being quite satisfied (MD:4.3, IQR:4-4.4) with the usability of the exoskeleton (Table 3). Participants were very satisfied (5/5) with the weight, sense of safety, durability and ease of use.

4 Discussion

The objective of this paper was to evaluate the physiological effect of a novel passive shoulder support exoskeleton on upper body muscle activity and on the development of fatigue during physically-demanding work. The muscular load during tool handling with arms above shoulder level can be significantly reduced by wearing the passive shoulder support exoskeleton evaluated in this study, relieving muscles in the upper arm, shoulder, neck and lower back. Our results are in line with previous studies evaluating the potential of passive devices to reduce muscle load during static tasks [7,10,14]. The DeltaSuit provided support within the ranges reported in the literature: Deltoid_{medial} activity reduced by 25.3% (11.1% [14] to 33.3% [10]), $\text{Deltoid}_{anterior}$ activity was reduced by 21.9% (18.2% [14] to 67.3% [7]) and Biceps Brachii activity was reduced by 31.8% (30.0% [14] to 58.1% [7]). A key difference between previously evaluated exoskeletons and the DeltaSuit is the attachment to the torso through a vest without having additional attachments at the hip. This design choice has several advantages as discussed in the previous sections, but it bears the potential risk that the ability to support the users shoulder is reduced as the attachment to the torso only might be less robust. Our findings confirm that a similar level of support for the shoulder and neck muscles can be achieved with such a design. The measurements also show that Erector Spinae activity was reduced by 12.1% compared to baseline, and thus refute concerns that a shoulder exoskeleton design without a dedicated fixation at the users' hip could increase the load on the back.

Besides reduction in muscle activity amplitude, a significant delay in the development of muscle fatigue was observed in the neck, shoulder and upper arm. Previous studies showed that such changes in median frequency correlate with perceived fatigue [5] and task endurance time [3], i.e. the time a task can be performed. To our knowledge this measure was only used by one other research group evaluating passive shoulder support exoskeletons [13]. Lee and colleagues showed that their exoskeleton reduced the development of fatigue in the Trapezius, Deltoid, Triceps Brachii and Biceps Brachii [13] and emphasized the importance of using this method when evaluating assistive devices. In our study, we observed a reduction in perceived exertion of 13%, changing the average rating from "hard" when performing the task without exoskeleton to "somewhat hard" when wearing the exoskeleton.

The changes in muscle activity amplitude did not only reduce the onset of muscular fatigue but likely also influenced perceived fatigue and cardiovascular load. During our task, the cardiac cost was reduced by 16%, which confirms our hypothesis that using such a passive exoskeleton reduces cardiac cost while working in an overhead position. Similar reductions in heart rate when working with passive shoulder support exoskeleton have been previously reported for tasks such as tightening screws/nuts (8.3% [9], 20.7% [15]) and drilling (28.0% [15]).

When interpreting these results one should consider that industry workers were not specifically recruited for this study and that the task was performed in controlled laboratory conditions. The sample consisted of individuals of working age (youngest: 20y, oldest: 65y) of both genders, but regular work above shoulder level was not an inclusion criteria. This may especially influence the interpretation of the QUEST item 8 "effectiveness (the extent to which needs are met)", since a need for shoulder support might have lacked in the professional life of the participants.

Finally, the usability of the novel exoskeleton presented in this paper was rated with the QUEST as high. Participants were especially satisfied with the weight, sense of security and ease of use, which reflects the simple and lightweight design which could be achieved through the use of textile springs. This overall supports the potential of passive shoulder support exoskeleton to already provide physiologically meaningful support during physically demanding tasks.

5 Conclusion

The DeltaSuit prototype significantly reduced the muscular, cardiovascular and perceived strain during work above shoulder level. The reduction in muscle activity led to a delay in the process of fatiguing. Quantifying changes in muscular fatigue using frequency analysis was shown to be a promising method for the evaluation of shoulder exoskeleton performance. This study shows that the novel exoskeleton design is promising and can result in a light, highly usable passive shoulder-support system, which offers relevant benefits to its users.

Acknowledgment. We thank Flavio Müller for his contribution to the exoskeleton development, Julia van Sluijs for the anatomical drawing and Tobias Luder and Cherilyn Camichel for their contribution to recruitment and data collection.

References

1. Barthelme, J., Sauter, M., Mueller, C., Liebers, F.: Association between working in awkward postures, in particular overhead work, and pain in the shoulder region in the context of the 2018 BIBB/BAuA Employment Survey. BMC Musculoskelet. Disord. **22**, 1–12 (2021). https://doi.org/10.1186/s12891-021-04482-4
2. Bureau of Labor Statistics, U.S.: Nonfatal occupational injuries and illnesses requiring days away from work. Press Office Bureau of Labor Statistics (2016). https://www.bls.gov/news.release/archives/osh2_11102016.pdf
3. Coorevits, P., Danneels, L., Cambier, D., Ramon, H., Vanderstraeten, G.: Assessment of the validity of the Biering-Sørensen test for measuring back muscle fatigue based on EMG median frequency characteristics of back and hip muscles. J. Electromyogr. Kinesiol. **18**(6), 997–1005 (2008). https://doi.org/10.1016/j.jelekin.2007.10.012
4. De Bock, S., et al.: Benchmarking occupational exoskeletons: an evidence mapping systematic review. Appl. Ergon. **98**, 103582 (2022). https://doi.org/10.1016/j.apergo.2021.103582

5. Dedering, Å., Németh, G., Harms-Ringdahl, K.: Correlation between electromyographic spectral changes and subjective assessment of lumbar muscle fatigue in subjects without pain from the lower back. Clin. Biomech. **14**(2), 103–111 (1999). https://doi.org/10.1016/s0268-0033(98)00053-9
6. Demers, L., Weiss-Lambrou, R., Ska, B.: Quebec user evaluation of satisfaction with assistive technology (QUEST). Assist. Technol. **12**(2), 96–105 (2000). https://doi.org/10.1080/10400435.2000.10132015
7. Desbrosses, K., Schwartz, M., Theurel, J.: Evaluation of two upper-limb exoskeletons during overhead work: influence of exoskeleton design and load on muscular adaptations and balance regulation. Eur. J. Appl. Physiol. **121**(10), 2811–2823 (2021). https://doi.org/10.1007/s00421-021-04747-9
8. Gilotta, S., Spada, S., Ghibaudo, L., Isoardi, M., Mosso, C.O.: Acceptability beyond usability: a manufacturing case study. In: Bagnara, S., Tartaglia, R., Albolino, S., Alexander, T., Fujita, Y. (eds.) IEA 2018. AISC, vol. 824, pp. 922–934. Springer, Cham (2019). https://doi.org/10.1007/978-3-319-96071-5_95
9. Grazi, L., Trigili, E., Proface, G., Giovacchini, F., Crea, S., Vitiello, N.: Design and experimental evaluation of a semi-passive upper-limb exoskeleton for workers with motorized tuning of assistance. IEEE Trans. Neural Syst. Rehabil. Eng. **28**(10), 2276–2285 (2020). https://doi.org/10.1109/TNSRE.2020.3014408
10. Hyun, D.J., Bae, K.H., Kim, K.J., Nam, S., Lee, D.H.: A light-weight passive upper arm assistive exoskeleton based on multi-linkage spring-energy dissipation mechanism for overhead tasks. Rob. Auton. Syst. **122**, 103309 (2019). https://doi.org/10.1016/j.robot.2019.103309
11. Kok, J., et al.: Work-related MSDs: prevalence, costs and demographics in the EU. Publ. Off. Eur. Union (2019). https://doi.org/10.2802/66947
12. Lamers, E.P., Soltys, J.C., Scherpereel, K.L., Yang, A.J., Zelik, K.E.: Low-profile elastic exosuit reduces back muscle fatigue. Sci. Rep. **10**(1), 1–16 (2020). https://doi.org/10.1038/s41598-020-72531-4
13. Lee, Y., Chee, Y.: Evaluation of the effectiveness of muscle assistive device using muscle fatigue analysis. In: Annual International Conference of the IEEE Engineering in Medicine and Biology Society, pp. 2112–2115. IEEE Press, New York (2013). https://doi.org/10.1109/EMBC.2013.6609950
14. Pacifico, I., et al.: An Experimental evaluation of the proto-MATE: a novel ergonomic upper-limb exoskeleton for reducing the worker's physical strain. IEEE Robot. Autom. Mag. **16**(23), 54–65 (2020). https://doi.org/10.1109/MRA.2019.2954105
15. Schmalz, T., et al.: Biomechanical and metabolic effectiveness of an industrial exoskeleton for overhead work. Int. J. Environ. Res. Public Health **16**(23), 4792 (2019). https://doi.org/10.3390/ijerph16234792
16. Sood, D., Nussbaum, M.A., Hager, K.: Fatigue during prolonged intermittent overhead work: reliability of measures and effects of working height. Ergonomics **50**(4), 497–513 (2007). https://doi.org/10.1080/00140130601133800
17. Spada, S., Ghibaudo, L., Carnazzo, C., Gastaldi, L., Cavatorta, M.P.: Passive upper limb exoskeletons: an experimental campaign with workers. In: Bagnara, S., Tartaglia, R., Albolino, S., Alexander, T., Fujita, Y. (eds.) IEA 2018. AISC, vol. 825, pp. 230–239. Springer, Cham (2019). https://doi.org/10.1007/978-3-319-96068-5_26
18. Spada, S., Ghibaudo, L., Gilotta, S., Gastaldi, L., Cavatorta, M.P.: Investigation into the applicability of a passive upper-limb exoskeleton in automotive industry. Procedia Manuf. **11**, 1255–1262 (2017). https://doi.org/10.1016/j.promfg.2017.07.252

Virtual Prototyping of a Leg Exoskeleton for Human Persons with Neuromotor Deficiencies

Sorin Dumitru, Nicolae Dumitru, Cristian Copilusi(✉), Ionut Geonea, and Leonard Gherghe-Ciurezu

University of Craiova, 200512 Craiova, Romania
cristian.copilusi@edu.ucv.ro

Abstract. Through this research it was designed a robotic system used for persons with neuromotor locomotion problems, especially the ones that have suffered AVC, and needs special recovery therapy for society integration and to perform daily living activities. The robotic system has in its own structure a patient lifting system, an exoskeleton equipped with proper sensors and actuators, a treadmill and a command & control unit. The exoskeleton legs were designed with special mechanisms which have adapted orthotic systems for hips, knees and ankles. These mechanisms were actuated based on achieved results from an experimental human walking analyses performed by 30 healthy persons. Thus, it was performed an inverse kinematic analysis for obtaining the proper angular variations necessary to control the proper drive joints. The research core was focused on a comparative analysis of the obtained results through virtual prototyping and processing the mathematical models, which validate the desired prototype. The obtained prototype was tested on specific laboratory conditions in two main stages, namely experimental tests with and without a patient.

Keywords: Neuromotor Rehabilitation · Human Walking · Kinematics and Dynamics · Human Lower Limb · Leg Exoskeleton

1 Introduction

Nowadays there are designed many rehabilitation systems dedicated to human locomotion recovery and these are addressed to adults and elderly persons. These have in their main structure an exoskeleton designed for different rehabilitation purposes. By having in sight a particular segment of persons, namely the ones with neuromotor deficiencies, it can be remarked that these rehabilitation systems are limited. By referring at this segment, it can be remarked a similar research work in [1–3]. Taking these systems as a research starting point it can be observed that most of them have actuation systems only for hips and knee joints. The ankle joints motions were considered passive ones and it can be substitute by devices with elastic elements.

Others like [4, 5] have an extended motion at the ankle joint level in order to have a fully actuated human locomotion systems. From this category it can be remarked

D. Tarnita et al. (Eds.): MESROB 2023, MMS 133, pp. 198–207, 2023.
https://doi.org/10.1007/978-3-031-32446-8_22

complex systems dedicated to the human walking rehabilitation process. By having in sight previous research developed in [6], especially the state-of-the art, it can be remarked the idea to design rehabilitation systems especially dedicated to persons with neuromotor problems based on simplicity, easy-operation features and also an affordable price. In previous researches like [7, 8], there were designed several exoskeleton solutions based on cam mechanisms and linear actuators for entire human locomotion system joints, which are presented in second section of these research. By having these systems as research references and in order to design new concept solutions, it is necessary to have an input database represented by the human anthropometry and experimental analysis of the human gait. These input data are summary presented in third section of this research. With these, it was achieved a new leg exoskeleton concept presented in fourth section of this research and a well done structural description can be found in [6]. The proposed leg exoskeleton has on its structure mechanisms actuated through chain transmissions by servomotor units. This configuration has on its background a complex research work, which consists on kinematic and dynamic analyses. The main objective of this research is to validate the leg exoskeleton concept through virtual simulations accomplished with MSC Adams software presented in fifth section. Thus the obtained prototype was experimentally tested and at the end it can be conclude that the designed exoskeleton can be used for persons with neuromotor deficiencies, which these can have a negative impact on their locomotion system.

2 Human Lower Limb Kinematic Models

By having in sight the human locomotion system main tasks, it can be recognized that the major one is represented by walking. Thus, in past researches like [7, 8] human walking was analyzed from experimental viewpoints in order to identify the absolute and relative angular variation depending on time for hip, knee and ankle joints. These represent the input data for elaborating several kinematic mechanisms for actuating a human lower limb in special recovery processes during walking. From this viewpoint it can be mentioned two main constructive solutions presented in Fig. 1 and Fig. 2.

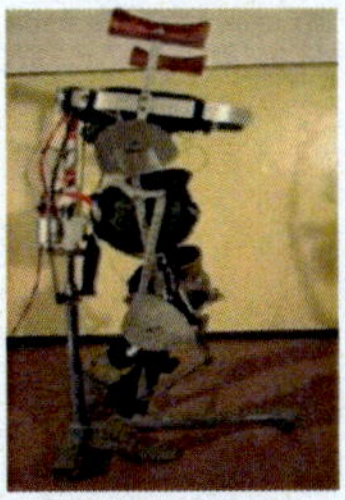

Fig. 1. Exoskeleton with cam mechanisms

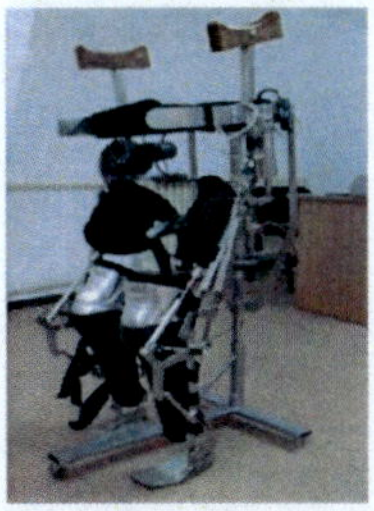

Fig. 2. Exoskeleton with linear actuators

These solutions have in common planar parallel mechanisms for actuating the knee and ankle joints for one leg. Based on these mechanisms, there were elaborated three actuation modes of the desired drive joints, respectively cam mechanisms, linear actuators and planetary servomotors. The cam mechanisms design was started from the cam follower motion law, in order to determine the cam profiles. For this it was considered as input data the angular variations obtained through experimental analyses performed on human healthy subjects groups, for knee and ankle joints. The exoskeleton leg control, performed by cam mechanisms, will affect in time the kinematic precision during motion, and the angular variations of the actuated joints have a restricted domain of use, because these depends on the cam profile. Due to this fact, there were analyzed the proposed leg exoskeleton solutions by having in sight several design criteria like: kinematic precision, command & control simplicity, reliability and functional safety during therapeutically specific procedures. Thus, the suitable solution was the one based on actuating the leg exoskeleton with planetary servomotors. From this viewpoint it was developed a virtual prototyping analysis of a complex robotic system especially designed for persons with neuromotor locomotion problems.

3 Human Walking Analysis for Exoskeleton Programming and Control

In order to have input data mark as gait patterns, for exoskeleton programming and control, it was developed an experimental analysis of human locomotion system. The analysis aim was to have a database with different gait patterns developed by healthy persons during walking activity. This will also give important reference elements in designing the exoskeleton mechanical structure. For this, it was used a high-speed motion analysis equipment called VICON [9], which can be found in one of the University of Craiova laboratories. The equipment has on its own structure 14 infrared high-speed cameras which can records video sequences together with VICON Data acquisition hardware. The experimental analyses workflow is summarized in Fig. 3, and an experimental test can be done by attaching a set of 57 markers with reflective properties on some characteristic points of a human body.

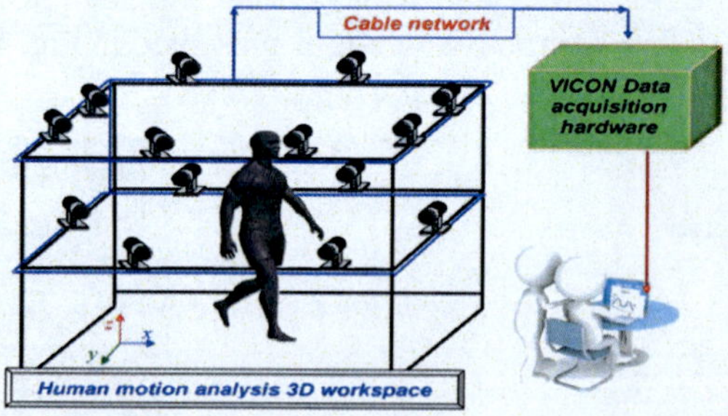

Fig. 3. VICON equipment workflow for developing experimental analyses [9]

By having in sight, the presented workflow from Fig. 3, which characterizes an experimental analysis of human gait, it was created two major databases, namely one of 30 human subjects (male and female) and 5 persons with neuromotor deficiencies.

The chosen human subjects have ages between 24 and 60 years old and anthropometric data known like 55 to 94 kg, height between 1.5 m and 1.9 m. The performed experimental tests of human gait were obtained in laboratory conditions for a 4 to 6 complete gait cycles.

The experimental data analysis was done with VICON – Nexus software for a single and complete gait cycle. In Fig. 4 there are shown some snapshots during human gait analysis performed by a healthy person. Thus, there were obtained the angular variations of hips, knees and ankles. A part of the acquired results can be found in Fig. 5 and 6. In these figures there are plotted diagrams developed by the analyzed healthy persons which will be used in further researches.

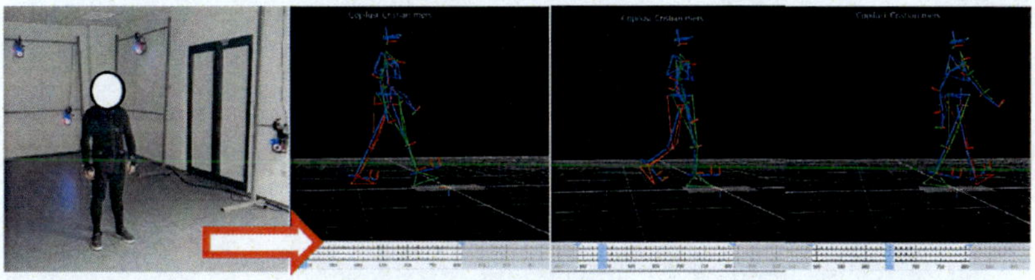

Fig. 4. Snapshots during experimental analysis of a human gait during walking

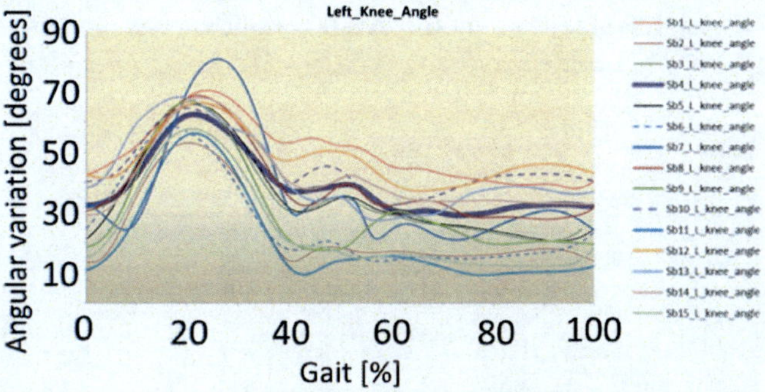

Fig. 5. Left knee angular variations [degrees] of the healthy persons for a complete gait cycle [100%]

From the diagram reported in Fig. 5, it can be identify the selected angular variation of the left knee, retained for the input data used in proposed exoskeleton dynamic analysis. Thus, it was recorded angular variation values between 35.398° and 78.861°. This corresponds to healthy subject no.4, from the acquired database. One it can be conclude that the angular amplitude will reach an approximate value of 43.463°. Similar with this, was obtained a database for right knee joints and it was selected the angular trajectory of the same human subject, which can be found in Fig. 6. In this case it can be remarked an angular variation between 18.445°and 65.806°. Thus it was resulted an angular amplitude of 47. 361°. The obtained results corresponds to the reference data reported in special literature [10].

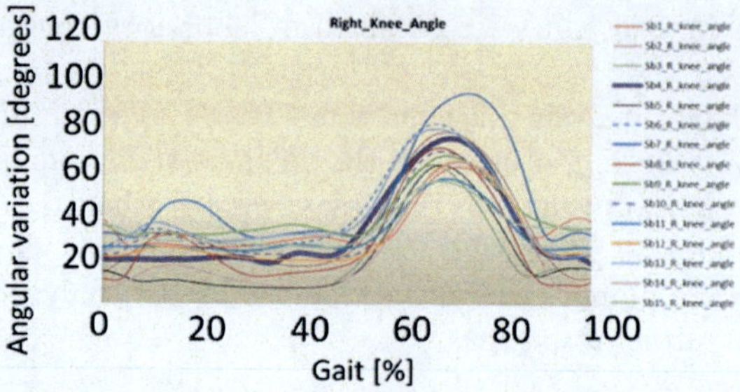

Fig. 6. Right knee angular variations [degrees] of the healthy persons for a complete gait cycle [100%]

4 Mathematical Models for Exoskeleton Mechanism Dynamic Analysis

In order to perform a mechanism dynamic analysis it is necessary to establish the structural solution of the robotic system mechanical part. Thus, in Fig. 7 it is shown the structural scheme of this and more details can be found in [6]. From Fig. 7 it can be identify the main components of the proposed conceptual solution: **ASD** – right hip servomotor; **APD** – right ankle servomotor; **AGD** – right knee servomotor; **ASS** – left hip servomotor; **APS** – left ankle servomotor; **AGS** – left knee servomotor.

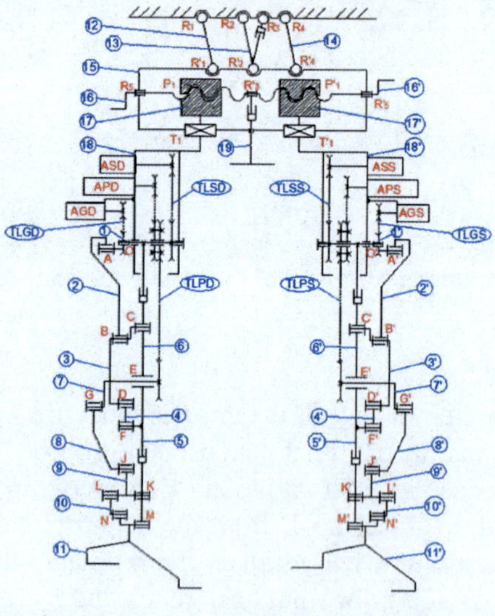

Fig. 7. Exoskeleton structural scheme used in human locomotion system recovery for persons with neuromotor deficiencies

The exoskeleton was designed with a mechanical device for width adjustment situated at the patient pelvic zone. This has power screws, which can be actuated manually for moving the exoskeleton legs close to the patient body through elements 16 and 16’.

These power screws were characterized by two thread sectors mirrored one to the other, namely P1 and P1'. These power screws are fixed by the base frame 15 through ball bearing R5, R3 and R5'. In this structural scheme it is identified component 19 which has an important role to sustain the patient body in an orthostatic position for performing the desired walking recovery procedures. The exoskeleton legs are articulated onto the main frame through connection elements 12, 13, and 14 (revolute joints R1, R2, R3, R4 and R1', R2', R3' and R4'). These elements will allow the exoskeleton to perform oscillations which occurs during walking in a vertical plane.

For each equivalent lower limb, the exoskeleton leg mechanism consists of two planar parallel mechanisms, which will assure the actuation at the knee level joint respectively at the ankle joint level. The proper kinematic schemes of these mechanisms are shown in Fig. 8.

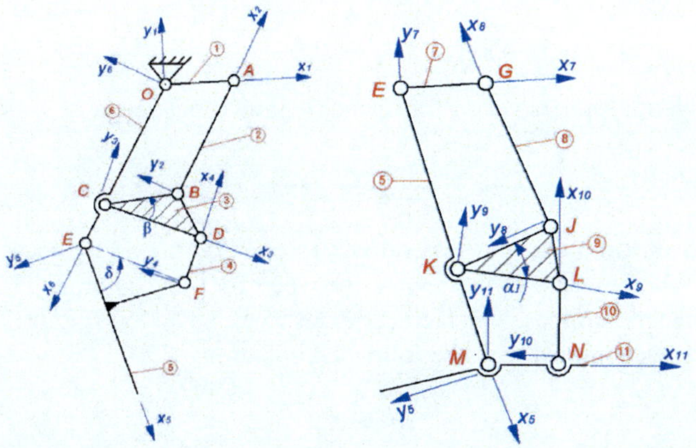

a. b.

Fig. 8. Kinematic scheme of the actuation mechanism from the analyzed leg exoskeleton structure: a – knee equivalent actuation mechanism; b – ankle equivalent actuation mechanism

For the knee joint equivalent actuation mechanism from Fig. 8a, the corresponding generalized coordinate's vector has the following form:

$$q_k = \{X_E, Y_E, \phi_{06}, X_F, Y_F, \phi_{65}, X_B, Y_B, \phi_{63}, X_A, Y_A, \phi_{01}, \phi_{32}\}^T \tag{1}$$

This vector has in its own structure the proper coordinates for E, F, B and A revolute joints. The kinematic constraints equations for the ankle joint actuation are:

$$\varphi_k(q_k, t) = 0, \; k = \overline{1, 16} \tag{2}$$

The Lagrange multipliers vector, which corresponds to the knee joint can be expressed as:

$$\lambda_k = J_{q_k}^{-1}\left[Q^k - M_k \ddot{q_k}\right] \tag{3}$$

where: M_k is the mass matrix, λ_k – Lagrange multipliers, $\ddot{q}_k$ accelerations, Q^k- active generalized forces vector, J_{qk} – Jacoby matrix which corresponds to the kinematic constraints equations. The connection forces, which will be developed during motion inside of the revolute joints, for the knee mechanism are:

$$F_k^i = \lambda_k^i, i = \overline{1, 16} \tag{4}$$

For the ankle joint actuation mechanism presented in Fig. 8b, the generalized coordinate's vector has the following form:

$$q_a = \begin{Bmatrix} X_M, Y_M, \phi_{65}, X_N, Y_N, \phi_{511}, X_L, Y_L, \\ \phi_{1110}, X_J, Y_J, \phi_{59}, X_G, Y_G, \phi_{57}, \phi_{98} \end{Bmatrix}^T \tag{5}$$

The kinematic constraints equations are:

$$\varphi_a(q_a, t) = 0, \;\; a = \overline{1, 16} \tag{6}$$

The Lagrange multipliers vector for the ankle joint mechanism is:

$$\lambda_a = J_{q_a}^{-1}\left[Q^a - M_a\, \ddot{q}_a\right] \tag{7}$$

It is well to mention that the generalized force structure - Q^a, it was considered a proper force which occurs at the contact between foot and ground. Thus, the kinematic joints connection forces, which corresponds to the ankle joint equivalent actuation mechanism can be processed with the following equation:

$$F_a^j = \lambda_a^j \tag{8}$$

The connection forces obtained through mathematical models were computed with a proper MAPLE algorithm. These were compared with the ones obtained through virtual prototyping with the aid of MSC Adams software. An example of this comparison can be found in Fig. 10, where are shown the connection forces diagram for ankle joint during simulations with MSC Adams software versus the one obtained with the developed mathematical models.

5 Robotic System Virtual Prototyping

Based on the kinematic scheme from Fig. 8 it was realized a virtual model of the exoskeleton mechanism. This model was imported in MSC Adams/AdamsView software where it was defined the proper kinematic model. This model consists in: kinematic links articulated through revolute joints, mobile reference systems connected with the links, revolute joints centered reference systems material properties and inertial characteristics. By knowing the angular variations of knee and ankle joints, obtained through experimental analyses, it is possible to perform an inverse kinematic analysis which allow to identify the drive joints angular variations, namely O and E, O' and E' from Fig. 8.

By taking into account the multibody systems theory and having in sight the Newton-Euler formalism, completed with Lagrange multipliers, there were obtained joint connection forces variations for a complete gait. The walking activity simulation was performed for 10 complete gaits (15 s), according with Fig. 9.

By comparing the results obtained through mathematical models process and the ones obtained from numerical simulations with MSC Adams software, as it can be remarked in Fig. 10, it result a complete feasibility study for creating a prototype of the robotic structure exoskeleton.

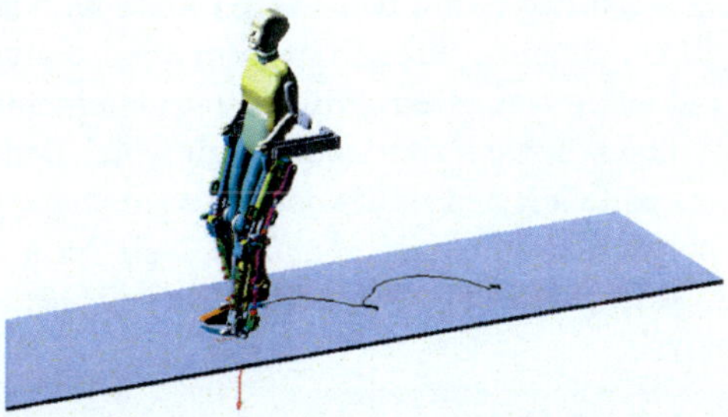

Fig. 9. Exoskeleton virtual model imported in MSC Adams software. Snapshot during virtual simulations.

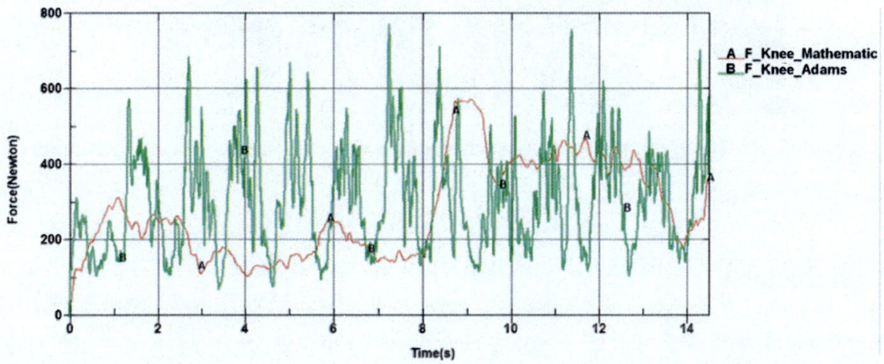

Fig. 10. Knee connection forces variation [Newton] vs. time [sec]

The connection forces variation presented in Fig. 10, path A, are generated by the dynamic model by considering the contact force between ground and foot, where a huge influence has the dumping coefficient. It was designed the command and control system which was made from two major parts: one hardware (the central unit for robotic system command & control) and other namely software in the sight of monitoring the commands and exoskeleton motions. There were manufactured, adjusted and assembled specific parts for the prototype in order to obtain a robust structure, well prepared for robotic system experimental tests developed in laboratory conditions and endurance specific to medical training programs.

6 Exoskeleton Experimental Tests

The exoskeleton experimental tests were performed in accordance with a specific kineto-therapeutically protocol addressed to patients with neuromotor disorders. This protocol was created and adapted only for walking activity and consists of two major tests: experimental evaluations of the exoskeleton prototype without patient, respectively experimental evaluations of the exoskeleton prototype with patient at a payload of 40% from its total capacity. This research frame will allow summarizing only the exoskeleton experimental evaluations performed without patient, other tests can be found in [6]. Thus, in command&control hardware unit was loaded a file with specific motion laws of the left and right hip joints obtained through experimental analysis, respectively the motion laws for knees and ankle processed through inverse kinematic analysis. These were applied in a tandem mode for each servomotor unit which controls the four planar parallel mechanism dedicated to left and right knees and ankles.

During tests it was performed an experimental analysis for a complete gait cycle which was occurred on a time period of 1.45 s. Thus, in Fig. 11, it can be seen some snapshots during this analysis.

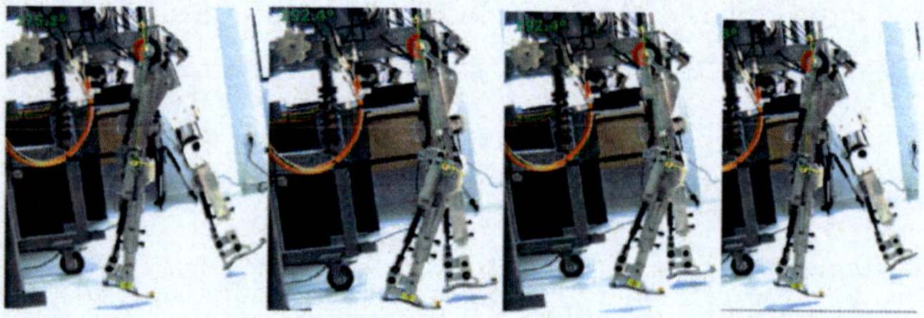

Fig. 11. Snapshots during robotic system experimental tests performed in laboratory conditions

7 Conclusions

The conceptual solution of the complex robotic system was analyzed from different viewpoints namely structural, kinematic and dynamic ones and through elaborating some mathematical models, with the aid of special algorithms and programs for numerical processing. From these there were obtained significant results used in the mechanical structure design and command & control unit achievement. There were obtained motion variation laws depending on time for a complete walking phase for point of interest, specific to hips, knees and ankles. These are mandatory for a good human walking recovery. Based on kinematic function obtained through experimental analysis of human lower limb motions, it was conceived an exoskeleton type mechanism composed by kinematic linkages which allow the actuation of the three main joints from human lower limb structure. It was elaborated a mathematical algorithm based on Newton Raphson method in order to perform a kinematic analysis of the proposed exoskeleton mechanism. Based on this algorithm it was created a program, with a flexible character, which allow the user to determine the kinematic parameters motion laws during time, on proper models developed through an inverse kinematic analysis. For these were also used, as input data, human anthropometric data and geometry characteristics acquired experimentally.

There were identified the angular variation laws and angular speeds from the drive revolute joints. These laws were used for robotic system program and control and are specific to walking phases in order to create a proper and complete gait.

The inverse dynamic analysis permit to obtain the revolute joints connection forces variation during time for a complete gait. These were obtained by considering input data the generalized coordinates variation, mechanism geometry, mass and inertia characteristics and generalized forces.

It can be remarked that were obtained numerical results which were validated through a comparative analysis through two methods namely computer mathematical modelling and numerical simulation with the aid of MSC Adams software. The numerical simulation was done through virtual simulations which allow validating the complex robotic system concept.

There were performed preliminary experimental tests, but also ones in laboratory specific conditions and the obtained results validate the conceptual solution. The experimental tests were done according with the respect of kineto-therapeutically protocol, for rehabilitating the human gait, specific to patients with neuromotor problems.

References

1. Esquenazi, A., Talaty, M., Jayaraman, A.: Powered exoskeletons for walking assistance in persons with central nervous system injuries: a narrative review. PM&R **2017**(9), 46–62 (2017)
2. Ghobrial, G.M., Wang, M.Y.: The next generation of powered exoskeleton use in spinal cord injury. Neurosurg. Focus **42**, E16 (2017)
3. Louie, D.R., Eng, J.J.: Powered robotic exoskeletons in post-stroke rehabilitation of gait: a scoping review. J. Neuroeng. Rehabil. **13**, 1–10 (2016)
4. Varela, M.J., Ceccarelli, M., Flores, P.: A kinematic characterization of human walking by using CaTraSys. Mech. Mach. Theory **86**, 125–139 (2015)
5. Shepherd M.K., Rouse E.J.: Design and validation of a torque-controllable knee exoskeleton for sit-to-stand assistance. IEEE/ASME Trans. Mechatron. **22**(4) 1695–1704, (2017)
6. Copilusi, C., Dumitru, S., Geonea, I., Ciurezu, L.G., Dumitru, N.: Design approaches of an exoskeleton for human neuromotor rehabilitation. Appl. Sci. **12**(8), 3952 (2022)
7. Dumitru, N., Copilusi, C., Geonea, I., Tarniţa, D., Dumitrache, I.: Dynamic analysis of an exoskeleton new ankle joint mechanism. In: 5th European Conference on Mechanism Science. Portugal (2014)
8. Dumitrache, I., Dumitru, N., Geonea, I.: Human locomotion system design based on cam mechanism. In: Proceedings of World Congress on Engineering, WCE 2012, London, U.K.,Tome 1, pp. 2032–2037 (2012)
9. Vicon Nexus Product Guide for Motion Analysis Equipment. Edited by VICON Industries (2016)
10. Bertomeu-Motos, A.: Biomechanics of human walking and stability descriptive parameters. Rev. Dr. UMH **1**, 4–8 (2015)

Biomechanics

An Experimental Testing Procedure for Validating a Passive Upper-Limb Exoskeleton

Jhon F. Rodríguez-León[1,2], Francesco Lago[2], Elio Matteo Curcio[2], Francesco Lamonaca[3], Juan A. Flores-Campos[4], and Giuseppe Carbone[2](✉)

[1] Centro de Investigación en Ciencia Aplicada y Tecnología Avanzada Unidad Querétaro, Mecatrónica, Instituto Politécnico Nacional, 76090 Querétaro, Mexico
[2] Department of Mechanical, Energy and Management Engineering, University of Calabria, 87036 Rende, Italy
giuseppe.carbone@unical.it
[3] Department of Computer Science, Modelling, Electronic and System Science, University of Calabria, 87036 Rende, Italy
[4] Interdisciplinary Professional Unit in Engineering and Advanced Technologies, UPIITA-IPN Instituto Politécnico Nacional, 07340 Mexico City, Mexico
jaflores@ipn.mx

Abstract. This paper proposes a low-cost experimental testing procedure to assess the effectiveness of an upper-limb exoskeleton. The proposed measurement methodology has been specifically designed to evaluate the performance of a passive self-locking magnetic spring exoskeleton that has been designed and built at University of Calabria. The proposed measurement system is based on the use of two commercially available low-cost cameras that allow to identify the moving joints during a holding task. Each of the cameras allows to identify three markers with different colors as attached on the human limb. Additionally, an external force sensor system has been included to determine the effort that a person is generating during a holding task.

Keywords: Exoskeleton · Experimental validation · Measurement test bed

1 Introduction

Recent years have seen a significant increase in the use of exoskeletons, particularly for military, industrial, and medical purposes [1]. Also, these are designed to increase the wearer's strength and endurance to lessen tiredness. Industrial exoskeletons are primarily used to prevent musculoskeletal problems and lower the risk of trauma [2]. Physical human-robot interaction is a transfer of force to overcome human physical limitations and enhance them. Since the user and robotic device interact significantly, it is important to evaluate the device's effectiveness and effectiveness in terms of force exchange [3]. The performance and impacts of the exoskeleton are often compared to the scenario when the exoskeleton is not worn in order to evaluate human-robot interactions [4].

D. Tarnita et al. (Eds.): MESROB 2023, MMS 133, pp. 211–219, 2023.
https://doi.org/10.1007/978-3-031-32446-8_23

Different methods are used to assess the forces and movement of the human body. A method is the use of kinetic analyses of human-exoskeleton interactions, which are essential and provide indispensable evaluation indices. The methodology is based on data collected through Electromyography (EMG) and motion capture systems. It works by calculating kinetic parameters, such as torque and power, without the need to measure ground reaction force. The method combines data from the literature with data collected in the laboratory [5]. Another estimation method for assessing the interaction force between the human lower limbs and the passive exoskeleton links during walking on level ground is based on kinematic data. Unlike conventional methods, this method does not require force sensors and is computationally cheaper to obtain the calculation results. The interaction force is evaluated by a spring model, which is used to simulate the binding behavior between the human limbs and the exoskeleton links, [6]. In addition, devices were used to capture the positions and movements of skeletal joints of the human body using depth cameras based on Infrared (IR) sensor inputs. Using machine learning algorithms with convolutional neural networks, they segmented human subjects and limb positions in 2D and combined them with depth information to estimate joint positions in 3D [7]. Motion tracking using depth cameras was also considered to detect the joints of the human skeleton for the performance evaluation of different types of industrial exoskeletons while a user performs a series of simulated industrial task poses. Experimented with different depth camera body tracking systems for performance testing of industrial exoskeletons. In addition, the consistency of human joint measurement was evaluated. These results were compared with data collected by an Optical Tracking Systems (OTS) [8].

This study aims to assess, with a low-cost set up, the performance of a user while performing a predefined task with the upper limbs, first without the exoskeleton and then while wearing it. The measurement method is based on markers using OTS positioned on the user and filmed by two cameras. In addition, there is a load cell to measure the required holding force while the user performs the operation with and without the exoskeleton.

2 Approach Measurement System

The measurement system implemented in this paper is based on a strategy of processing images in real time by identifying three markers with different color, in addition, a force measurement system has been used, which allows to evaluate the performance of the exoskeleton with a low-cost setup.

2.1 Marker Detection Strategy

To validate the trajectory performance, a strategy on marker detection was used to identify the position of the three important point through image processing; this strategy was explained in reference [9]. Figure 1 shows the position of camera 1 and 2 within the test scenario. Additionally, the position that the user should have during the tests has been defined. The measurement system using two cameras (Logitech 1080pp) was developed in Python, this system allows to know the real time (every 3 s) the x, y and z coordinates of each of the marker. This data has been sent to MATLAB to be processed and plotted. The test stage has been illuminated with LED light to control the brightness variable. In addition, two white boards have been incorporated that allow to identify with quality the colors of the markers.

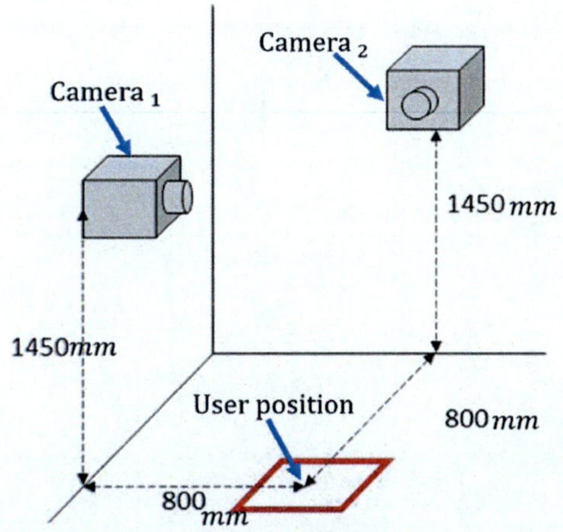

Fig. 1. Test scenario: position of camera 1 and 2 and the position of the user during the tests.

2.2 Payload Measurement System

The U9C force transducer was used, see the Fig. 2. The most important characteristics are: Tensile/compressive force transduce, accuracy class 0.2, nominal (rated) forces 50 N – 50 KN, non-rusting, protection class IP67, high rigidity, particularly suited for dynamic measurement tasks.

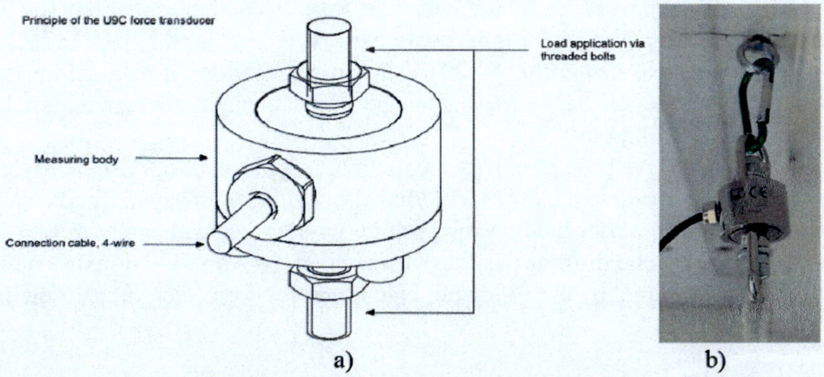

Fig. 2. The selected U9C force transducer: a) a scheme; b) the installed sensor.

The load measurement system was used to validate the performance of the exoskeleton in terms of forces and physical strain during a specific application consisting of ceiling-surface drilling tasks. This system was located at the top and center of the test scenario. Figure 3 shows the test scenario explaining the location of the force sensor, the cameras and the user position.

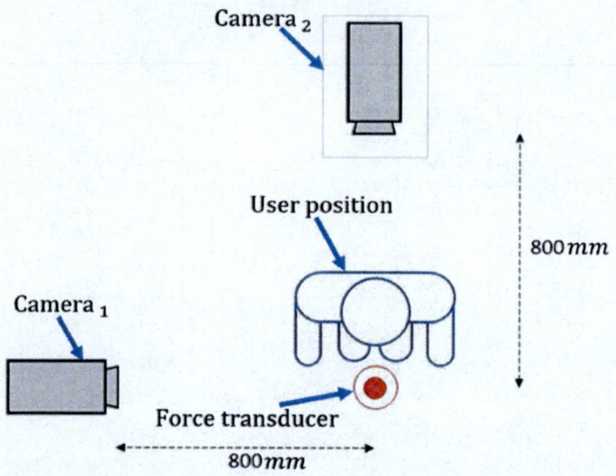

Fig. 3. Load measurement system: test scenario explaining the location of the force sensor, the two cameras and the user position.

3 Experimental Setup

The test scenario is shown in Fig. 4 and the positions of the cameras and force sensor can be identified. In addition, LED light is used which allows for brightness control. A computer is also used to acquire and process data from experiments. For better identification of the colors used as markers, a white background has been defined.

A passive exoskeleton was used in the experimental evaluation, this prototype was developed in [10]. This paper explores the use of cameras as contactless position sensors and a force sensor to measure the effects when using an exoskeleton during a drilling task. The aim of the experimental was to measure the position and physical strain required by a user to maintain a drilling task.

Four experiments have been proposed: the user holding the position without payload and without wearing exoskeleton; the user holding the position with payload and without wearing exoskeleton; the user holding the position without payload and with wearing exoskeleton and the user holding the position with payload and with wearing exoskeleton. During the four experiments, the following characteristics were measured to the test person, shown in Table 1.

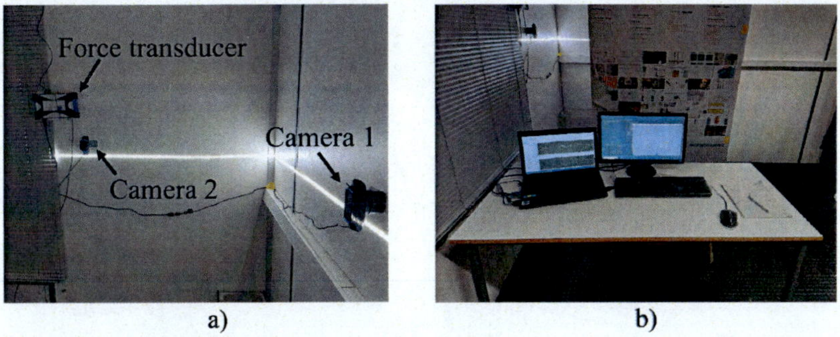

Fig. 4. Test scenario with positions of the cameras and force sensor: a) the location of the sensors; b) the PC and user interface for sensor monitoring.

Table 1. Anthropometric sizes.

Users	Weight [kg]	Length of ARM [cm]	Height [cm]
User 1	85	35	175
User 2	87	30	180
User 3	95	32	190

4 Experimental Evaluation

The proposed experimental set up is specifically designed for a passive exoskeleton that has been designed and built at University of Calabria according to the scheme shown in Fig. 5. During the test, each of the markers have been fixed in the same position during the four experiments. Also, each camera was able to identify the three colors and presents the identification of the center of each marker allowing to generate a triangle with each of the identified centers. Four experiments were carried out as in Figs. 6, 7, 8 and 9.

4.1 First Tests – User Without Wearing the Exoskeleton and Without Payload

The first experiment has been performed and its result is shown in Fig. 6. The results show that the person could support the indicated position for 3 min, also it can be observed as the posture of the column is changing by increasing the physical effort applied to hold the required position.

4.2 Second Tests – User Without Wearing the Exoskeleton Holding a Payload

In the second experiment it can be seen how the person supports 1.25 min, which indicates that it supports less time compared to the first experiment as shown in Fig. 7. Figure 8 shows a detail of the measured displacements and holding force.

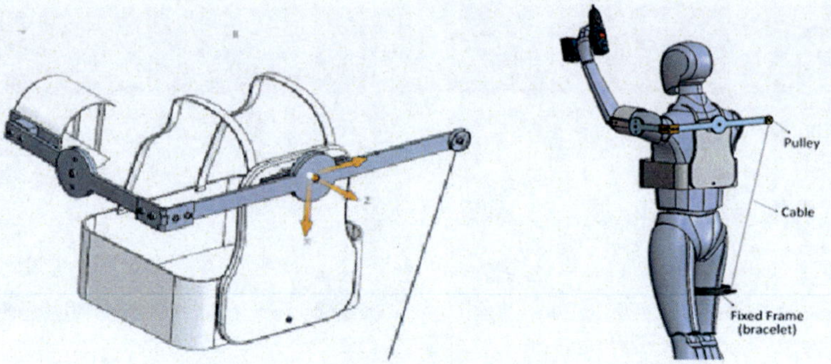

a) b)

Fig. 5. The proposed passive exoskeleton that has been designed and built at University of Calabria: a) a 3D CAD model; b) a model of its human body installation.

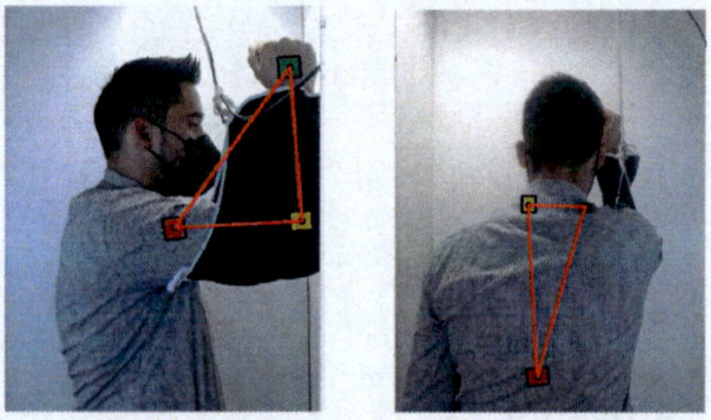

Fig. 6. The user holding the position without payload and without wearing the exoskeleton.

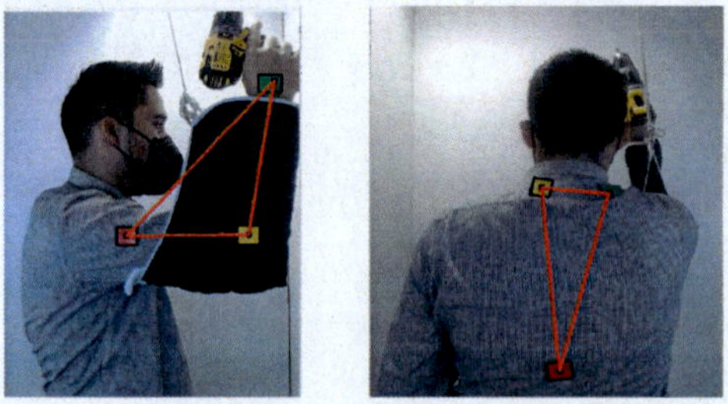

Fig. 7. The user holding the position with payload and without wearing the exoskeleton.

4.3 Third Tests – User Wearing the Exoskeleton Without Holding a Payload

Figure 8 shows the results that indicate the user was able to support the final position for 15 min, which indicates that he was able to support the posture a longer time compared to tests one and two. In the third experiment it can be observed that the assistance of the exoskeleton allows to increase the support time during the proposed task, this is because the mechanical system allows to distribute the forces along the body and especially in the user's leg as shown in Fig. 9.

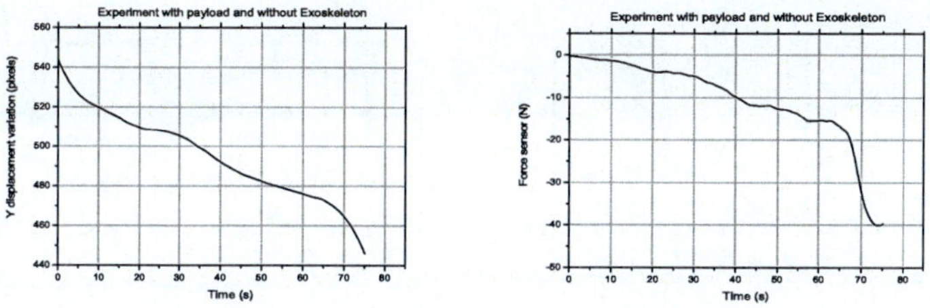

Fig. 8. Y-displacement of the green marker of camera 1 and variation in force detected.

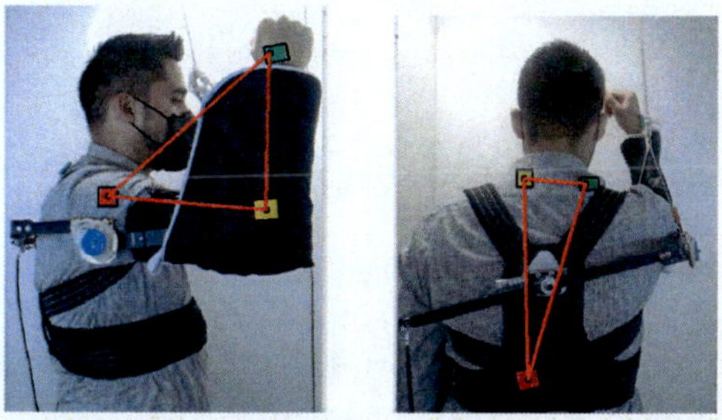

Fig. 9. The user holding the position without payload and wearing the exoskeleton.

4.4 Fourth Tests - User Wearing the Exoskeleton and Holding a Payload

In the four of can observe how the user can hold the load of the drill longer time compared to test number two, in addition the support time for this scenario was 12 min, which indicates that the exoskeleton allows to help the user to maintain the desired holding posture. This experiment is shown in Fig. 10. Figure 11 shows a detail of the measured displacements and holding force. A comparison of the plots in Fig. 11 with Fig. 8 allows to compare the obtained motion trajectory with a proper position holding and a reduction of the holding force due to the use of the exoskeleton. Future work will include the implementation of more sensors to the test scenario allowing to monitor the behavior of the arm muscles by using EMG (Electromyography signals) and cables to apply external forces such as proposed for example in [11].

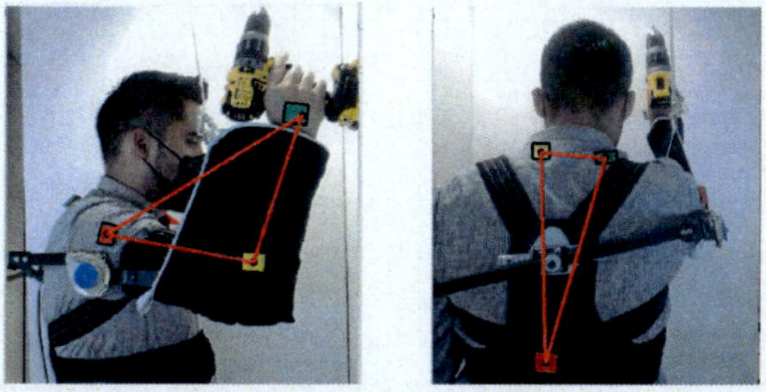

Fig. 10. The user holding the position with payload and wearing the exoskeleton.

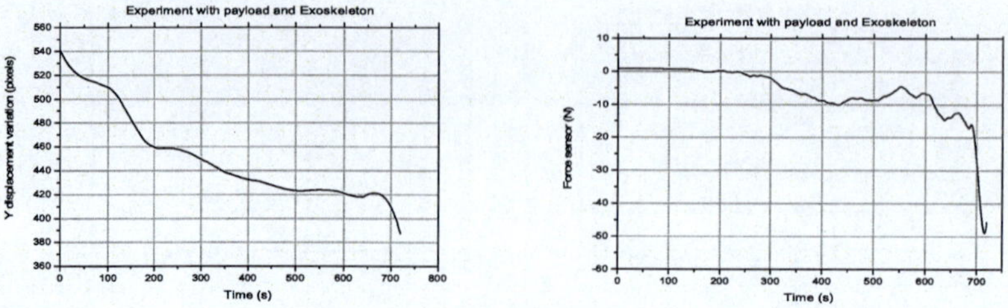

Fig. 11. Y-displacement trajectory of the green marker of camera 1 and variation in force detected by the force sensor.

5 Conclusions

This paper proposes a new experimental testing procedure for validating a passive upper limb exoskeleton. The results of the imaging system made it possible to identify the user's change of posture during the proposed task. In addition, it could identify the time that the user can keep in the four different test scenarios. Data from an external force sensor allow to determine the user effort showing the effectiveness of the proposed testing procedure for assessing a passive exoskeleton.

Acknowledgements. We acknowledge financial support from: PNRR MUR project PE0000013-FAIR.

References

1. Bai, S., et al.: User-centered development and performance assessment of a modular full-body exoskeleton (AXO-SUIT). Biomimetic Intell. Robot. **2**(2), 100032 (2022)
2. Pinto-Fernandez, D., et al.: Performance evaluation of lower limb exoskeletons: a systematic review. IEEE Trans. Neural Syst. Rehabil. Eng. **28**(7), 1573–1583 (2020)
3. Li, J., et al.: Influence of a compatible design on physical human-robot interaction force: a case study of a self-adapting lower-limb exoskeleton mechanism. J. Intell. Rob. Syst. **98**(2), 525–538 (2019). https://doi.org/10.1007/s10846-019-01063-5
4. Maurice, P., et al.: Objective and subjective effects of a passive exoskeleton on overhead work. IEEE Trans. Neural Syst. Rehabil. Eng. **28**(1), 152–164 (2020)
5. Vasco, F., et al.: Assessment methodology for human-exoskeleton interactions. kinetic analysis based on muscle activation. Front. Neurorobot. **16** (2022)
6. Pang, M., et al.: Estimation of the interaction force between human and passive lower limb exoskeleton device during level ground walking. Biomimetic Intell. Robot. **2**(3), 100056 (2022)
7. Wang, J., Liu, T., Wang, X.: Human hand gesture recognition with convolutional neural networks for K-12 double-teachers instruction mode classroom. Infrared Phys. Technol. **111**, 103464 (2020)
8. Soocheol, Y., et al.: Feasibility of using depth cameras for evaluating human-exoskeleton interaction. In: Proceedings of the Human Factors and Ergonomics Society Annual Meeting, vol. 66, no. 1, pp. 1892–1896. Sage CA: Los Angeles, CA: SAGE Publications (2022)
9. Rodríguez-León., J.F., Chaparro-Rico, B.D.M., Russo, M., Cafolla, D.: An autotuning cable-driven device for home rehabilitation. J. Health Eng. (2021)

10. Rodríguez-León., J.F., Lago., F., Castillo-Castañeda., E., Carbone, G.: Preliminary design of a magnetic-locking system for specific exoskeleton-assisted holding tasks. In: IEEE International Conference on Dependable, Autonomic and Secure Computing, International Conference on Pervasive Intelligence and Computing, International Conference on Cloud and Big Data Computing, International Conference on Cyber Science and Technology Congress (DASC/PiCom/CBDCom/CyberSciTech), Falerna, Italy, 2022, pp. 1–6 (2022). https://doi.org/10.1109/DASC/PiCom/CBDCom/Cy55231.2022.9928011
11. Hernández-Martínez, E.E., Ceccarelli, M., Carbone, G., López-Cajún, C.S., Jáuregui-Correa, J.C.: Characterization of a cable-based parallel mechanism for measurement purposes#. Mech. Based Des. Struct. Mach. **38**(1), 25–49 (2010)

A New Bio-Inspired Joint with Variable Stiffness

Christine Chevallereau[1], Philippe Wenger[1(✉)], and Anick Abourachid[2]

[1] Nantes Université, Ecole Centrale de Nantes, CNRS, LS2N, 44000 Nantes, France
{Christine.Chevallereau,Philippe.Wenger}@ls2n.fr
[2] UMR 7179 CNRS/MNHN, MECADEV, Département Adaptations du Vivant, Muséum National d'Histoire Naturelle, 75000 Paris, France

Abstract. This paper addresses stiffness modulation and antagonistic actuation in light-weight tendon-driven bio-inspired manipulators suitable for safe interactions. Designing manipulators with variable stiffness is of great interest in human-robot collaboration tasks. Remote actuation with tendons allows inertia reduction and, if the tendons are properly routed, makes it possible to tune joint stiffness. The way in which the tendons are connected to the bodies for their actuation requires attention. Pulleys are often used to ensure a constant lever arm. However this approach does not allow antagonistic forces to change the joint stiffness. The condition for allowing an increase in stiffness via an increase in antagonistic forces is established. Then this condition is used to propose a new bio-inspired variable-stiffness joint.

Keywords: antagonist actuation · stiffness · tendon driven manipulator · pulley

1 Introduction

The scope of this work is the design of bio-inspired collaborative robots suitable for safe interactions, i.e. allowing joint stiffness modulation. Biological organs constitute interesting models of inspiration for the roboticist. Indeed, they propose frugal solutions both in matter and energy.

To mimick the joint between two animal vertebrae, the simplest mechanism is a revolute joint but, if the center of rotation is not fixed like in the knee joint [1], an anti-parallelogram mechanism would be more appropriate. Biological joints are actuated by antagonistic muscles. Most of the time, two antagonistic muscles work in opposite ways: when one contracts, the other relaxes, so that energy consumption is minimized [2]. However, simultaneous activation of antagonistic muscles may occur for a short time. This so-called *coactivation* principle aims to increase the stiffness of the joint [2]. Moreover, energy consumption should be minimized and one should be able to increase joint stiffness when needed. Variable stiffness actuators (VSA) have been developed to allow for joint stiffness modulation in applications involving interactions, such as in robots and biped [3]. Stiffness modulation in VSA can be achieved through software or hardware. Several different hardware implementations of VSA have been proposed with appropriate spring arrangement and properties [4–6] or by changing

D. Tarnita et al. (Eds.): MESROB 2023, MMS 133, pp. 220–227, 2023.
https://doi.org/10.1007/978-3-031-32446-8_24

transmission angle with cams [7]. Other solutions use antagonistic cable actuation together with springs [8]. In such solutions, several pulleys are needed and stiffness modulation uses rather complex solutions.

In this paper, a simple solution is proposed to allow for stiffness modulation in tendon-actuated joints. This solution uses a elliptical pulley. This rest of this paper is organized in two parts. Section 2 studies and compares coactivation of antagonistic forces in a circular pulley and in a X-joints. The proposed solution, called E-pulley, is proposed in Sect. 3. Section 4 concludes this paper.

2 Joints Actuated by Antagonist Tendons

In biological systems, the joints are often modeled with revolute joints actuated by antagonistic tendons and/or muscles [9]. However, it was shown recently that stiffness descreases when antagonistic tendon forces increase in simple revolute joints [10]. When designing tendon-driven joints, the attachment points of the tendons must be defined carefully to avoid singularities when the tendon line crosses the joint. Accordingly, tendons can be attached via pulleys. Not only this solution avoids singularities but it also produces a constant lever arm and it mimics bones swelling at their extremities [11].

Some biological joints such as the knee joint [1] or intervertebrae joints in the bird neck [12] can be modeled by crossed four-bar joints or *X-joints*. On the other hand, we observed that the knee and ankle joints can be modelled as pulleys, with antagonistic muscles being used to modulate stiffness. Measurements on the bones suggest that the pulleys may not be circular. In the work presented here, we compare the coactivation of X-joint solutions with circular and elliptical pulleys, which could be found in the osteo-muscular system of birds.

We first compare the two joints actuated with antagonistic tendons shown in Fig. 1: the P-module (for pulley) on the left and the X-module (for anti-parallelogram joint) on the right. The P-module (resp. the X-module) is defined by parameter R (resp. b and L). The moving link is attached to the pulley or to the upper bar of the anti-parallelogram.

2.1 Joint Stiffness

Let U be the potential energy of a module: $U = U_g + U_k + F_1 l_1 + F_2 l_2$, where U_g (resp. U_k) is the contribution of gravity (resp. of the springs if any), l_1, l_2 are the cable lengths and F_1, F_2 are the forces applied by the cables (see Fig. 1). The equilibrium condition of a module is $\frac{\mathrm{d}U}{\mathrm{d}\alpha} = 0$, that is:

$$G + \frac{\mathrm{d}l_1}{\mathrm{d}\alpha} F_1 + \frac{\mathrm{d}l_2}{\mathrm{d}\alpha} F_2 = 0 \tag{1}$$

where $G = \frac{\mathrm{d}U_g}{\mathrm{d}\alpha} + \frac{\mathrm{d}U_k}{\mathrm{d}\alpha}$. From fig. 1, it is apparent that $\frac{\mathrm{d}l_1}{\mathrm{d}\alpha} \leq 0$ and $\frac{\mathrm{d}l_2}{\mathrm{d}\alpha} \geq 0$ around $\alpha = 0$ (this will be detailed later). The equilibrium solution with minimal forces s.t. $0 \leq F_{min} \leq F_i \leq F_{max}$ is therefore obtained when one of the forces is at F_{min}. For simplicity, we take $F_{min} = 0$.

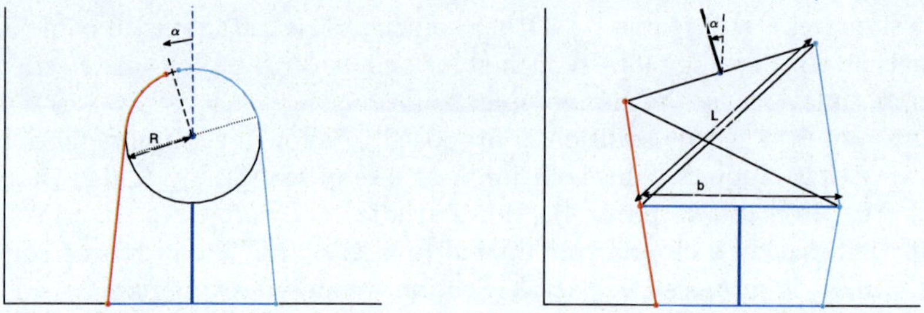

Fig. 1. Two possible ways to build a rotating joint actuated by antagonistic tendons: a P-module (left) and a X-module (right)

Suppose that we want to reach a desired configuration α^d such that $G(\alpha^d) < 0$. Then, the minimum force solution denoted by F^* is:

$$F_2^* = -\frac{G(\alpha^d)}{\frac{\mathrm{d}l_2}{\mathrm{d}\alpha}}, \qquad F_1^* = 0 \tag{2}$$

Other solutions, which would involve coactivation, can be defined in terms of F_2 as follows:

$$F_2 = -\frac{G(\alpha^d) + \frac{\mathrm{d}l_1}{\mathrm{d}\alpha}F_1}{\frac{\mathrm{d}l_2}{\mathrm{d}\alpha}} = F_2^* - \frac{\frac{\mathrm{d}l_1}{\mathrm{d}\alpha}}{\frac{\mathrm{d}l_2}{\mathrm{d}\alpha}}F_1 \tag{3}$$

The joint stiffness, for given cable forces F_1, F_2 is defined by :

$$K = \frac{\mathrm{d}^2U}{\mathrm{d}\alpha^2} = \frac{\mathrm{d}G}{\mathrm{d}\alpha} + \frac{\mathrm{d}^2l_1}{\mathrm{d}\alpha^2}F_1 + \frac{\mathrm{d}^2l_2}{\mathrm{d}\alpha^2}F_2 \tag{4}$$

For the equilibrium with minimal forces, the stiffness is :

$$K^* = \frac{\mathrm{d}G(\alpha^d)}{\mathrm{d}\alpha} - \frac{\frac{\mathrm{d}^2l_2}{\mathrm{d}\alpha^2}G(\alpha^d)}{\frac{\mathrm{d}l_2}{\mathrm{d}\alpha}} \tag{5}$$

The impact of a non-zero force F_1 on the system stiffness is written using equation (4):

$$K = K^* + D_1F_1 \tag{6}$$

with

$$D_1 = \left(\frac{\frac{\mathrm{d}^2l_1}{\mathrm{d}\alpha^2}\frac{\mathrm{d}l_2}{\mathrm{d}\alpha} - \frac{\mathrm{d}^2l_2}{\mathrm{d}\alpha^2}\frac{\mathrm{d}l_1}{\mathrm{d}\alpha}}{\frac{\mathrm{d}l_2}{\mathrm{d}\alpha}}\right) \tag{7}$$

To be able to change the joint stiffness by the antagonistic forces, when must have $D_1 \neq 0$. Finding a behavior similar to that observed in biological systems implies that $D_1 > 0$ for values of α s.t. $G(\alpha^d) < 0$. Let C be the numerator of D_1. Since $\frac{dl_2}{d\alpha} > 0$, this condition can be written:

$$C = \frac{\mathrm{d}^2 l_1}{\mathrm{d}\alpha^2}\frac{\mathrm{d}l_2}{\mathrm{d}\alpha} - \frac{\mathrm{d}^2 l_2}{\mathrm{d}\alpha^2}\frac{\mathrm{d}l_1}{\mathrm{d}\alpha} > 0 \tag{8}$$

A similar condition can be written for values of α s.t. $G(\alpha^d) > 0$. It can be shown that this leads to the same conditions (8).

2.2 Joint Stiffness Modulation for the P-module

For the P-module shown in Fig. 1, when the output rotates of an angle $\delta\alpha$, the length variation of the left tendon is obviously the length of an arc of circle of angle $\delta\alpha$, namely, $R\delta\alpha$. Note that the point of contact of the cable around the pulley does not move since it is defined by the point where the tendon is tangent to the pulley. The length variation of the left tendon is: $R\delta\alpha$.

Accordingly :

$$\frac{\mathrm{d}l_1}{\mathrm{d}\alpha} = R, \quad \frac{\mathrm{d}l_2}{\mathrm{d}\alpha} = -R, \quad \frac{\mathrm{d}^2 l_1}{\mathrm{d}\alpha^2} = \frac{\mathrm{d}^2 l_2}{\mathrm{d}\alpha^2} = 0, \quad C = 0 \tag{9}$$

This shows that stiffness modulation is not possible with a P-module and additional devices must be used, see [7] for example.

2.3 Joint Stiffness Modulation for the X-module

The cable lengths l_1, l_2 are:

$$l_1 = l_{10} + l - bsin(\frac{\alpha}{2}), \qquad l_2 = l_{20} + l + bsin(\frac{\alpha}{2}) \tag{10}$$

where l_{10}, l_{20} are constant values, and l is the distance between the midpoints of bottom and top bars [12]:

$$l = \sqrt{L^2 - b^2\cos^2(\frac{\alpha}{2})} \tag{11}$$

Upon successive differentations, we obtain:

$$\frac{\mathrm{d}l_1}{\mathrm{d}\alpha} = \frac{b^2\cos(\frac{\alpha}{2})\sin(\frac{\alpha}{2})}{2\sqrt{L^2 - b^2\cos^2(\frac{\alpha}{2})}} - \frac{b}{2}cos(\frac{\alpha}{2}) \tag{12}$$

$$\frac{\mathrm{d}l_2}{\mathrm{d}\alpha} = \frac{b^2\cos(\frac{\alpha}{2})\sin(\frac{\alpha}{2})}{2\sqrt{L^2 - b^2\cos^2(\frac{\alpha}{2})}} + \frac{b}{2}cos(\frac{\alpha}{2}) \tag{13}$$

$$\frac{\mathrm{d}^2 l_1}{\mathrm{d}\alpha^2} = \frac{b^2(L^2\cos(\alpha) - b^2\cos^4(\frac{\alpha}{2}))}{4(L^2 - b^2\cos^2(\frac{\alpha}{2}))^{3/2}} + \frac{b}{4}\sin(\frac{\alpha}{2}) \tag{14}$$

$$\frac{d^2 l_2}{d\alpha^2} = \frac{b^2(L^2\cos(\alpha) - b^2\cos^4(\frac{\alpha}{2}))}{4(L^2 - b^2\cos^2(\frac{\alpha}{2}))^{3/2}} - \frac{b}{4}\sin(\frac{\alpha}{2}) \tag{15}$$

Thus :

$$C = \frac{b^3(L^2 - b^2)\cos^3(\frac{\alpha}{2})}{4(L^2 - b^2\cos^2(\frac{\alpha}{2}))^{3/2}} \tag{16}$$

Since $\cos(\frac{\alpha}{2}) > 0$ within the joint limits and since $L > b$, C is always positive.

3 A Novel Module: The E-module

From the previous study, we observe that an increase in stiffness by forces coactivation requires that the cable length expression be non-linear in α and this condition is not satisfied with a classical pulley. We now show that it can be the case if the pulley is elliptical For more simplicity, we are interested in a symmetrical joint with a rotation center fixed at the center of the ellipse. We call this joint and its antagonistic actuation a E-module (for ellipse). Figure 2 shows an example with $a = 0.045$ m, $b = 0.06$ m, base point at $A = (0.02, -0.1)$ m for the right tendon and a symmetric base point for the left tendon.

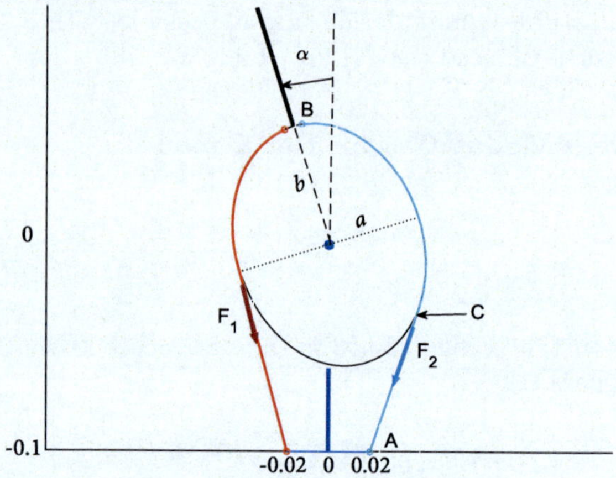

Fig. 2. A E-module is a rotating joint actuated by antagonistic tendons attached to an elliptical pulley.

Each tendon is attached to the ellipse at a certain point (indicated as B for the right tendon) and passes through a certain base point (A for right tendon). We now need to express the tendon lengths as functions of α. To this goal, we calculate the coordinates of the point of tangency between the ellipse and the tendon (at point C for the blue tendon) as a function of α. For the ellipse, no closed form expression of the arc length CB exists, we thus proceed by numerical integration.

Let us consider the E-module of Fig. 2. The plots of the tendon lengths l_1 and l_2 (resp. of their derivatives $\frac{dl_1}{d\alpha}$, $\frac{dl_2}{d\alpha}$, $\frac{d^2l_1}{d\alpha^2}$, $\frac{d^2l_2}{d\alpha^2}$) are shown in Fig. 3, top left (resp. top right and bottom left). The coefficient C is calculated using Eq. (8) and its plot is shown in Fig. 3, bottom right. It turns out that C is positive in the range -0.70 rad $< \alpha < 0.70$ rad. This means that coactivation is possible within this range. We call this range *coactivation range.*

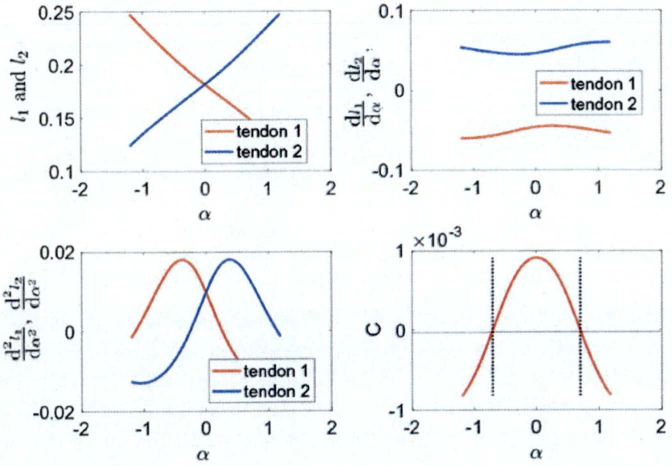

Fig. 3. Plot of tendon length (top left) and of their successive derivatives (top right, bottom left). Bottom right: plot of coefficient C showing the coactivation range.

3.1 Design Parameters of the E-module

We first study the effect of the ellipse shape on the coactivation range. We fix b and the attachment points of the tendons as in Fig. 2 and we investigate several values of a, namely, $a = 0.03$ m, $a = 0.045$ m (as in Fig. 2), $a = 0.06$ m (i.e. a circle) and $a = 0.075$ m. For each case, C is plotted against α in Fig. 4. When $a = 0.03$ m and $a = 0.045$ m, coactivation around $\alpha = 0$ is possible and the coactivation range is similar for these two values. However, coactivation is not possible when $a = 0.075$. This means that the orientation of the ellipse axes plays a central role: the long axis must be vertical at $\alpha = 0$ to have coactivation. However, the length of the semi-axis has little influence on the coactivation range. We also notice the special case $a = b$ (circle) for which $C = 0$, as expected.

A second study is the effect of the direction of the antagonistic tendons. Considering the symmetric E-module of Fig. 2, the lateral distance of point A x_A is varied from 0 to 0.08 m, and the corresponding variation of $C(\alpha)$ is plotted in Fig. 5. It appears that for coactivation to exist, x_A must be lower than a certain value. In fact, we have observed that this value is the length of the horizontal semi-axis but this result needs to be proved. In other words, the limit is when

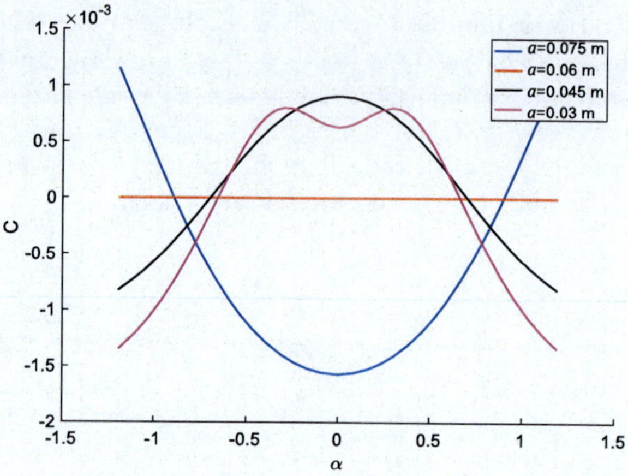

Fig. 4. Influence of the ellipse shape on coactivation range for a E-module.

the two tendons are vertical at $\alpha = 0$. Besides, decreasing x_A does not change the range of coactivation. In conclusion, the choice of the tendon base points also affects coactivation.

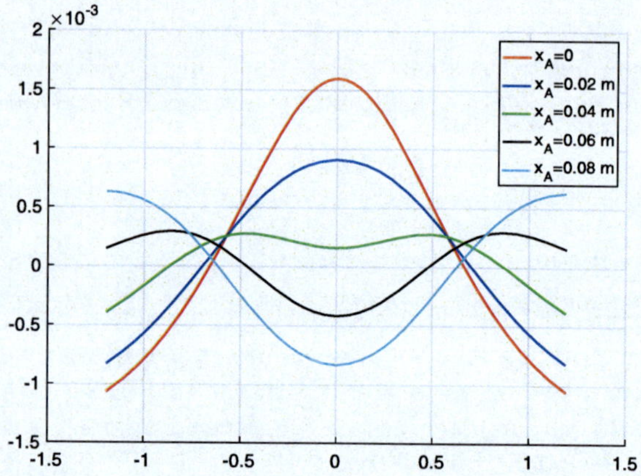

Fig. 5. Influence of the location of tendon base points on coactivation for a E-module.

4 Conclusion

The ability to modulate joint stiffness is an important property in collaborative robotics. To move safely with low energy consumption, it is desirable to provide low stiffness. In contrast, it can be necessary to increase stiffness by coactivation when needed, such as, e.g., during process tasks. In this study, we have proposed a new way to design a rotating joint with variable stiffness via the E-module. This new design can have applications in the design of variable stiffness SEA joints in robotics and for studying biological joints. Interesting avenues of study include studying non-symmetrical pulleys, eccentric or moving rotation axis.

References

1. Hamon, A., Aoustin, Y.: Cross four-bar linkage for the knees of a planar bipedal robot. In: 10th IEEE-RAS International Conference on Humanoid Robots, pp. 379–384 (2010)
2. Latash, M.: Muscle coactivation: definitions, mechanisms, and functions. J. Neurophysiol. **120**, 88–104 (2018)
3. Vanderborght, B., et al.: Variable impedance actuators: a review. Robot. Autonom. Syst. **61**(12), 1601–1614 (2013)
4. Jafari, A., Tsagarakis, N.G., Caldwell, D.G.: Awas-ii: a new actuator with adjustable stiffness based on the novel principle of adaptable pivot point and variable lever ratio. In: 2011 IEEE International Conference on Robotics and Automation, pp. 4638–4643 (2011)
5. Esteveny, L., Barbé, L., Bayle, B.: A novel actuation technology for safe physical human-robot interactions. In: 2014 IEEE International Conference on Robotics and Automation, pp. 5032–5037 (2014)
6. Medina, J., Lozano, P., Balaguer, C.: Design and characterization of a novel mechanism of multiple joint stiffness (MMJS). In: 2016 IEEE/RSJ International Conference on Intelligent Robots and Systems (IROS), pp. 2444–2451 (2016)
7. Ham, R.V., et al.: Compliant actuator designs. IEEE Rob. Aut. Magazine **16**(3), 81–94 (2009)
8. Zhou, X., Jun, S.-K., Krovi, V.: A cable based active variable stiffness module with decoupled tension. J. Mech. Robot. **7**(02), 011005 (2015)
9. Biewener, A., Patek, S.: Animal Locomotion. Oxford University Press, Oxford (2018)
10. Muralidharan, V., Wenger, P.: Optimal design and comparative study of two antagonistically actuated tensegrity joints. Mech. Mach. Theor. **159**, 104249 (2021)
11. Elmas , V., et al.: Toute l'UE 5-Anatomie-Cours+ QCM: Organisation des appareils et des systèmes-Aspects morphologiques et fonctionnels. Elsevier Health Sciences (2019)
12. Fasquelle, B., et al.: Identification and control of a 3-X cable-driven manipulator inspired from the bird neck. J. Mech. Robot. 1–25 (2021)

Parametric Identification of Postural Control Models in Humans Challenged by Impulse-Controlled Perturbations

Carlo De Benedictis(✉), Maria Paterna, Andrea Berettoni, and Carlo Ferraresi

Department of Mechanical and Aerospace Engineering, Politecnico Di Torino, Torino, Italy
carlo.debenedictis@polito.it

Abstract. The study of postural control system is relevant by academic and clinical points of view, and it can be improved by considering model-based approaches. In this framework, to improve the understanding of the underlying mechanism of balance control, it is often necessary to apply external perturbations to the body of a patient. This work deals with the parametric identification of postural control models by fitting with experimental data collected with a custom-made automated perturbation device. The results of model optimization are discussed and provide a preliminary validation of the methodology.

Keywords: Postural Control · Balance · Biomechanical Modeling · Posturography · Impulse

1 Introduction

Balance is a challenging task that involves the continuous action of the postural control system, even in a quiet stance. The human body is inherently unstable and tends to fall under the gravitational force action. The dorsi/planta flexors muscular tone and the viscoelasticity of the ankle joint tissues provide about 60–90% of the necessary corrective torque needed to maintain balance [1–3]. Therefore, an active modulation of the ankle and hip muscle contractions is required to produce stability. The active joint torques magnitudes, and the multi-joint coordination are managed by the central nervous system thanks to the afferences provided by the somatosensory, visual, and vestibular systems.

In order to study the human postural reaction, it could be useful to analyze the patient's response to external mechanical stimuli. However, the physiological and biomechanical responses strongly depend on the perturbation's characteristics [4], which can be classified by application point or dynamics. The perturbation can be applied to the base of support or to the trunk. In the first case, shifting [5, 6] or rotating [7] platforms are employed; in the second, pulling or pushing forces are imparted to the patient by releasing pendulum [8] or weight connected to the body via a cable [9], by pneumatic [10, 11] or electric [12] actuators, or through the action of manual devices which record the impact force [13]. Despite the wide variety of tests available, the complex interaction between physiological systems that contribute to the balance makes the interpretation

D. Tarnita et al. (Eds.): MESROB 2023, MMS 133, pp. 228–237, 2023.
https://doi.org/10.1007/978-3-031-32446-8_25

of experimental results difficult. In this sense, model-based analyses [8, 14–17] could be a helpful tool to achieve information about not easily monitored variables, such as joint angles and torques. Generally, human stance is modelled as a single-link inverted pendulum (SIP) pivoting on the ankle. Healthy subjects standing on a stable surface, in fact, prefer the ankle strategy to recover or maintain balance. On the other hand, the adopted strategy also depends on the previous experience of the subject and the entity of the disturbance, therefore ankle and hip strategies may be both present in postural control, with one dominating the other. In this regard, a double-link inverted pendulum (DIP) could provide additional information and more realistic kinematic result about postural response with respect to the single-link model.

This work aims to present the parametric identification of SIP and DIP models based on experimental data collected during dynamic posturography trials. These analyses have been possible thanks to a custom-made automatic device used to perturb balance in healthy subjects with appropriate control of the magnitude and duration of the perturbations. The aim of this study is to provide customizable and robust models that can help in the investigation of the mechanisms underlying postural control.

2 Materials and Methods

2.1 Experimental Trials with Automated Perturbation Device

Posturographic analyses have been conducted on 11 healthy subjects (age = 22.82 ± 2.18 years; weight = 62.45 ± 9.50 kg; height = 171 ± 11 cm; BMI = 21.36 ± 1.76 kg/m^2) with a custom-made prototype of an automated perturbation device (AP). Each analysis consisted in multiple perturbations with selectable impulse (i.e., time integral of the force profile) exerted to the back of the subject at a defined location between the scapulae. Due to prior research, two impulse levels, 6 Ns and 10 Ns, were considered to elicit responses of different amplitudes without running into the risk for falling or evoking step responses in any subject. The two levels were obtained by fixing the magnitude of the perturbation force at 40 N and by changing its duration between 150 ms and 250 ms. Each subject was standing on a force platform and faced in the opposite direction with respect to the operator handling the AP, to ensure the unpredictability of the perturbation. The signals recorded by the force platform were processed to estimate the center of pressure (CoP) displacement over the base of support.

The perturbation device (Fig. 1d, [10]) consisted of a double-acting linear pneumatic actuator controlled by two flow-proportional valves and was directly handled by a human operator. The accuracy, repeatability and scalability of the perturbations enabled by the device have already been discussed in previous works and proved to be adequate for this application [10, 11]. Examples of the force and CoP signals obtained during a session with a 10 Ns impulse reference are shown in Fig. 1a-b, along with a scheme of a typical trial set-up (Fig. 1c). The signals were digitally filtered (Butterworth low-pass filter, 8th order – 150 Hz cut-off frequency for the force signal, 4th order – 20 Hz for the CoP) and segmented in order to get a consistent set of data that included 5 consecutive perturbations at each impulse level.

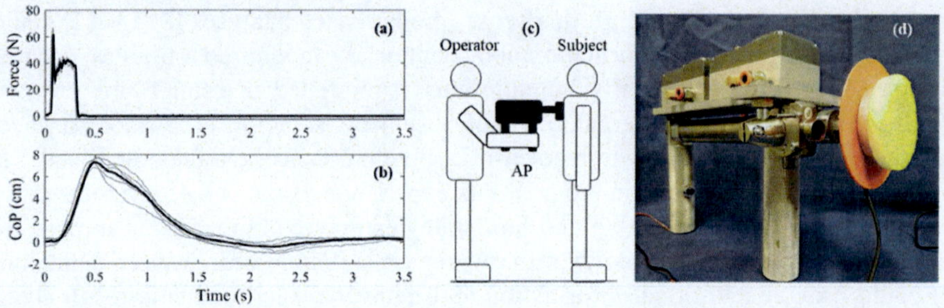

Fig. 1. Force (a) and CoP (b) signals for 10 Ns stimuli. Each plot shows 5 consecutive stimuli and the average signal in bold line. (c) Set-up of a trial, AP is the automatic perturbator (d).

2.2 Single-Link and Double-Link Inverted Pendulum Models

The segmented experimental data were used to fit two models for postural control based on inverted-pendulum formulation. A single (SIP) and a double (DIP) link models have been implemented in MATLAB-Simulink® to assess the dynamics of the human body in perturbed balance conditions. The non-linear analytical description of the plant has been considered in both cases, differently from the linearized version that is commonly used in similar works [14, 16, 17], to take into account those postural responses whose magnitude does not fall in the small displacement hypothesis. Figure 2 shows a representation of the free-body diagrams used to derive the mathematical formulation of the dynamics of both models.

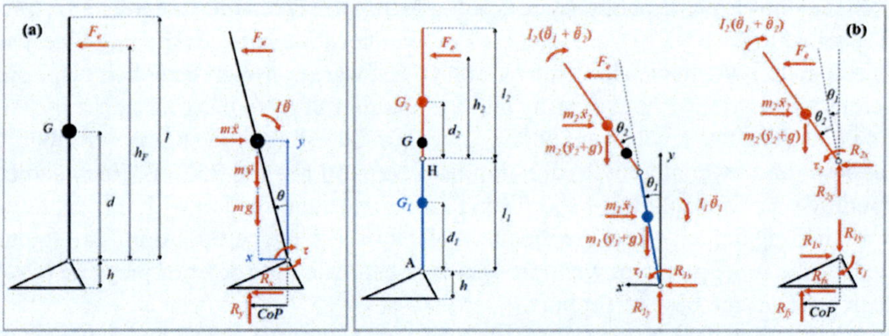

Fig. 2. Free-body diagrams for SIP (a) and DIP (b) models.

The diagrams clearly show the role of the correcting torques τ_i at each joint that are critical to achieve the stabilization of the system. Each torque has been modelled as the sum of a passive (intrinsic) and an active contribution, the former being dependent on the constraints and the visco-elastic behavior of tissues surrounding the joint, the latter being the result of the neuro-muscular control performed by the central nervous system (CNS) along with the afferences provided by the sensory systems through their respective feedback paths. In particular, the passive control can be generally described by the sum of an elastic and a viscous term, whereas the active control is often implemented as a delayed, proportional-derivative (PD) action [15, 17]. The torques included in SIP and DIP models have been implemented according to this approach, which requires the knowledge of the rotation angles and angular velocity at each joint. That information is part of the dataset that the CNS handles when posture is adjusted in quiet standing or during and after a perturbation. To account for errors in such estimation from the CNS, pink noise has been included in the model and tuned according to the literature (magnitude = $4 \cdot 10^{-3}$ rad [17]). The time delay setting for the active control action is necessary to take into account the finite response time of CNS coordinating the musculoskeletal system in the development of the postural reaction. Finally, as suggested by previous works [18], the muscle activation dynamics has been implemented by means of a second order transfer function ($\omega_n = 15.7$ rad/s, $\beta = 0.7$) in series with the neural controller to filter out the high-frequency components of the controller output that are not compatible with the dynamics of the musculoskeletal system.

Some authors suggest the adoption of a term proportional to the acceleration within the active control logic when muscle activation dynamics is considered [19, 20]. This approach has been tested in the SIP model, however it did not seem to be reasonable for the application considered. This result will be discussed later and motivated the exclusion of acceleration-related terms in the active control for the DIP model. In the latter, additional (indirect) terms considering the coupling between the two segments were added, as shown in [17], that link the torque at one joint to the rotation and angular velocity occurring at the other joint. A scheme reporting the general configuration of balance control system as implemented in the current work is presented in Fig. 3.

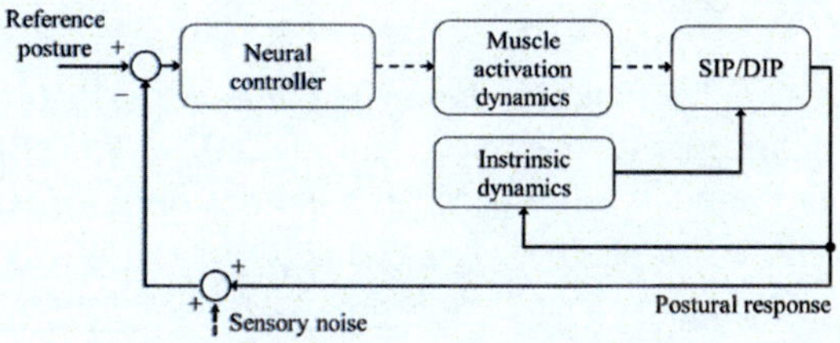

Fig. 3. Modeling of postural control system.

2.3 Parametric Identification of Balance Control Models

Optimization techniques for the parametric identification of SIP and DIP models have been investigated to achieve the best fit with the experimental dataset discussed in Sect. 2.1. A nonlinear least-squares solver (*lsqnonlin* in MATLAB®) has been selected as an adequate tradeoff between computational time and goodness of fit. This method requires an initial guess of the unknown parameters as input, that were derived from previous works [8], and it enables the possibility of setting lower and upper boundaries for each parameter. These limits were selected as large as possible to avoid over-constrained optimization, but still they helped in avoiding unrealistic sets of parameters (e.g., negative time delays) that could potentially lead to not feasible local minima of the objective function. The latter was designed as the root-mean-square error (RMSE) between the average CoP signal measured during experimentation (CoP_e) and the one predicted by the model (CoP_m).

Before the optimization could be performed, the body mass and height of each subject were used to estimate the anthropometric parameters required by the models according to the formulation presented in the literature [21]. The point of application of the perturbation was set at the same height measured during trials (T4-T5 level), while its magnitude was set equal to the force signal averaged over 5 consecutive stimuli.

Due to the different formulations, the parameters included in the optimization algorithm were different between SIP and DIP models. Regarding SIP model, the active control proportional K_p and derivative K_d terms, the time delay T_d, the acceleration-proportional gain K_a, and the passive viscous gain B were subjected to optimization, whereas the passive elastic gain K was set to the 60% of the critical stiffness of the ankle joint [22]. The same logic was applied to the DIP model, leading to the following set of parameters to optimize (1 refers to the ankle joint, 2 refers to the hip joint): the active control gains K_{p11}, K_{d11}, K_{p22}, K_{d22}; the time delays T_{d1} and T_{d2}; the passive viscous gains B_1 and B_2. The indirect terms of the active control action (K_{pij}, K_{dij}) were fixed and set according to the literature [17], while the passive elastic gains K_1 and K_2 were respectively set to the 60% and to the 100% of the respective joint critical stiffness, in agreement with the literature [22].

The optimization was performed separately for each subject and for each impulse level (6 Ns and 10 Ns). Each simulation led to an optimal set of parameters and to a corresponding value of RMSE between experimental and estimated CoP signals.

3 Results and Discussion

Figure 4a-c shows an example of the simulation outcomes on a single subject. Figure 4d shows the RMSE normalized with the maximum of CoP_e (NRMSE) for each subject and for both SIP and DIP models, considered as a metrics for goodness of fit.

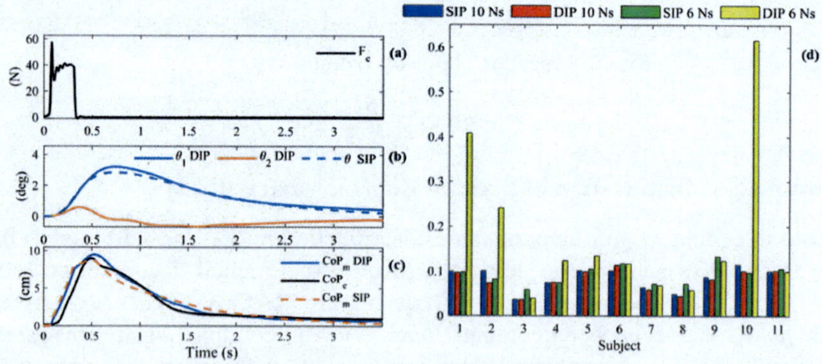

Fig. 4. Force signal (a), rotation angles (b) and CoP (c) fit for a single subject in SIP and DIP models. (d) Normalized RMSE values (NRMSE) for all subjects tested.

A qualitative assessment of fitting accuracy for a specific subject can be observed by the curves shown in Fig. 4c. In this particular case, the RMSE values obtained for both SIP and DIP models were lower than 5 mm, with the latter performing slightly better. This result was not confirmed for all the subjects as shown by data presented in Fig. 4d, since fitting for the DIP model at 6 Ns impulse level was sub-optimal for three subjects (#1, #2 and #10). This outcome may depend on multiple factors: (1) *lsqnonlin* algorithm performs local optimization, therefore the minimum of the objective function might be elsewhere; (2) low level impulse perturbations might evoke small oscillations in those subjects that compromise the usage of a double-link model. The latter hypothesis is motivated by the fact the DIP model still fits correctly in those subjects for 10 Ns perturbations. However, in-vivo data about kinematics or muscle activation would be necessary to confirm this deduction.

The values of optimized parameters obtained for both models are shown in Fig. 5.

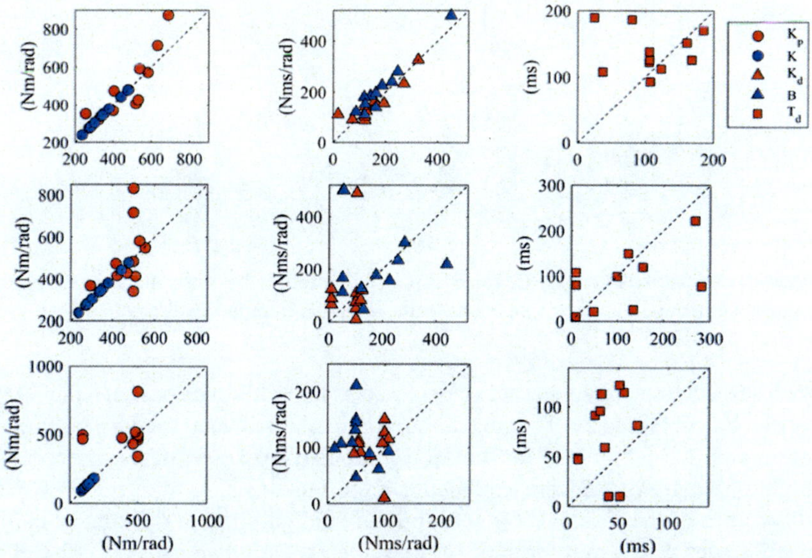

Fig. 5. Balance control parameters obtained after optimization: SIP model (top); DIP model, ankle joint (center); DIP model, hip joint (bottom). For each plot, *x*-axis presents the parameters obtained at 6 Ns, *y*-axis shows the corresponding values obtained at 10 Ns.

Only K_a (acceleration-proportional feedback in SIP model) was not included in the figure since it was forced to the lower boundary (0 Nms^2/rad) by the optimization algorithm for most of the subjects. This result is in contrast with the findings of some authors in the literature [20], however this might be explained by the significantly different features of the perturbation considered. In our work, the direct application of an impact force to the body of the subject causes a sudden increase of the body acceleration that is likely superior to the one considered in previous works. Therefore, the implementation of an acceleration-proportional feedback results in an overestimation of the control torque that does not allow accurate fit of the model. Data presented in Fig. 5 show quite a large variability of the optimized parameters among the different subjects, nonetheless they are coherent with similar results presented in the literature [8, 17, 20]. Those differences might be related to inter-subject variability and could be in some way considered for a subject-specific characterization of postural control. However, further work has to be done to assess the robustness and physical or clinical significance of these parameters.

Finally, the same set of parameters obtained at the lower level (6 Ns) was used for simulating the behavior of the system when subjected to higher impulse level (10 Ns) perturbations, to investigate the ability of each tuned model to predict the postural response without falling into unrealistic behavior or instability. Figure 6 shows the results of these simulations, in which ΔRMSE was used as an indicator of the worsening in the quality of fit.

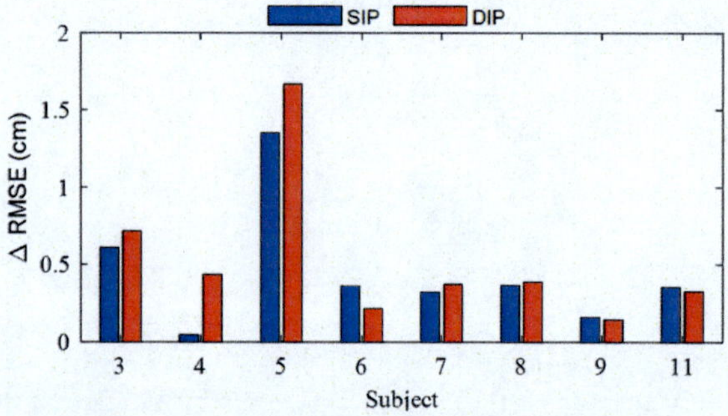

Fig. 6. Increase of residuals (ΔRMSE) for SIP and DIP models by selecting the sub-optimal configuration of control parameters. The results refer to 10 Ns impulse level.

For each subject, this parameter was calculated as the difference between the RMSE values respectively obtained by choosing the sub-optimal (estimated for the 6 Ns impulse level) and the optimal (estimated for the 10 Ns impulse level) sets of parameters. The outliers highlighted in Fig. 4d were excluded from this analysis. As shown in Fig. 6, the increased variance of the residuals for sub-optimal configuration of the control parameters was still lower than 5 mm for most of the subjects. Only two subjects (#3 and #5) showed large ΔRMSE due to significant differences between the sub-optimal and the optimal sets of control parameters provided by the algorithm. No significant difference was observed by comparing SIP and DIP results. This result provided a preliminary validation of the methodology and confirmed that both models, after tuning, were able to predict the postural response with a good level of accuracy for most of the subjects considered.

4 Conclusion

This work showed the application of a nonlinear optimization technique to parametric identification of postural control models. Those were fit to experimental data obtained during dynamic posturographic analyses performed with a custom-made automated perturbation device, which was able to exert perturbations with controlled impulse level. The accuracy of fitting was good for most of the subjects tested, leading to a preliminary validation of the methodology and to a set of optimized models that could effectively predict the postural reactions in terms of CoP displacement over the base of support.

Compared to the previous work from the authors [11], the muscle activation dynamics implementation allowed for smoother CoP behavior in line with the measured signal, whose component frequencies are less than 20 Hz. Moreover, the identification of passive elastic and viscous gains unique for each subject allows for taking into account the influence of the anthropometric characteristics within the passive contribution. In this way, the active contribution should be influenced just by different postural control strategies. Finally, a double-link model has been developed to consider a hip strategy that could play a significant role, especially in response to greater impulses.

However, neither SIP nor DIP model has proven to be indisputably optimal in terms of quality of fitting, hence their suitability to predict the correct behavior of postural control system remains under discussion. Of course, they allow for different observations since kinematics and dynamics variables refer to systems with single (SIP) or multiple (DIP) degrees of freedom. Therefore, the choice of the optimal model surely depends on the entity of the research questions to be answered.

Parametrized models of balance control can help in the investigation of the mechanisms and strategies developed to maintain the equilibrium, due to the simplified yet detailed description they allow of postural control system. The implementation of optimized postural control models can support the physical interpretation of parameters collected by experimentation (as the maximum CoP displacement, or the latency between perturbation and response) and improve the understanding of how those parameters are influenced by the characteristics of the subjects in a wider scenario than the one that can be feasibly investigated with experimental trials.

However, it is fundamental to obtain good fitting with experimental data to consider a model reliable and accurate enough. In this sense the outcomes of our study are promising but, to further improve the quality of the results, future work should consider: (1) adding sensory feedback pathways to the models; (2) implementing more sophisticated models for neural controller, as suggested by recent literature [23, 24]; (3) testing global optimization techniques to improve the goodness of fit; (4) expanding the experimental dataset.

References

1. Loram, I., Lakie, M.: Direct measurement human ankle stiffness during quiet standing: the intrinsic mechanical stiffness is insufficient for stability in most subjects. J. Physiol. **545**(3), 1041–1053 (2002). https://doi.org/10.1113/jphysiol.2002.025049
2. Casadio, M., et al.: Direct measurement of ankle stiffness during quiet standing: implications for control modelling and clinical application. Gait Posture **21**(4), 410–424 (2005). https://doi.org/10.1016/j.gaitpost.2004.05.005
3. Vlutters, M., et al.: Direct measurement of the intrinsic ankle stiffness during standing. J. Biomech. **48**(7), 1258–1263 (2015). https://doi.org/10.1016/j.jbiomech.2015.03.004
4. Diener, H.C., et al.: Influence of stimulus parameters on human postural responses. J Neurophysiol **59**(6), 1888–1905 (1988). https://doi.org/10.1152/jn.1988.59.6.1888
5. Potocanac, Z., et al.: A robotic system for delivering novel real-time, movement dependent perturbations. Gait Posture **58**, 386–389 (2017). https://doi.org/10.1016/j.gaitpost.2017.08.038

6. Robinson, C.J., et al.: Design, control, and characterization of a sliding linear investigative platform for analyzing lower limb stability (SLIP-FALLS). IEEE Trans. Rehabil. Eng. **6**(3), 334–350 (1998). https://doi.org/10.1109/86.712232
7. Grassi, L., et al.: Quantification of postural stability in minimally disabled multiple sclerosis patients by means of dynamic posturography: an observational study. J. Neuroeng. Rehabil. **14**, 4 (2017). https://doi.org/10.1186/s12984-016-0216-8
8. Davidson, B.S., et al.: Neural control of posture during small magnitude perturbations: effects of aging and local-ized muscle fatigue. IEEE Trans. Biomed. Eng. **58**(6), 1546–1554 (2011). https://doi.org/10.1109/tbme.2010.2095500
9. Martinelli, A.R., Coelho, D.B., Magalhães, F.H., Kohn, A.F., Teixeira, L.A.: Light touch modulates balance recovery following perturbation: from fast response to stance restabilization. Exp. Brain Res. **233**(5), 1399–1408 (2015). https://doi.org/10.1007/s00221-015-4214-z
10. Maffiodo, D., et al.: Pneumo-tronic Perturbator for the Study of Human Postural Responses. In: Berns, K., Görges, D. (eds.) RAAD 2019. AISC, vol. 980, pp. 374–383. Springer, Cham (2020). https://doi.org/10.1007/978-3-030-19648-6_43
11. Paterna, M., et al.: Center of pressure displacement due to graded controlled perturbations to the trunk in standing subjects: the force–impulse paradigm. Eur. J. Appl. Physiol. **122**(2), 425–435 (2021). https://doi.org/10.1007/s00421-021-04844-9
12. Pacheco Quiñones, D., et al.: Automatic electromechanical perturbator for postural control analysis based on model predictive control. Appl. Sci. **11**(9), 4090 (2021). https://doi.org/10.3390/app11094090
13. Dvir, Z., et al.: Linearity and repeatability of postural responses in relation to peak force and impulse of manually delivered perturbations: a preliminary study. Eur. J. Appl. Physiol. **120**(6), 1319–1330 (2020). https://doi.org/10.1007/s00421-020-04364-y
14. Peterka, R.J.: Sensorimotor Integration in Human Postural Control. J Neurophysiol **88**, 1097–1118 (2002). http://dx.doi.org/10.1152/jn.00605.2001
15. van der Kooij, H., et al.: Comparison of different methods to identify and quantify balance control. J. Neurosci. Methods **145**, 175–203 (2005). https://doi.org/10.1016/j.jneumeth.2005.01.003
16. van der Kooij, H., Peterka, R.J.: Non-linear stimulus-response behavior of the human stance control system is predicted by optimization of a system with sensory and motor noise. J Comput Neurosci **30**, 759–778 (2011). https://doi.org/10.1007/s10827-010-0291-y
17. Goodworth, A.D., Peterka, R.J.: Identifying mechanisms of stance control: a single stimulus multiple output model-fit approach. J. Neurosci. Methods **296**, 44–56 (2018). https://doi.org/10.1016/j.jneumeth.2017.12.015
18. Pasma, J.H., et al.: Changes in sensory reweighting of proprioceptive information during standing balance with age and disease. J Neurophysiol **114**, 3220–3233 (2015). https://doi.org/10.1152/jn.00414.2015
19. Welch, T.D.J., Ting, L.H.: A feedback model reproduces muscle activity during human postural responses to support-surface translations. J Neurophysiol **99**, 1032–1038 (2008). https://doi.org/10.1152/jn.01110.2007
20. Pasma, J.H., et al.: Assessment of the underlying systems involved in standing balance: the additional value of electromyography in system identification and parameter estimation. J. Neuroeng. Rehabil. **14**, 97 (2017). https://doi.org/10.1186/s12984-017-0299-x
21. Winter, D.A.: Biomechanics and Motor Control of Human Movement, Fourth Edition. John Wiley and Sons, pp. 1–370 (2009)
22. Morasso, P., et al.: Quiet standing: the single inverted pendulum model is not so bad after all. PLoS ONE **14**(3), e0213870 (2019). https://doi.org/10.1371/journal.pone.0213870
23. Mengarelli, A., et al.: A Sliding Mode Control Model for Perturbed Upright Stance in Healthy Subjects. In: Lhotska, L., Sukupova, L., Lacković, I., Ibbott, G.S. (eds.) World Congress on

Medical Physics and Biomedical Engineering 2018. IP, vol. 68/2, pp. 719–724. Springer, Singapore (2019). https://doi.org/10.1007/978-981-10-9038-7_133
24. Wang, H., van den Bogert, A.J.: Identification of postural controllers in human standing balance. J. Biomech. Eng. **143**(4), 041001 (2021). https://doi.org/10.1115/1.4049159

Nonlinear Dynamics Used to Study the Influence of Treadmill Speed and Incline on the Human Hip Stability

Daniela Tarnita[1](✉), Ionut Geonea[1], Marius Georgescu[1], Dan B. Marghitu[2], Gabriela Marinache[1], and Danut-Nicolae Tarnita[3]

[1] Faculty of Mechanics, University of Craiova, Craiova, Romania
daniela.tarnita@edu.ucv.ro
[2] Department of Mechanical Engineering, Auburn University, Auburn, USA
[3] University of Medicine and Pharmacy, Craiova, Romania

Abstract. This study uses the tools of nonlinear dynamics and the maximum Lyapunov exponents (LEs) are estimated to measure quantify the human hip stability starting from the experimental data of both hips' flexion-extension (fl-ext) angle and abduction-adduction (abd-add) angle of 6 healthy subjects (HS) and 5 patients (P) affected by the osteoarthritis of knee. HS performed 9 walking tests on treadmill (TM) with 3 speeds and 3 incline angles, while the patients performed 3 walking tests on plane TM, before surgery (BS) and two months after surgery (AS). Rosenstein-Kantz algorithm and TISEAN software are used to analyze the 336 collected time series with methods and tools of nonlinear dynamics.

Keywords: human hip · walking tests · treadmill · Lyapunov exponents · stability

1 Introduction

Gait stability represents the individual's ability to maintain a functional gait even if small kinematic disturbances or control errors occur [1]. Walking is a daily dynamic activity, and its instability constitutes a high risk of falling. Among the elderly population, falls occur as the effects of several factors, like: osteoarthritis, stroke, Parkinson's disease, obstacles or slopes [2-5]. Statistics show that worldwide, one in three people over 65 falls at least once a year [5, 6]. The instability of an individual can be caused by musculoskeletal disorders and one of the frequently met cause is osteoarthritis, which involves a degenerative process of joints' cartilages leading to their loss [6]. Aspects regarding the variability, stability of gait and the risk of falling in patients affected by osteoarthritis have been addressed in previous scientific articles [6-9]. In the last stage of the disease, a total joint replacement is usually required, reducing pain and increasing mobility and improving the quality of life [9]. Because of a greater risk of falling, for individuals with unstable gait it's important to quantify dynamic local stability during walking, using nonlinear dynamic tools, as researchers showed in [10-16].

D. Tarnita et al. (Eds.): MESROB 2023, MMS 133, pp. 238–250, 2023.
https://doi.org/10.1007/978-3-031-32446-8_26

Chaoticity has been observed and studied in several biomedical fields, particularly highlighting electrocardiogram to the identification and examination of cardiac disorders [17], electroencephalogram signals and kinematic gait data [14, 18, 19].

The evaluation of the chaotic behavior of the joints of the lower legs during walking can be done by quantifying the local dynamic stability during walking, that is the degree of resistance of the walking control to infinitesimally small perturbations that manifest as natural kinematic variability [1, 10, 11]. These perturbations, which cause step-to-step differences in kinematic measurements, can be attenuated by the musculoskeletal system to maintain a stable gait pattern [1].

In this paper, the stability of the human hip joint is quantified with help of LE-s, which are estimated based on the experimental time series of the hip fl-ext angle and abd-add angle of 6 HS walking on plane and inclined TM with 3 different speeds and 3 different incline angles, and of 5 patients suffering of knee osteoarthritis walking on plane TM with 3 speeds.

2 Experimental Protocol

Experimental Tests. The subjects performed nine walking tests on TM at different speeds and inclines, while the patients performed only first three experimental tests (T1, T2 and T3) in two different stages: one day before osteoarthritic knee surgery (**BS**) and, respectively, two months after knee surgery (**AS**). A total number of 336 experimental time series from which: 216 series of subjects (9 tests*2 hips*2 planes*6 subjects) and 120 series (3 tests*2 hips*2 planes*2 stages*5) of patients were collected and processed.

Subjects. A group of 6 healthy subjects and a group of 5 patients suffering of knee osteoarthritis were selected for the present study. All the 9 tests were performed by HS in the Biomechanics Research Laboratory of the University of Craiova, while the patients performed the walking tests, before and after surgery, at the Emergency Hospital of Dolj County (Table 1).

Table 1. Experimental tests performed by the subjects

Test name	T1	T2	T3	T4	T5	T6	T7	T8	T9
Speed [Km/h]	2,5	5	7,5	2,5	5	7,5	2,5	5	7,5
Incline [degrees]	0	0	0	7	7	7	11	11	11

Equipment. The biomechanical time series were acquired and processed by using Biometrics system [20], usually found in research, as equipment based on wearable sensors, in fields like: biomechanics, biomedical engineering, movement analysis, clinical rehabilitation and sports [4, 6, 8, 21-25]. Two twin electrogiometers SG 150 were mounted on the both hips of each participant in experimental tests, in order to acquire, at a frequency of 500 Hz, synchronized biomechanical data of fl-ext angles in the sagittal plane and of abd-add angles in the frontal plane. The subjects agreed and they had written their consent to participate in the experiment. The Ethics Committee of the University of Craiova approved all tests (Fig. 1).

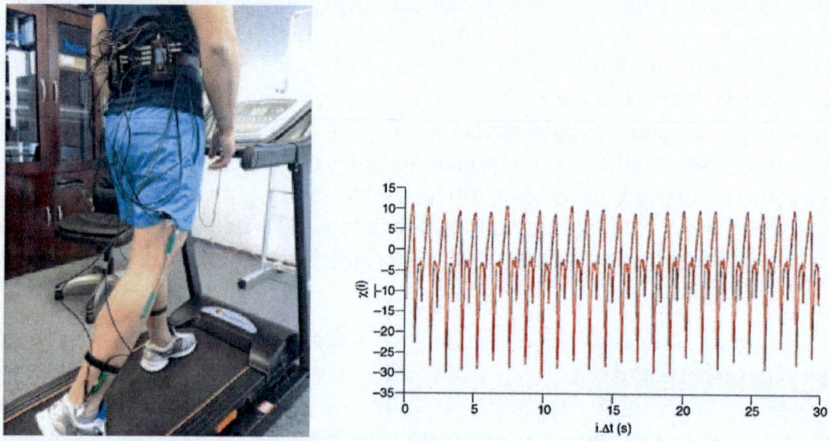

a) b)

Fig. 1. Acquisition system mounted on a subject during experimental test and Kinematic data series representing the variation of the fl-ext angle of hip - Subject1, Test T1.

In Table 2 the anthropometric data of healthy subjects and patients samples is presented.

Table 2. Healthy subjects' and patients' average anthropometric data

	Age [years]	Weight [kg]	Height [cm]	Leg length [cm]
Subjects	32,5	80,00	187	95,7
Patients	65,2	67,4	163	81,3

3 Nonlinear Dynamic Analysis

3.1 State Space Reconstruction (SSR)

Determination of SSR Parameters. To estimate the local dynamic stability of the human hip joint, LEs must be calculated based on experimental data series collected in both planes from all participants in the experiment. The first step in nonlinear time series analysis involves the appropriate SSR from the collected biomechanical data to estimate the invariant properties of the embedded attractor. It has been shown in previous research that a correctly SSR is topologically identical to the original state space and many of its important properties, such as the LEs of a trajectory, are preserved. The parameters of the SSR (time delay and reconstruction dimension) must be first estimated for each of the 336 time series.

Time Delay Selection. When the time delay, T, is selected to be used for SSR it is very important that, for very small T, X(t) must be very similar to X(t + T). Thus, the coordinates m in each of the delay vectors are highly correlated, which makes the embedded dynamics to be found near the main diagonal of the SSR. The most known and used method of SSR is the *Method of delays* [26]. For choosing an appropriate T for each collected and analyzed time series, the *mutual* routine from the TISEAN package [27], which implements the *Average Mutual Information* (AMI) method [28], is used. AMI states that an adequate choice for *T* is the one that, given *X(t)*, it provides new information with measurement *X(t + T)*. An example of plots of AMI is shown in Fig. 2.

To obtain SSR of human hip joint's dynamical system, the vectors constituted from T values of a single measured time series were used to create a trajectory in the new space:

$$x_n = \{s(t_0 + nT_s), s(t_0 + nT_s + T), \ldots, s(t_0 + nT_s + (m - 1)T\}; \quad (1)$$

where *m* is the embedding dimension, s(.) is a measured scalar function, *Ts* is the sampling time, $n = 1,.., m$ and $T = dT_s$ is a good chosen T [29].

Embedding Dimension Selection. To estimate the embedding dimension (m), the False Nearest Neighbor (FNN) method [30], one of the most known methods for determining the minimal sufficient m, is used. The criterion that shows that m is adequate is when the fraction of FNN is close to zero, or at least is sufficiently small (in this case, m is chosen for a percentage of FNN falls below 10%). The FNN routine from the TISEAN package is used to determine m.

Plots of *FNN* of the left hip fl-ext Subject 4, T2 are graphically represented in Fig. 2b).

Phase-plane portraits are two-dimensional state spaces, having as axes the time derivative ϕ'(deg/s) (on ordinate) and, respectively, ϕ (deg) (on abscissa). In Fig. 3, the phase plane portraits of the left hip time-series corresponding to each test performed by Subject 5 are shown. Similar graphs are obtained for HS and patients for all time series. Phase plane portraits are usually used to compare the kinematics of Healthy Subjects' joints with patients' joints or to compare the kinematics of a joint, depending on different parameters.

In Fig. 4, 3D-Plots of SSR of fl-ext left hip of Subject 5 (Test 7) and Patient 3 (Test 1) time-series are shown.

It can be seen that the graphs corresponding to HS show small divergence of their trajectories, confined to a narrower space, compared to those of the patients. Phase plane curves and reconstructed state spaces are more compact for subjects than for patients whose curves are more divergent and do not overlap.

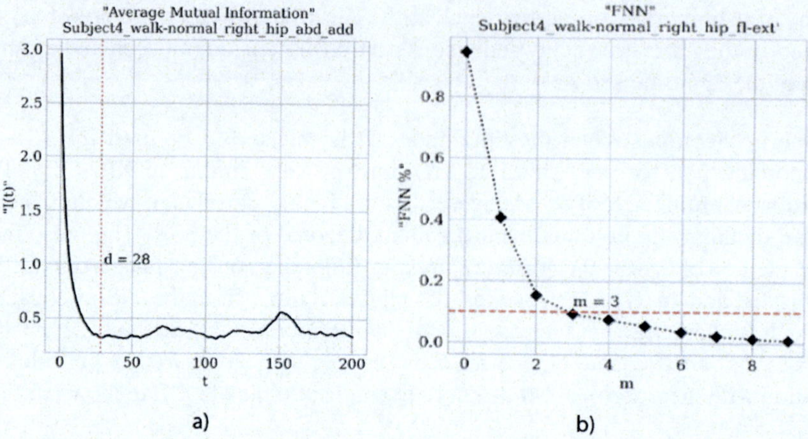

Fig. 2. a) Plots of AMI function of the abd-add; b) Plots of FNN of the fl-ext - right hip, Subject 4, Test T2.

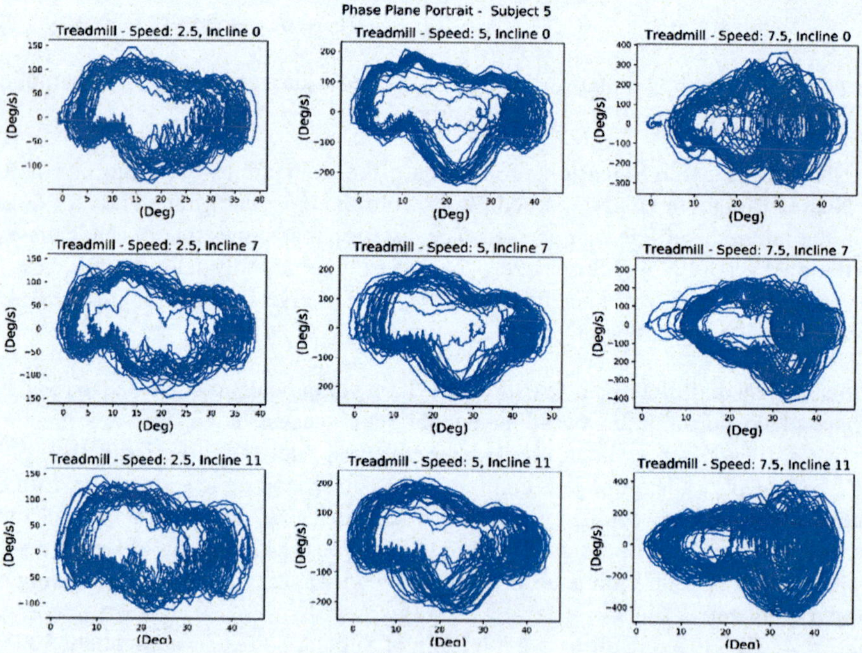

Fig. 3. Phase-plane plots of the left hip time-series of Subject 5 for each test.

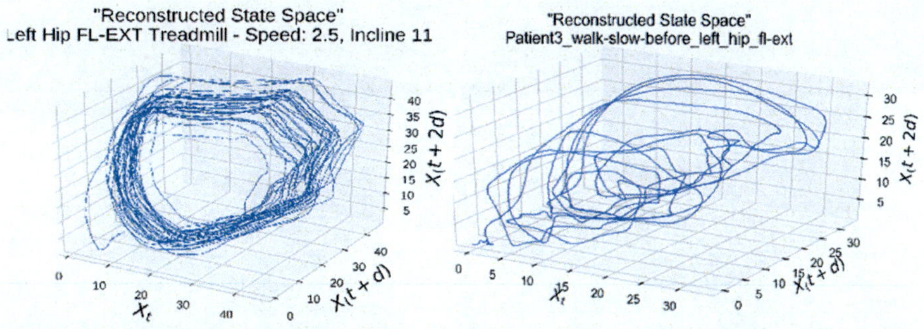

Fig. 4. 3D-Plots of SSR of the left hip time-series measured on: a) T7- Subject 5; b)T1-Patient 3.

Lyapunov Exponents. To estimate the LEs, we used the Rosenstein-Kantz algorithm [31] which monitors the average distance between the reference point and a set of neighbors. It selects N reference points (states) in the SSR, and for each of them it identifies all neighbors such that the distance between them and the reference point is less than ε. Tracks the reference point and all neighbors for some distance in time τ and averages the neighbors' distances from the reference point until it is greater than ε. Then choose a new reference point and repeat the procedure described above until the end of the trajectory. If $\delta(0) = \delta_o$ is a small initial perturbation from the initial condition, the space state vector is defined by:

$$x_n = x_0 + \delta_o \tag{2}$$

The exponential rate of expansion or contraction, which means stability, or instability, respectively, defines the LEs, for a correct value of δ_o:

$$LE_i = \lim_{t \to \infty} \frac{1}{t} \ln\left(\frac{\|\delta(t)\|}{\|\delta_0\|}\right) \tag{3}$$

where ||.|| represents the vector norm operator [29].

For a state space with 3 dimensions, there will be an exponent for each dimension: all negative exponents will indicate the presence of a fixed point; one zero and the other negative indicate a limit cycle; for at least one positive LE and for a purely deterministic system, then the system is "chaotic", indicating a chaotic attractor. In order to be able to analyze the effect of speeds and incline of the TM on the walking stability in the dynamic nonlinear analysis, the LEs were estimated for all 336 time series, based on TISEAN soft. The graphs of mean curves of logarithmic divergence corresponding to the nine fl-ext time-series of left hip collected from Subject 5 are plotted in Fig. 5.

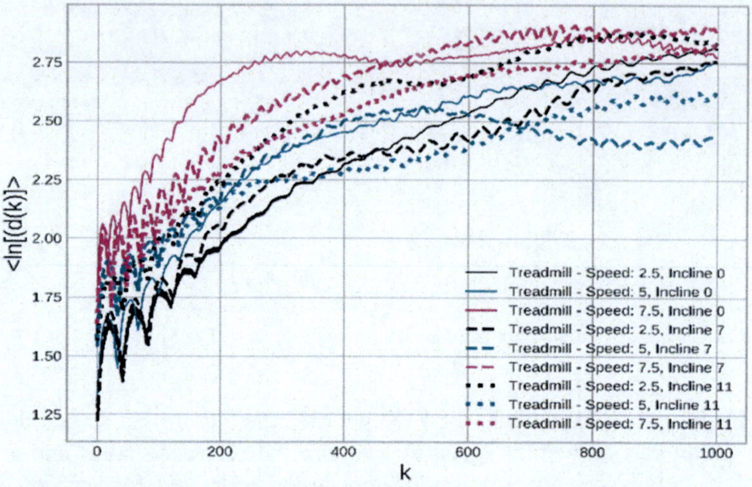

Fig. 5. Average fl-ext time-series logarithmic divergence < [ln[d(k)]] left hip–all tests, Subject 5.

4 Results

Table 3 and Fig. 6 show the average values of LEs, corresponding to the 216 time series collected in all experimental tests performed by healthy subjects. For fl-ext in sagittal plane, the values of LEs varied from 0.228 to 0.338, while for the movement in the frontal plane, the values of LEs varied from 0.251 to 0.349 so the values are bigger for the movement in frontal plane than the one in the sagittal plane.

Table 3. Average values of LEs corresponding to the hip at the level of the subjects' sample.

Angle	Incline	Speed [km/h]	Left Hip	Right Hip
abd-add	0 deg	2.5	0.343	0.375
		5	0.336	0.343
		7.5	0.349	0.381
	7 deg	2.5	0.302	0.327
		5	0.275	0.284
		7.5	0.298	0.295
	11 deg	2.5	0.286	0.298
		5	0.251	0.255
		7.5	0.290	0.292
fl-ext	0 deg	2.5	0.338	0.331

(continued)

Table 3. (*continued*)

Angle	Incline	Speed [km/h]	Left Hip	Right Hip
		5	0.309	0.325
		7.5	0.326	0.337
	7 deg	2.5	0.290	0.324
		5	0.228	0.247
		7.5	0.291	0.275
	11 deg	2.5	0.309	0.331
		5	0.227	0.245
		7.5	0.233	0.257

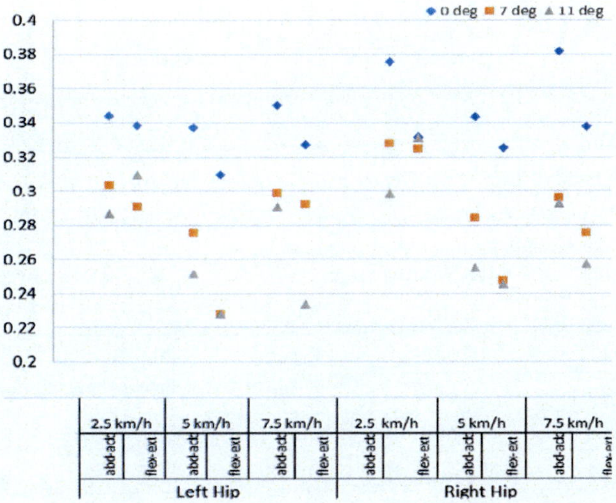

Fig. 6. Graph of average values of LEs for the entire sample of subjects for each test.

Figure 7 a) and b) show the average values of the Les related to the frontal and lateral movement of both hips of the subjects'sample for each incline and speed, respectively.

În Table 4 and Fig. 8 the mean values of LEs obtained for the three tests performed by patients before surgery (BS) and, respectively, after surgery (AS) are presented.

It can be seen that the patients obtained, on average, higher values for the hip joint of the leg affected by osteoarthritis (left) compared to the hip joint of the healthy leg (right). In plus, the values of the LEs computed for the both hip joints before surgery varied in the interval [0.671, 0.872] for the osteoarhritic leg and in [0.522, 0.755] for the healthy leg, beeing higher than the values obtained for the hip joints after total replacement surgery, which varied in the interval [0.318–0.629] for the hip of the affected leg and in [0.211–0.430] for the hip of the other leg.

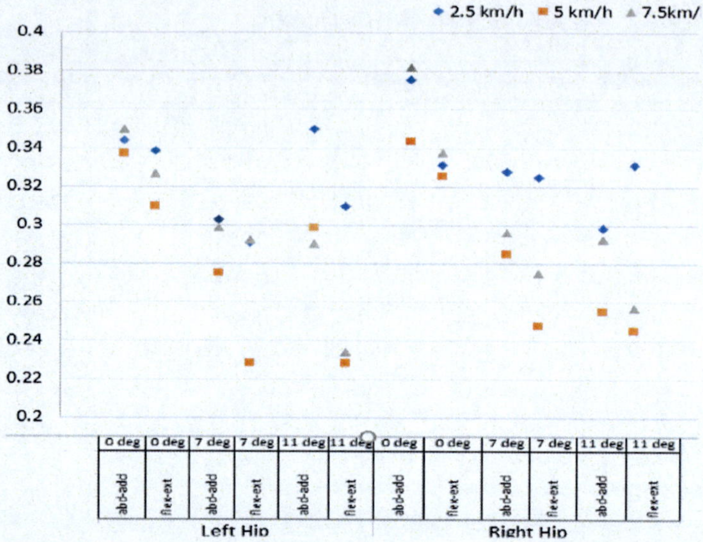

Fig. 7. Average values of LEs for entire subjects' sample a) for each incline; b) for each speed.

Table 4. Average values of LEs for patients' sample before surgery and after surgery, for both movements.

Test	Angle	AS (after surgery)		BS (before surgery)	
		Left	Right	Left	Right
T1	fl-ext	0.558	0.348	0.683	0.688
	abd-add	0.629	0.430	0.872	0.755
T2	fl-ext	0.579	0.211	0.671	0.560
	abd-add	0.404	0.338	0.829	0.645
T3	fl-ext	0.377	0.312	0.696	0.522
	abd-add	0.318	0.343	0.711	0.549

In Fig. 9, comparative plots of average LEs computed for both movements of both hips of patients and subjects (all tests) are shown.

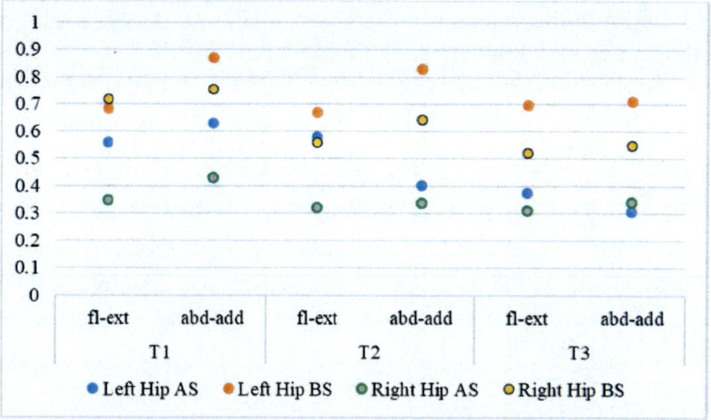

Fig. 8. Average values of LEs all tests for patients' sample Before (BS) and After surgery (AS)

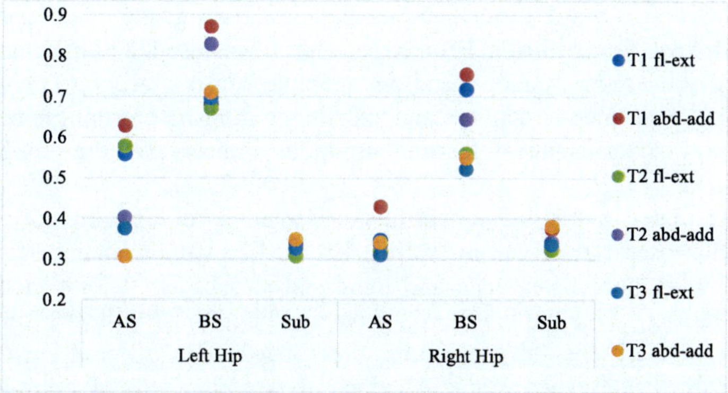

Fig. 9. Comparative plots of average LEs obtained for subjects and patients (BS and AS).

5 Discussions

All values obtained for LEs of both subjects and patients were positive values suggesting that human joint movements exhibit chaotic characteristics, On average, for all walking tests and for both samples, the highest values were obtained for T1 test for abd-add. For the leg affected by osteoarthritis the values are higher than those obtained on the other leg of the patients. These can be explained by the influence of pain, but also of the change in the integrity of the joint. From Fig. 6, it can be seen that for each individual walking speed, the subjects obtained on average lower values as the inclination increases. In general, for each test, the higher values are those in the frontal plane, and the lower ones are those in the sagittal plane.

The average values of LEs obtained for the sample of HS ranged from 0.379 to 0.796. From Fig. 7 we can see that, in general, lower values were obtained for walking at a normal speed of 5 km/h, values between 0.253 and 0.349, compared to walking at a reduced or fast speed. The highest values are obtained for 2.5 km/h. For walking with a speed equal to 2.5 km/h the values vary between 0.279 and 0.429, while for walking with 7.5 km/h the values vary between 0.257 and 0.482.

For T1, T2 and T3 tests, the average values of LEs of the subjects were lower compared to the values of the patients, both before and after the operation. Also, the average values of LEs in the two planes, frontal (abd-add) and sagittal (fl-ext), of the patients before surgery were higher than those obtained after the surgical intervention. They vary between 0.327 and 0.513, being lower than those of patients, which vary between 0.589 and 0.989 before surgery and between 0.291 and 0.601 after surgery.

For T1, T2 and T3 tests, the average values of LEs for the right hip, that of the non-operated leg, were lower, varying between 0.542 and 0.643, than for the left hip, varying between 0.657 and 0.989.

6 Conclusions

In this study, 336 time series corresponding to both hip joints were collected in 9 experimental tests on the treadmill, processed and analyzed for a group of HS and a group of patients with knee osteoarthritis. Biometrics system was used, a biomechanical data acquisition and processing system based on wearable sensors, accurate performance, easy to use. The experimental data are analyzed using the LEs of both movements (in sagittal plane and frontal plane) in the human hip, as a measure of the stability of hip dynamical system.

The LEs calculated in this study quantified the sensitivity of hip joint motion to local perturbations that characterize gait instability. Higher LEs values obtained for patients are associated with more divergence and increased variability of joint motion, with higher risk of falling, while the lower values obtained by the HS reflect local stability, small divergence, small sensitivity to perturbations. The results are similar to the results reported in previously published articles. Hip flexion-extension and abduction-adduction movements during locomotion are important for the study of the bipedal locomotion applied to humanoid robots, to measure the balance control of human walking. The results can be used for future work to compare normal and abnormal hip joint motion, to develop devices for rehabilitation, or in bio-inspired robots, to study the complex process of locomotion. The quantification of dynamic gait stability is extremely important for the evaluation and monitoring of people who present a higher risk of falling. For the future work, we propose to apply this type of analysis to the time series collected for the evaluation of walking disorders caused by other types of neurological or musculoskeletal disorders, taking into account other additional parameters, such as the size of the correlation and the approximate entropy.

References

1. England, S.A., Granata, K.P.: The influence of gait speed on local dynamic stability of walking. Gait Posture **25**, 172–178 (2007)
2. Hausdorff, J.M.: Gait dynamics, fractals and falls: finding meaning in the stride-to-stride fluctuations of human walking. Hum. Mov. Sci. **26**(4), 555–589 (2007)

3. Kannus, P.: Prevention of falls and consequent injuries in elderly people. Lancet **366**(9500), 1885–1893 (2005)
4. Kronfol, N.: Biological, medical and behavioral risk factors on falls. World Health Organisation (2012). http://www.who.int/ageing/project/falls_prevention_older_age/en/inded.html
5. Haawley Hauge, H.: Older adults' perceptions of technologies aimed at falls prevention, detection or monitoring: a systematic review. Int. J. Med. Inform. **83**(6), 416–426 (2014)
6. Tarnita, D., Marghitu, D.: Nonlinear dynamics of normal and osteoarthritic human knee. Proc. Rom. Acad. **18**(4), 353–360 (2017)
7. Gustafson, J.A.: Alterations in walking knee joint stiffness in individuals with knee osteoarthritis and self-reported knee instability. Gait Posture **43**, 210–215 (2016)
8. Pisla, D., Tarnita, D., et al.: A parallel robot with torque monitoring for brachial monoparesis rehabilitation tasks. Appl. Sci. **11**, 9932 (2021)
9. Yakhdani, H.R.F.: Stability and variability of knee kinematics during gait in knee osteoarthritis before and after replacement surgery. Clin. Biomech. **25**(3), 230–236 (2010)
10. Dingwell, J.B., et al.: Local dynamic stability versus kinematic variability of continuous overground and treadmill walking. J. Biomech. Eng. Transact ASME **123**, 27–32 (2001)
11. Dingwell, J., Cusumano, J.: Nonlinear time series analysis of normal and pathological human walking. Chaos **10**, 848–863 (2001)
12. Tarnita, D., Georgescu, M., Tarnita, D.N.: Application of nonlinear dynamics to human knee movement on plane and inclined treadmill. In: Wenger, P., Chevallereau, C., Pisla, D., Bleuler, H., Rodić, A. (eds.) New Trends in Medical and Service Robots, vol. 39, pp. 59–73. Springer, Cham (2016). https://doi.org/10.1007/978-3-319-30674-2_5
13. Georgescu, M., et al.: Analysis of human hip movement using nonlinear time-series analysis methods. Acta Technica Napocensis: Appl. Math. Mech. Eng. **64**(1-S2) (2021)
14. Terrier, P., Deriaz, O.: Kinematic variability, fractal dynamics and local dynamic stability of treadmill walking. J. Neuroeng. Rehabil. **8**, 12 (2011)
15. Broomhead, D.S., King, G.P.: Extracting qualitative dynamics from experimental data. Physica D. **20**, 217–236 (1986)
16. Bradley, E., Kantz, H.: Nonlinear time-series analysis revisited. Chaos **25**(9) (2015)
17. Chen, Ch.-K., Lin, Ch.-L., Chiu, Y.-M.: Individual identification based on chaotic electrocardiogram signals. In: 6th IEEE Conference on Industrial Electronics and Applications, pp. 1765–1770 (2011)
18. Josiński, H., Michalczuk, A., Świtoński, A., Mucha, R., Wojciechowski, K.: Quantifying chaotic behavior in treadmill walking. In: Nguyen, N.T., Trawiński, B., Kosala, R. (eds.) ACIIDS 2015. LNCS (LNAI), vol. 9012, pp. 317–326. Springer, Cham (2015). https://doi.org/10.1007/978-3-319-15705-4_31
19. Cohen, M.E.: Chaos. Wiley Encyclopedia of Biomedical Engineering (2006)
20. Biometrics LTD. www.biometricsltd.com. https://www.biometricsltd.com/
21. Tarnita, D., Berceanu, C., Tarnita, C.: The three-dimensional printing–a modern technology used for biomedical prototypes. Materiale Plastice **47**(3), 328–334 (2010)
22. Geonea, I.D., et al.: Dynamic analysis of a spherical parallel robot used for brachial monoparesis rehabilitation. Appl. Sci. **11**, 11849 (2021)
23. Tarnita, D., Geonea, I., Petcu, A.: Experimental human walking and virtual simulation of rehabilitation on plane and inclined treadmill. In: Herisanu, N., Marinca, V. (eds.) Acoustics and Vibration of Mechanical Structures—AVMS-2017. SPP, vol. 198, pp. 149–155. Springer, Cham (2018). https://doi.org/10.1007/978-3-319-69823-6_18
24. Tarniţă, D., Geonea, I., Petcu, A., Tarniţă, D.-N.: Experimental characterization of human walking on stairs applied to humanoid dynamics. In: Rodić, A., Borangiu, T. (eds.) RAAD 2016. AISC, vol. 540, pp. 293–301. Springer, Cham (2017). https://doi.org/10.1007/978-3-319-49058-8_32

25. Tarnita, D., Geonea, I., Petcu, A., Tarnita, D.N.: Numerical simulations and experimental human gait analysis using wearable sensors. In: Husty, M., Hofbaur, M. (eds.) MESROB 2016. MMS, vol. 48, pp. 289–304. Springer, Cham (2018). https://doi.org/10.1007/978-3-319-59972-4_21
26. Takens, F.: Detecting strange attractors in turbulence. In: Rand, D., Young, L.S. (eds.) Dynamical Systems and Turbulence, pp. 366–381. Springer, Heidelberg (1981). https://doi.org/10.1007/BFb0091924
27. Hegger, R., Kantz, H.: Practical implementation of nonlinear time series methods: the TISEAN package. Chaos Interdisc. J. Nonlinear Sci. **9**(2), 413–415 (1999)
28. Fraser, A.M., Swinney, H.L.: Independent coordinates for strange attractors from mutual information. Phys. Rev. A **33**, 1134–1140 (1986)
29. Packard, N.H., Crutchfield, J.P., Farmer, J.D., Shaw, R.S.: Geometry from a time series. Phys. Rev. Lett. **45**, 712–716 (1980)
30. Kennel, M.B., Brown, R., Abarbanel, H.D.I.: Determining minimum embedding dimension using a geometrical construction. Phys. Rev. A **45**, 3403–3411 (1992)
31. Rosenstein, M.T., Collins, I.J., Deluca, C.J.: A practical method for calculating largest Lyapunov exponents from small data sets. Phys. D **65**, 117–134 (1993)

Numerical Analysis of a Testbed Used for Liver Tissue of Biomechanical Behavior

A. Y. Prieto-Vázquez[1], L. A. Guerrero-Hernández[1], E. Gomez-Apo[2], and C. R. Torres-San Miguel[1](✉)

[1] Instituto Politécnico Nacional, Escuela Superior de Ingeniería Mecánica y Eléctrica, Sección de Estudios de Posgrado e Investigación, Unidad Zacatenco Edificio, 07738 Ciudad México, Mexico
{aprietov1000,lguerreroh1300}@alumno.ipn.mx, ctorress@ipn.mx
[2] Hospital General de México, Jefatura de Patología Post-Mortem, 06720 Ciudad de México, Mexico

Abstract. This work presents a system for evaluating the mechanical properties of liver tissue. This system is composed of a three-stage mechanism. The first stage consists of an epicyclic gear train. The second stage consists of bevel gears and a rack and pinion system. The three stages generate the conversion from rotary to linear motion at four points. The system can generate a compression load on the surface of a liver tissue sample. Results show the deformation and displacement values of the components of the testbed.

Keywords: Biomechanics · Liver tissue testbed · FEM

1 Introduction

The analysis of the mechanical behavior of biological tissues represents a high degree of complexity. Tissues are a fundamental part of every living being. The mechanics of the continuous medium gives us a concept that encompasses that a material has specific properties that depend on its structure and internal composition. In the literature, it is found that tissues are composed entirely of collagen fibers and elastin, which form interlocking systems. In addition, the tissues have a coating or layer of proteoglycans. This layer has a specific function to cover the tissue [1]. Analyze the relationship between tissue leads' biological and mechanical behavior depending on how it is organized internally. Liver tissue has an anisotropy property that presents non-linearity and can be physically visible when the tissue shows a wavy pattern belonging to collagen fibers [2]. One aspect being highlighted is the structural composition of liver tissue since it has 80% water in its structure, which is why it has the characteristic of an incompressible material [3]. The question at this point is how to obtain the displacements that loads can cause. To determine the above, it is necessary to adapt equilibrium equations consistent with the load system and the efforts generated internally, in this case, in the liver tissue [4, 5]. There is a limitation in obtaining a solution because the relationship between stresses and deformations in biological tissues is unknown. This leads to applying a

D. Tarnita et al. (Eds.): MESROB 2023, MMS 133, pp. 251–259, 2023.
https://doi.org/10.1007/978-3-031-32446-8_27

hyperelastic model to liver tissue [6–8]. Liver tissue performs an essential function in the metabolic cycle. It weighs approximately 1,400 kg, the relationship being indistinct if it is a man or a woman [9]. This pathology is a common reaction of the liver tissue to chronic lesions produced by various factors, such as metabolic disorders, viral causes, alcoholism, drugs, or congenital anomalies [10]. In general, this pathology is associated with a sustained inflammatory process, causing the liver cells to become scar tissue, affecting the vital function of this tissue. It also promotes its hardening. It is the organism itself that generates fibrosis, which does not occur in acute illnesses. The research seeks to describe the biomechanical behavior of specific pathologies related to liver tissue and describe procedures to evaluate mechanical properties with in vitro studies [11], also providing information relevant to the diagnosis and treatment of liver cancer [12]. Lastly, Medical Robots determine the forces required for needle insertion during a medical liver procedure [13].

In the open literature, some investigations aim to get the mechanical properties of soft tissues using methodologies that go from imageology to universal testing machines and tests in vivo. The work aims to design a mechanical system to generate the compression load and obtain the mechanical properties to verify the computational liver model.

2 Methods

Figure 1 explains the methodology used for this work for the design test bed for liver tissue.

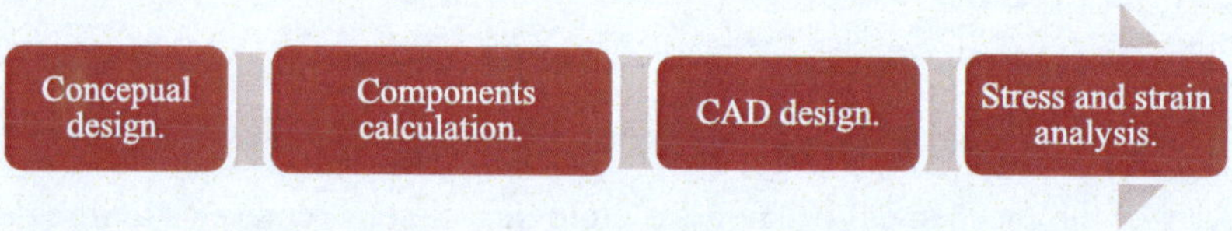

Fig. 1. Methodology of design test bed for liver tissue.

The conception of the device design comes from the problem of carrying out compression tests with equipment that offers portability because the study requires that the equipment be inserted into a tomograph. For this reason, the kit must not contain metal parts or electronics to avoid interference in the TAC. Table 1 lists the systems used to test biological tissues, but none are designed to be inserted into a tomograph. The mechanical properties of liver tissue will be studied through an automated system capable of generating a compression load to a post-mortem sample. Ten post-mortem liver tissue samples are required to have acceptable results. In particular, the results obtained from this experimental configuration are intended to provide data for creating simulator software for diagnostic procedures such as biopsies or processes that require surgery caused by common pathologies such as fibrosis.

The compression system will be introduced to a computerized axial tomography to obtain tomography. This 3D model will be analyzed with image processing tools and

Table 1. Tissue testing machines [14–16].

Test	Manufacturing	Electronic parts	Image	Reference
Tension /compres-sion	Metallic structure	Yes, non-removable parts	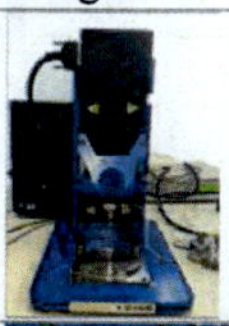	[14]
Compression	Metallic structure	Yes, non-removable parts	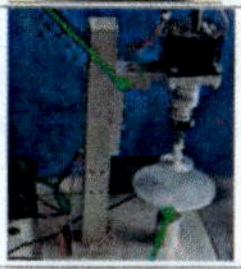	[15]
Compression	Metallic structure	Yes, non-removable parts	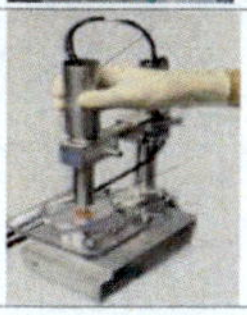	[16]

a hyperelastic model to get the properties. The compression system is characterized by comprising the following mechanism that is described below.

In Fig. 1, three stages of motion are shown to obtain a linear motion; below each step is described:

- The first stage consists of using an epicyclic gear train using a configuration where the satellite carrier is locked, and the satellite gears rotate simultaneously in four points.
- The second stage transmits the movement in four points through perpendicular axes. A system was implemented of bevel gears. The bevel gear is pressure coupled to the gear of the satellite carrier
- A linear movement generates the third stage. A gear-rack system is implemented to achieve a rotary motion to the rack, coupled to the clamping element to the platform, allowing it to move vertically and generating a compression load.

Figure 2 shows the compression system. It used ABS plastic as construction material for the device, and the plates of the compression platforms are acrylic with a 5 mm thickness, which gives us a device that does not generate interferences within the computerized axial tomography. This system has the following dimensions 485 mm in height and a width of 200 mm. It is designed for soft tissue with maximum dimensions of 260 mm long by 240 mm wide and 220 mm high. These measurements are the average of liver tissue. The force that the machine can generate is 28 Kgf. The operation of the proposed system requires one operator. First, the operator activates the function to advance or retreat the device. This is because the compression load has been exerted on the sample of liver tissue. The operator must start the device and stop once this is done. Next, the operator uncouples the engine. The device has a brake that retains the mechanism to prevent it from recoiling and losing the compression load. It will be introduced into the CT scanner to scan the tissue sample with compression load.

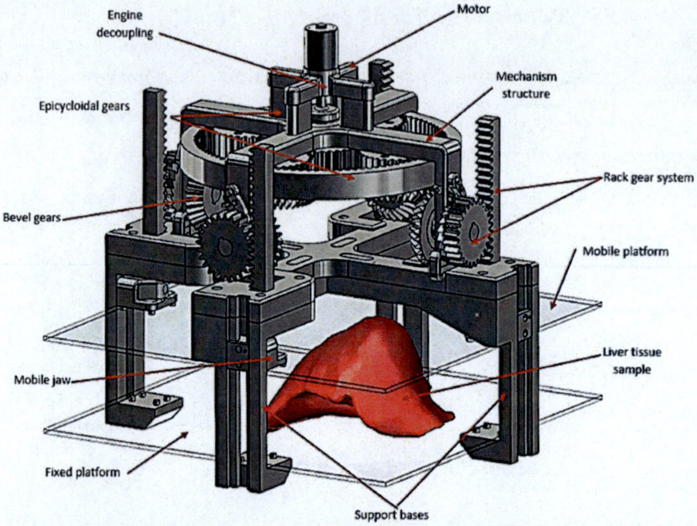

Fig. 2. Testbed design for assessment of liver tissue properties.

Figure 3 shows the methodology to obtain the tissue compression displacement.

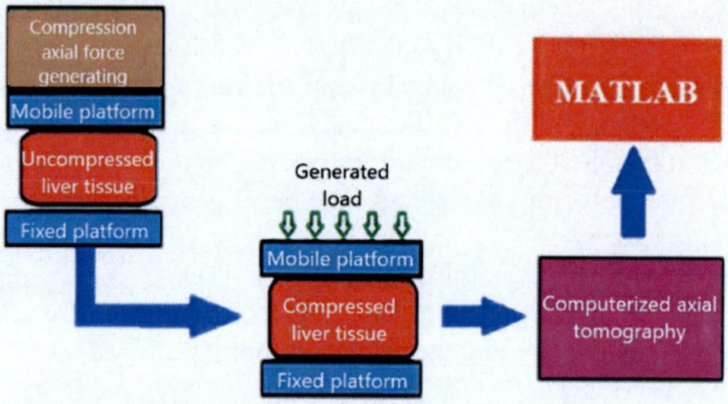

Fig. 3. Experimental methodology.

The sample of the liver tissue without compression load is used as a reference, and it must be tomography and generate a three-dimensional model. Once the topographies of the tissue sample with compression load have been carried out, a three-dimensional model is developed in the same way to be later analyzed in Matlab®. For the model that shows displacement and deformations, an image processing tools with the Matlab® computer program were coded. Figure 4 shows the coded tools, with the data obtained from the analysis of deformations and displacements will be analyzed by the Mooney-Rivlin hyperelastic model.

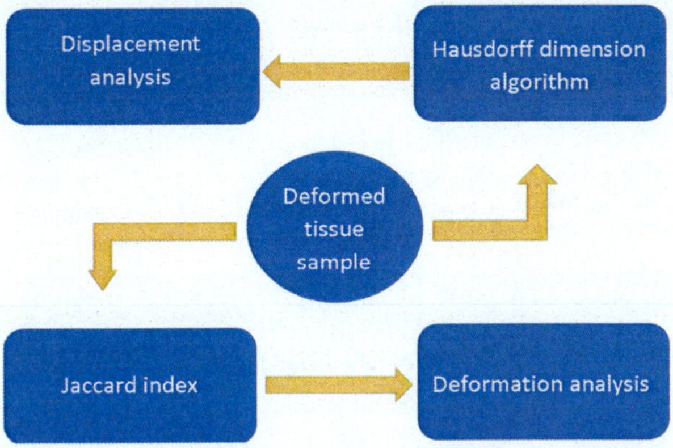

Fig. 4. Image Processing Tools

3 Results

The result obtained is based on the requirements described in Sect. 2. Regarding the mechanism responsible for generating the compression load, the following was determined, the first stage has the following characteristics the gearmotor selected for the orientation of the rotary movement in the epicyclic gear train has the elements shown in Table 2.

Table 2. Characteristics calculated for the geared motor.

Geared motor
Material: Aluminum Alloy
Mechanical torque: 100 Kgf - cm
Angular velocity: 3.059 $\frac{rad}{s}$

The epicyclic gear train has the following parameters for the development of the epicyclic gear train, it was taken into account that the planet gear is modulo 3 with a primitive diameter of 120 mm, and for the satellite gears they will have a modulus of 3 with a diameter primitive 90 mm and in the case of the primitive diameter of the crown is 300 mm in order to be able to perform tests with complete liver tissues with approximate dimensions of 260 mm long by 240 mm wide and 220 mm high, the characteristics obtained for the gear train are shown in Table 3.

The second stage consisted of coupling conical gears under pressure in the satellite gears of the epicycloidal gear train. The calculated characteristics are shown in Table 4. This stage guarantees that when generating compression in the tissue, there is no setback in the direction of actuation of the mechanism and is implemented a ratchet system coupled to the shaft of the bevel gear.

Finally, a rack and pinion system was used to obtain the linear movement. Although the calculated characteristics are shown in Table 5, this system was developed based

Table 3. Characteristics calculated for the Epicyclic gear train.

Epicyclic gear train		
Planet Number of teeth: 40 Angular velocity: 4.71239 $\frac{rad}{s}$	Satellite Number of teeth: 30 Angular velocity: 1.34638189 $\frac{rad}{s}$	Crown Number of teeth: 100 Angular velocity: 1.88496 $\frac{rad}{s}$

Table 4. Characteristics calculated for the bevel gears.

Bevel gears	
Bevel gear 1 Number of teeth: 40 Type: 90°	Bevel gear 2 Number of teeth: 30 Type: 90°

on average measurements of complete liver tissue. In other words, the platform and the racks generate a 220 mm stroke.

Table 5. Characteristics calculated for the rack and pinion system.

Rack and pinion system	
Pinion Number of teeth: 30 Angular velocity: 1.34638189 $\frac{rad}{s}$	Rack Number of teeth: 24 Stroke: 202 mm

The motor is coupled to the mechanism, and a ratchet system was used as a brake and anti-return system. The characteristics determined for this system are shown in Table 6.

Table 6. Characteristics calculated for the Ratchet system.

Ratchet system	
Ratchet Number of teeth: 30 The direction of rotation: clockwise	Pawl Pawl angle: 61.43° Activation direction: clockwise Locking direction: counterclockwise

Figure 5 shows a FEM study of the device structure, specifically where loads are generated by the mechanism that produces the linear displacement. This study aimed to determine if the design supports the applied loads during a compression test. The results show micro deformations concentrated in the central part where the case of the mechanism joins the base. The deformations in this area are 5.47×10^{-5} MPa, and on the upper side of the base are present micro deformations of 6.38×10^{-5} MPa. Finally, perceptible micro deformations in the lower lateral part of 2.74×10^{-5} MPa.

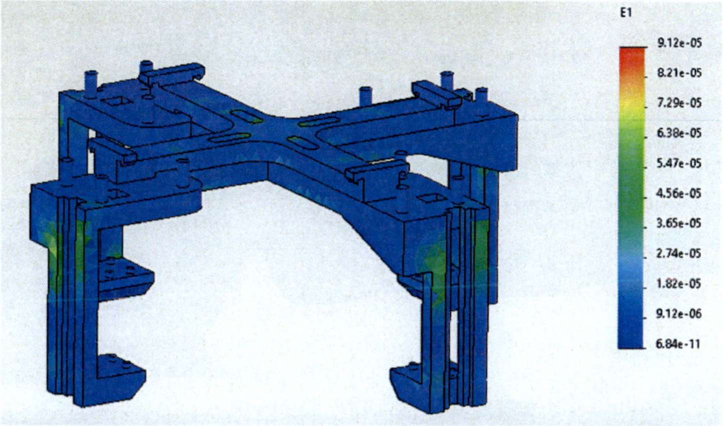

Fig. 5. Deformations on the structure.

Figure 6 shows the displacements. In this case, the displacements are generated in the base unions. This displacement ranges from 2.68×10^{-2} mm to 8.95×10^{-2} mm, and the displacements on the upper side of the base range from 1.79×10^{-2} mm to 2.68×10^{-2} mm. From the above, it is concluded that the chassis of the proposed device has an adequate resistance level for experimental tests in future works.

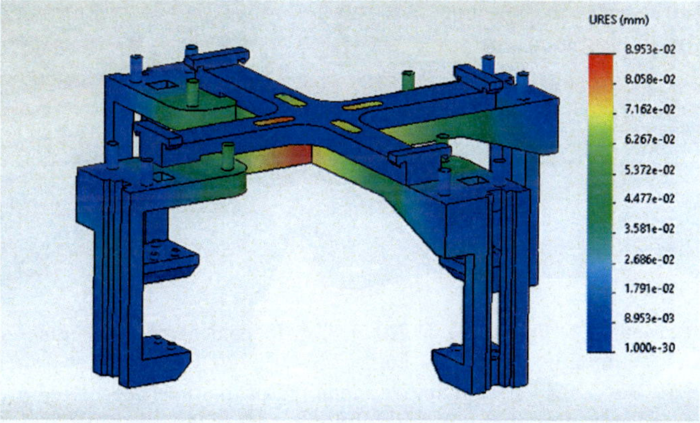

Fig. 6. Displacements on the structure.

Figure 7 shows the testbed proposed is in the assembly process, and the first tests with tissue will be carried out when the required sensors and motors are fitted in the device.

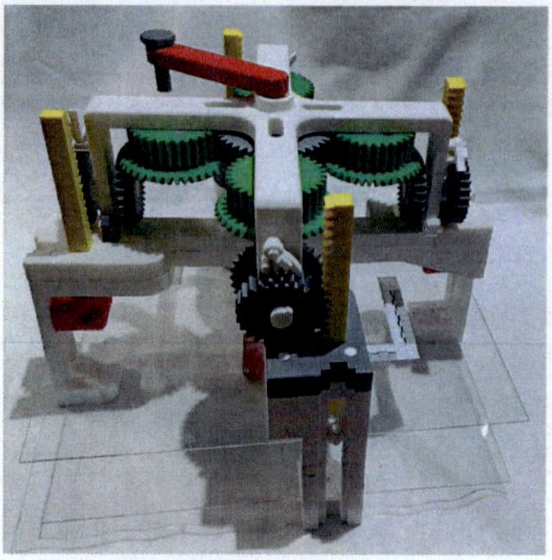

Fig. 7. 3D Printed Testbed with ABS.

4 Conclusion

The proposal presented above was developed as an experimental validation method intended to use a simplified measurement system of mechanical properties for liver tissue. The testbed can generate an axial compression force that gradually increases on the surface of the liver tissue sample, which is expected to obtain constant displacements in three directions (X, Y, Z). The system presented above intends to generate a compression load in a sample of liver tissue with a cylindrical shape. The system is made of ABS plastic because it will be inserted inside a computerized axial tomography to avoid interference patterns that could cause a metallic material in its construction. This work is focused on obtaining future results towards generating a surgical simulator that increases the success rate of the specialist who executes the diagnoses and interventions of the liver tissue affected by pathologies.

Acknowledgments. The authors wish to gratefully acknowledge Consejo Nacional de Ciencia y Tecnologia (CONACyT) and the Instituto Politécnico Nacional. The authors acknowledge partial support from projects 20231625, 20231131 and an EDI grant provided by SIP/IPN.

References

1. Lin, J., Shi, Y., Men, Y., Wang, X., Ye, J., Zhang, C.: Mechanical roles in formation of oriented collagen fibers. Tissue Eng. Part B Rev. **26**(2), 116–128 (2020)
2. Bergstrom, J.S., Boyce, M.C.: Constitutive modeling of the time-depent and cyclic loading of elastomers and aplication to soft biological tissues. Mech. Mater. **33**(9), 523–530 (2001)
3. Miller, K.: Constitutive modelling of abdominal organs. J. Biomech. **33**(3), 367–373 (2000)
4. Bergstrom, J.S.: Mechanics of Solid Polymers: Theory and Computational Modeling: First Edition. Elsevier, USA (2015)
5. Chagnon, G., Ohayon, J., Martiel, J.L., Favier, D.: Hyperelasticity modeling for incompressible passive biological tissues. In: Biomechanics of Living Organs, vol. 1, no. 1, pp. 3–30. Elsevier (2017)

6. Meirmanov, A., Galtsev, O., Zimin, R.: A. Elements of continuum mechanics: In Free Boundaries in Rock Mechanics. De Gruyter Series in Applied and Numerical Mathematics, vol. 1, no. 1, pp. 167–206
7. Oliver, X., and Agelet: Mecánica de Medios Continuos para Ingenieros, 2nd edn. Edicions UPC, Barcelona (2002)
8. Basaran, C.: Introduction to Unified Mechanics Theory with Applications, 2st edn. Springer, Cham (2021)
9. Lee, Y.A., Wallace, M.C., Friedman, S.L.: Pathobiology of liver fibrosis: a translational success story. Gut **64**, 1337–1337 (2015)
10. Trautwein, C., Friedman, S.L., Schuppan, D., Pinzani, M.: Hepatic fibrosis: concept to treatment. J. Hepatology **62**(1), S15–S24 (2015)
11. Chen, Y., et al.: Correlation analysis of structural and biomechanical properties of hepatocellular carcinoma tissue. J. Biomech. **141**, 111227 (2022)
12. Pei, W., et al.: Regional biomechanical imaging of liver cancer cells. J. Cancer **10**(19), 4481–4487 (2019)
13. Tucan, P., et al.: Design and experimental setup of a robotic medical instrument for brachytherapy in non-resectable liver tumors. Cancers **14**(23), 5841 (2022)
14. Griffin, M., Premakumar, Y., Seifalian, A., Butler, P.E., Szarko, M.: Biomechanical characterization of human soft tissues using indentation and tensile testing. JoVE J. Bioeng. **118** (2016)
15. Yu, L., Yang, J., Wang, L., Wang, W., Yan, Y.: Study on the effect and the eliminate method of preloading force on the compression tests of liver tissue. J. Med. Biol. Eng. **39**(4), 583–595 (2018). https://doi.org/10.1007/s40846-018-0438-2
16. Wellman, P.S., Howe, R.D., Kern, K.A.: Breast Tissue Stiffness in Compression is Correlated to Histological Diagnosis. Biol. Eng. (1999)

Check for updates

Experimental Evaluation of Respiration in Patients Undergoing Thoracic Surgery

Marco Ceccarelli[1](✉), Manuel D'Onofrio[2], Cristiano Casciani[2], Matteo Russo[1], and Vincenzo Ambrogi[2]

[1] Department of Industrial Engineering, University of Rome Tor Vergata, 00133 Rome, Italy
{marco.ceccarelli,matteo.russo}@uniroma2.it
[2] Department of Surgical Sciences, University of Rome Tor Vergata, 00133 Rome, Italy
ambrogi@uniroma2.it

Abstract. This paper provides insights for analysis of ribcage motions as a predictive diagnostic tool of complications after thoracic surgery. RESPIRholter, a novel Holter ventilatory device, is used to detect the biomechanics of a single rib as an indicator of respiration. The reported experimental campaign shows the ability of the RESPIRholter device to detect a respiratory insufficiency with numerical evaluations, even in advance to a rise of clinical complications in surgery-operated patients.

Keywords: Biomechanics · Medical Devices · Wearable Devices · Respiration · Testing

1 Introduction

This paper presents an investigation for analyzing the ribs motion using RESPIRholter, [1], a portable device based on an IMU sensor. The aim of the report is to broaden knowledge of how thoracic surgery affects rib cage movements.

Few researchers as in [2–6] have tried to develop new techniques to assess ventilatory health status. Limitations of these methodologies are high cost, difficult set up or continuous presence of a medical operator during the sampling. Likewise, SENSIRIB device [7, 8], from which RESPIRholter was derived, requires the presence of the operator during the sampling. The new Holter device provides a continuous monitoring of the rib motion without any requirement of physically present assistance, and therefore it can be used by patients on their own with cost effective, lightweight, and comfortable features as outlined in [8, 9].

The spirometry, as the standard in clinical practice to analyze the respiratory system status, requires a contribution from the subjects under testing. The proposed RESPIRholter device, [1, 10] is a passive diagnostic device that does not require an active contribution from the subject under testing and can be used in non-compliant patients, such as patient with dementia or children.

D. Tarnita et al. (Eds.): MESROB 2023, MMS 133, pp. 260–268, 2023.
https://doi.org/10.1007/978-3-031-32446-8_28

In this paper, results of implementing RESPIRholter, a holter device for respiration monitoring, are discussed coming from a campaign of tests with patients at the Thoracic Surgery unit of the University Hospital Policlinico Tor Vergata in Rome.

The outcomes of the reported experimental investigation will have interesting implications in preventing early postoperative complications in patients with major thoracic surgery as well as have a diagnostic device useful during preoperative assessment and in checking respiratory health status.

2 Issues in Patients with Thoracic Surgery

Patients with thoracic surgery are sensitive to several postoperative complications such as air leak due to an alveolar-pleural fistula (APF), atrial fibrillation, pneumonia, pulmonary edema, atelectasis, pulmonary insufficiency, [11, 12].

Preoperative ventilatory functional tests are performed to prevent complications during and after surgery and define the patient's fit. The incidence of postoperative complications in major thoracic surgery is approximately 25% [11] and pulmonary function analysis plays a key role in predicting it. In general, initial screening consists of anamneses, spirometry, diffusion capacity, if necessary 6-min walking test, and assessment of the cardiovascular status. The incidence of postoperative pneumonia is 2.2–20% according to diagnosis criteria. When it occurs, it is related to a significant morbidity and mortality (7.5%) [12]. Atelectasis is a common complication after thoracic surgery and when it involves a lung segment or more, there is a relevant risk for the onset of pneumonia. Poor cough, impaired pulmonary function, diaphragmatic dysfunction, and chest wall instability are risk factors for segmental atelectasis. The best treatment option is prevention by performing chest physiotherapy, walking at least three to four time daily, secretions hygiene, and coughing. Pulmonary insufficiency remains a postoperative complication, even with a positive preoperative evaluation. The difficulty usually occurs on day 2 or 3 of postoperative care, due to pneumonia, poor coughing, or pulmonary edema. Clinical signs precede the evidence from the radiograph, and a treatment is aimed to maximize the pulmonary mechanism through intense chest physiotherapy, intravenous fluid, bronchodilators, incentive spirometry, ambulation, and control of secretions. All the above can be more conveniently addressed using a regular check also of the respiration looking at the rib cage motion and functionality. A practical evaluation with numerical values can be worked out by analyzing the motion parameters of the ribcage during respiration such as the displacement of the ribcage reference points and motion quality such as acceleration ribcage response during respiration, as summarized in Fig. 1.

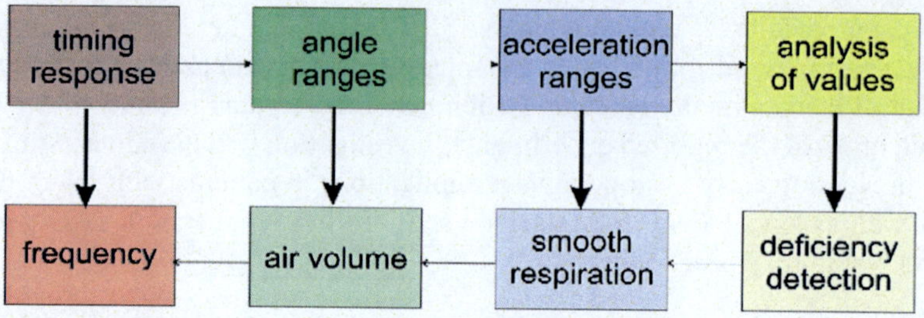

Fig. 1. A scheme of main parameters for respiration evaluation via ribcage biomechanics

3 RESPIRholter, the Monitoring Device

RESPIRholter, [1, 10] is an IMU sensor that detects the accelerations among the axes *x*, *y*, *z*, the Roll and the Pitch angles and the time references. The main element of the prototype is the box that contains an Arduino NANO 33 IoT breadboard equipped with the 6 axis LSM6DSL IMU sensor. A MicroSD module supports the placement of the storage unit microSD with 5V power input. The board communicates with the operator through blink sequences of a LED (low power led, 1W of power consumption) varying their frequency and period. The power supply is provided by a power bank using a micro-USB connector cable. The device is lightweight, at only 33g, and its size is 55 mm × 30 mm × 16 mm, Fig. 2.

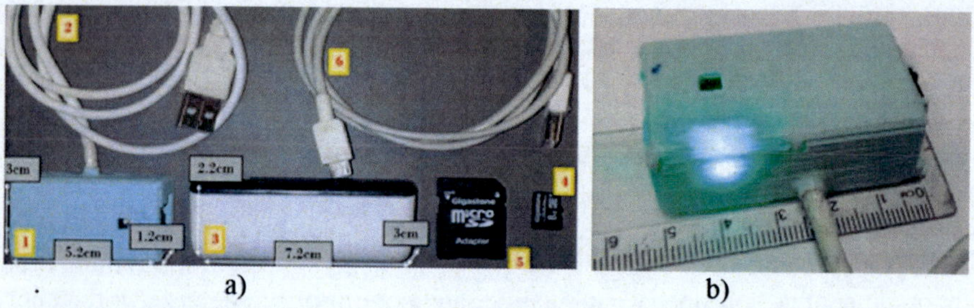

Fig. 2. RESPIRHOLTER design, [1, 10]: a) all the components (1- sensor box, 2- power cable. 3-power bank, 4-microSD, 5-microSD adapter, 6- connection cable); b) the used prototype.

Data analysis is performed through a specifically elaborated user-friendly RESPIRholter code in MATLAB that can be operated by the physician during the process. Clicking on preview, the physician can take a quick look at the acquisitions and eventually delete acquisitions that are not considered valid, and then, clicking on execute, code can be started for its autonomous operation.

In the post-sampling data elaboration, the first step is to divide each acquisition into five segments with same time duration and all the initial and final intervals with no data can be eliminated. Then, the RESPIRholter code automatically computes the averages of the five acquisitions for each parameter P according to the scheme in Fig. 3. When dealing with the roll and pitch angles, the displacement angles plots are obtained. Then, the average of all the acquisitions is computed as the average of the averages.

RESPIRholter code allows the physician to select a representative plot and a selected plot as per diagnosis purposes in a synthetic representation of the results. The representative plot is a part of a single acquisition that is representative of the entire sampling, and the selected plot let the physician insert in the final report a part of a single acquisition that is not representative of the entire acquisition, but that is worthy of attention for the diagnosis. RESPIRholter is set up to perform a 6-h long acquisition sampling 1 min each 20 min for each motion parameter, [10]. A diagnosis report can be generated thanks to the report generator package with data of the subject under testing, investigator data, a database of results, and a form to be filled by the physician with clinical analysis and diagnosis considerations.

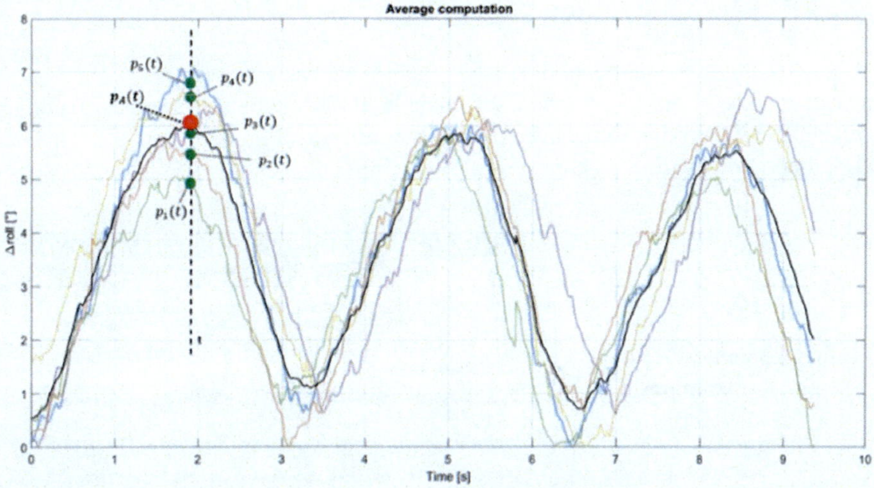

Fig. 3. A scheme of elaboration of the average results from RESPIRholter acquisitions, [10]

4 Testing Protocol

An experimental campaign has been carried out involving two different groups of subjects, namely patients and healthy people as control group for medical statistics.

The subjects of the patient group are patients undergoing pulmonary resection without distinction based on surgical access and type of surgery (wedge or lobectomy) due to the small number of cases. Subjects of the control group are healthy volunteers not affected by ventilatory disease such as asthma, COPD, pneumonia and without familiarity with pneumological disease.

The sampling is performed during the night between the first and second postoperative day while the patient sleeps. The device is placed at the intersection point between the anterior axillary line and the sixth rib of the hemithorax if interested in the surgery, Fig. 4 a). Figures 4.b) shows a model for the motion parameters that the IMU sensor (in

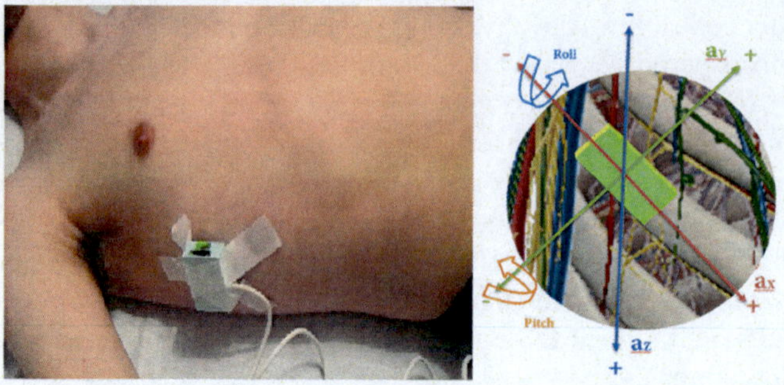

a) b)

Fig. 4. Installation of RESPIRholter: a) in a subject under testing; b) a scheme of the sensed parameters.

green) can acquire along its sensing axes, namely along x axis roll angle and along y axis pitch angle in addition to the acceleration components. Figures 5 lists the sequence of testing operations within an approved clinical protocol.

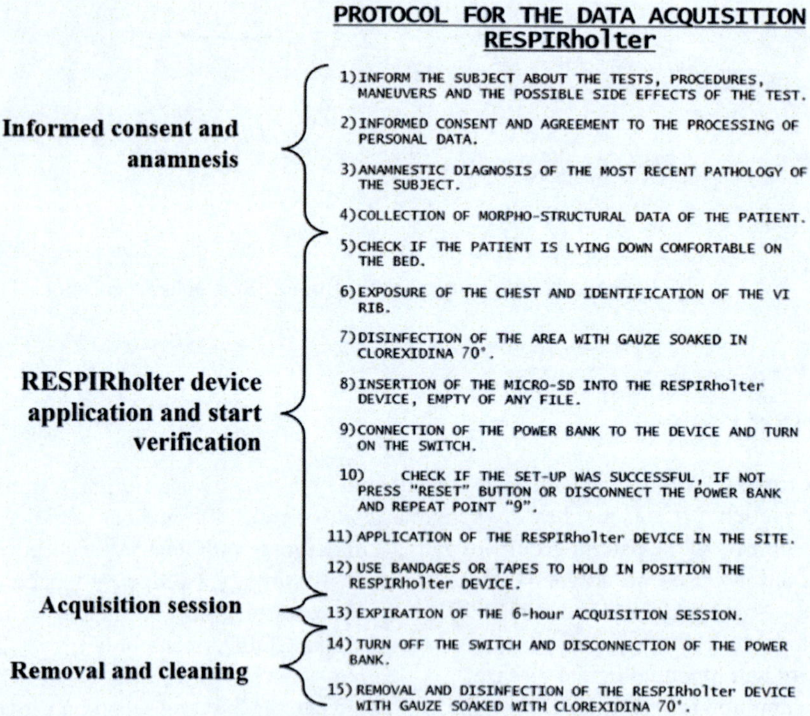

Fig. 5. The protocol workflow of RESPIRholter operation in the reported campaign

5 Results and Diagnosis Outputs

Sampling performed with a control group of 10 people has been used to define a refence range for healthy conditions as reported in the first rows of Tables 1 and 2 as an average range, since there is no previous work in scientific literature. For each acceleration component are considered the maximum and the minimum range values in g. The Roll and Pitch angles are measured as angles excursion. In patient group of 10 people the same statistical analysis has been elaborated and reference range has been identified similarly as reported in the second rows of Tables 1 and 2. The outcomes for the patient group when compared with results of the healthy group permits to identify how and how much thoracic surgery affects chest wall motion, and which early marker of postoperative complications can be detected.

Once the early motion critical markers are identified, physiotherapy could be intensified to move the secretions and to decrease the chances of respiratory infections [12] so that pain can be better handled to allow a more effective cough when in the first postoperative days, patients avoid coughing due to pain related to the chest drainage.

Table 1. Test results with healthy and patient subjects in terms of angles

	ΔRoll (deg)	ΔPitch (deg)
Healthy population	0.58–0.92	0.73–1.11
Patients	1.25–1.78	1.76–2.35

Table 2. Test results with healthy and patient subjects in terms of acceleration components

	a_x min (g)	a_x max (g)	a_y min (g)	a_y max (g)	a_z min (g)	a_z max (g)
Healthy population	−0.84–0.78	−0.80 – 0.81	−0.16–0.19	−0.12–0.12	−0.31–.63	−0.28–0.67
Patients	−0.71––0.69	−0.65 – −0.63	−0.40– −0.37	−0.33– −0.31	0.55–0.62	0.62–0.69

5.1 A Patient Case Study

The patient S01 is a 59-year-old male, non-smoker that was operated with a lobectomy in uniportal VATS. The first day after surgery he was clinically eupneic and performed the test between the first and the second day after surgery. The RESPIRholter detection has shown a dyspneic pattern as shown in Fig. 6–8 with a short superficial breathing.

From the plots in Fig. 6, a strong difference of rib acceleration can be noted between a healthy person (in red) and a patient S01(in blue), indicating a very significant motion change, although with small values, with loss of cyclic and regular timeline. In Figs. 7 and 8, the anomaly is even more evident in the respiration of the patient when compared with the reference behavior in a healthy patient, indicating an incomplete cycling of the respiration and a reduced rib motion variation. Thus, during the second postoperative

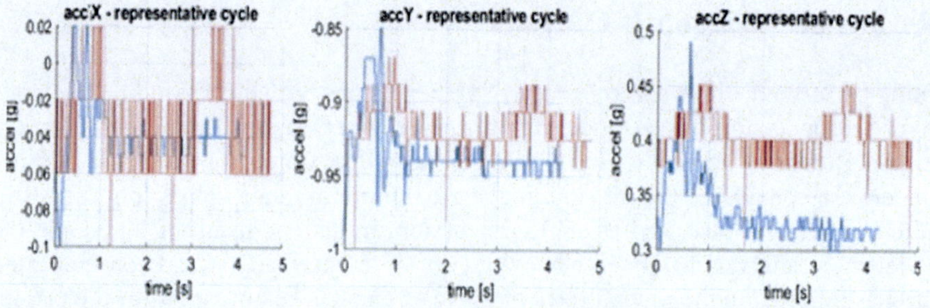

Fig. 6. Comparison of acquired results of rib acceleration along X, Y, and Z axes during test in a healthy patient (red line) and the example patient S01 (blue line)

day, the patient S01 was diagnosed with a light respiratory insufficiency that was treated with oxygen therapy through a nasal cannula, with a flow of 2 L/minute that mitigated the respiration deficiency.

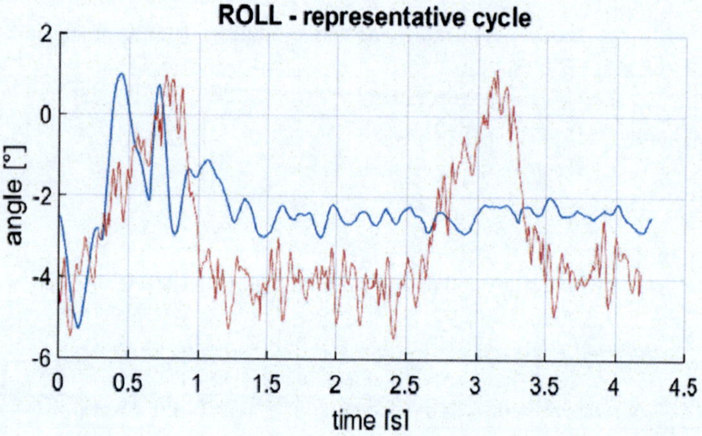

Fig. 7. Comparison of acquired results of rib roll angle during test in a healthy patient (red line) and the example patient S01 (blue line)

The abnormal thoracic motion that was detected during the first postoperative day could have been the cause of the upcoming respiratory insufficiency as consequences of what is discussed in Sect. 2 and therefore, thanks to the monitored respiration status, actions could be taken in due advance to mitigate those unexpected effects and to prevent a more critical situation.

This experience suggests that the device has the capability to identify subliminal complications in advance from the clinical onset of symptoms, providing the physicians with the potential to act in advance and avoid complications.

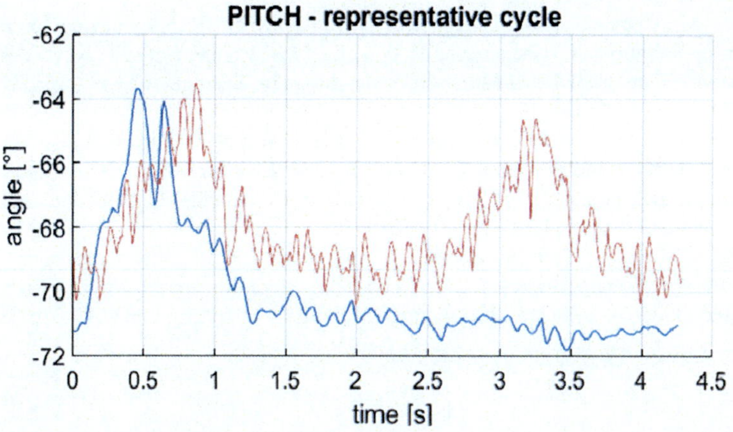

Fig. 8. Comparison of acquired results of rib pitch angle during test in a healthy patient (red line) and the example patient S01 (blue line)

6 Conclusions

The results of an experimental campaign for analysis of respiration using RESPIRholter device is presented to discuss the significance of the testing as diagnostic tool. Among the carried tests one is reported as case of study indicating that a proper evaluation of the results could detect critical rising issues in a thoracic surgery-operated patient much in advance that in the traditional diagnostics. The RESPIRholter device represents a promising new tool for respiratory monitoring and has the potential to improve patient outcomes in a variety of clinical settings.

References

1. Ceccarelli, M., Ambrogi, M., Puglisi, L., Aquilini, M.: Ventilatory holter device, patent no. IT102021000008585, Italy, 7 April 2021
2. Alfverti, A., Cesareo, A.: A wearable device for the continuous monitoring of the respiratory rate, patent WO 2019/012384, Italy, 11 January 2019
3. Ciocchetti, M., et al.: Smart textile based on fiber Bragg grating sensors for respiratory monitoring: design and preliminary trials. Biosensors **5**(3), 602–615 (2015)
4. Freeman J. F., et al.: Devices and methods for respiratory variation monitoring by measurement of respiratory volumes, motion and variability, patent WO2012021900A1, 16 February 2012
5. Gentili Biffi G.: Device for monitoring of respiration functions, patent IT1222263B, Italy, 21 June 1990
6. Ceccarelli, M.: Portable device for measuring the movement of human ribs, patent n. IT102021000005726, Italy, 13 March 2021
7. Ceccarelli, M., Puglisi, L., Mesiti, F., Aquilini, M., Ambrogi, V.: A device for experimental characterization of biomechanics of breathing and coughing. In: 26th ABCM Int. Congress of Mechanical Engineering, Florianópolis, paper COB-2021–0273 (2021)
8. Ceccarelli, M., Papuc, P.E., Taje, R., Aquilini, M., Ambrogi, V.: A biomechanics analysis of ventilation in thorax operated patients. Int. J. Clin. Stud. Med. Case Rep. **15**(1), 1–3 (2021)

9. Aquilini, M., Ceccarelli, M.: Design and testing of RESPIRholter device for respiratory monitoring. In: Niola, V., Gasparetto, A., Quaglia, G., Carbone, G. (eds.) Advances in Italian Mechanism Science - IFToMM Italy 2022, pp. 480–488. Springer, Cham. https://doi.org/10.1007/978-3-031-10776-4_55
10. Patterson, G.A., Cooper, J.D., Deslauriers, J., Lerut, A.E.M.R., Luketich, J.D., Rice, T.W.: Pearson's Thoracic and Esophageal Surgery, 3rd edn. Elsevier, Philadelphia (2008)
11. LoCicero, J., III., Feins, R.H., Colson, Y.L., Rocco, G.: Shields' General Thoracic Surgery, 8th edn. Wolters Kluwer, Philadelphia (2019)
12. Kendall, F., Abreu, P., Pinho, P., Oliveira, J., Bastos, P.: The role of physiotherapy in patients undergoing pulmonary surgery for lung cancer. A literature review. Revista Portuguesa de Pneumologia **23**(6), 343–351 (2006). https://doi.org/10.1016/j.rppnen.2017.05.003

Dynamic Functional Stability Analysis of Gait After Anterior Cruciate Ligament (ACL) Reconstruction

Mihnea Ion Marin, Dorin Popescu, Alin Horia Burileanu, and Ligia Rusu(✉)

University of Craiova, 13 A.I. Cuza, Craiova, Romania
ligiarusu@hotmail.com

Abstract. Dynamic functional stability during gait is a challenge. The aim of the paper is to analysis the lower limb joints pattern after anterior cruciate ligament (ACL) reconstruction, by analyze the gait parameters, using the symmetry indexes and range of motion. The research includes and the results demonstrate that for both lower limbs are developed the similar pattern for increase the balance and stability of the body during gait. The most important effect is under the hip joint which again seems to be the control key for lower limb.

Keywords: gait symmetry · pattern · reconstruction · compensatory mechanism

1 Problem Description

1.1 A Subsection Sample

One of the research problems is how selected gait parameters may change as a result of anterior cruciate ligament (ACL) deficiency and following ACL reconstruction. For this reason, one way for assess this aspect is gait analysis data analysed from heel strike until toe lift of the gait cycle.

In field of rehabilitation, orthopaedic and sport medicine the problem of dynamic functional stability is define as the conditions that assure joint stability during daily activities. From this point of view are many controversies regarding how we can do the analysis of dynamic stability.

Gait analysis is a challenge regarding dynamic functional stability and is a process that could integrate a lot of inputs, based on video acquisitions systems and facilitate to obtain movement patterns that are useful for clinical activity.

This analysis make sense is in relationship with the possibility to identify the abnormal movements by 3D analysis, in each movement, like knee joint.

Biomechanical analysis of gait is, in neuromuscular pathology, very important because we observe a great variability of functional stability and functional stability.

Hence a contradictory hypothesis has been proposed in which variability is described as "healthy flexibility. This approach is in the context of functional dynamic and could be explain through behaviours variability of biologic systems which allow and provide mechanism for adaptation to daily stress.

D. Tarnita et al. (Eds.): MESROB 2023, MMS 133, pp. 269–278, 2023.
https://doi.org/10.1007/978-3-031-32446-8_29

In this context knee injuries, we can speak about so called healthy flexibility, which could be associated with stiffness, decrease of daily adaptation to stress generated by locomotion and gait.

The ain of ACL reconstruction is to restore the ACL function as much as possible and these aspects have been studied in the last 30years. This because during time were developed a lot of surgical procedures and many biomechanics studies which give information about the dynamic knee stability during gait.

ACL is one of the most important knee ligament witch suffered injuries especially in sport activity. The impact of its injury is under gait, which is a movement that need coordination and muscle balance. This is a problem, because in the literature the authors speak about the decrease of knee stability even after 1years after surgical reconstruction.

The present researches speak about the great incidence of ACL lesion, which need surgical intervention to people with average age 30-40years. Because after ACL injury the risk of development the osteoarthritis (OA) is need to do a complex evaluation and monitoring the evolution. Also, an important aspect is to study the movement pattern of contralateral lower limb movement [1–6].

2 Application Field

ACL rupture is a frequent knee injury and is reconstruction is followed by rehabilitation process for restore the passive and dynamic knee stability. Usually, the evaluation of ACL status is made using arthrometer, but this is an evaluation during static position, knee rest position and is not allow to make the evaluation of knee behaviours during dynamic functionality. For this reason, gait analysis is the main process for evaluation the dynamic knee functional stability but also evaluation of whole kinematic lower limb, in specific conditions of knee injury. Also, this analysis helps to know more about the compensatory mechanism development during gait.

3 Research Stages-State of the Art in Biomechanics Assessment

Gait analysis is an advance process for laboratory analysis, which use inputs during gait. The present approach is stride-to-stride variability, define like patterns fluctuations during gait, which provide information for a qualitative evaluation of functional stability of lower limb after ACL reconstruction.

Biomechanics gait analysis after arthroscopy of knee, for ACL reconstruction, demonstrate an improvement of tibia rotation during swing phase.

The studies of Li et. al. [7] and Liu et.al. Propose an evaluation of gait in case of ACL injury during gait phases for build the rehabilitation program. They used for gait system Gait Measurement The Intelligent Device for Energy Expenditure and Activity (IDEEA, Mini Sun, LLC, Fresno, CA, USA) [8]. They patients have a comfortable gait speed, and the supplementary tasks were gait, fast gait, changes of gait directions, walking with dual task, upstairs, downstairs, and normal walking after warm-up. The parameters were: single support (ms), double support (ms), SLS/DLS (%), swing duration (ms), step duration (ms), cycle duration (sec), pulling accel (G), swing power (G), ground impact (G), foot fall (G), push off (G), speed (m/min), cadence (steps/min), step length (meters), and stride length (meters). Both studies included in their research people, after 3 weeks from knee injury interested ACL, till 1 year after injury. The results show that the stability restoration need on one side periodic evaluation of gait and observe also a disorder to contralateral knee during 1 year.

In their paper Sharafoddin et al. [9], speak about the factors that could predict a possibility of reinjury of ACL and development of functional sequelae that have functional impact according to other studies [10–12].

According with these authors the hypothesis are that reinjury of ACL is possible due to the decrease of muscle force and development of muscle balance of lower limb. Also is possible to develop the multi-planar asymmetry of lower limb, more to hip and knee and these could permit three times more the reinjury of ACL. Form kinetic and kinematic point of view asymmetry is associated with inter-segmentary compensatory mechanism [13, 14].

This occurs as knee extensor torque and hip extensor torque are respectively decreased and increased, causing a compensatory hip-dominant strategy within the limb [15].

Another inter-segmentary compensatory mechanism has been described by Butler and refers to the plantarflexion, hip flexion, moment of plantarflexion and ground reaction force during jumping. The author speaks about high level of asymmetry in this situation [11, 16].

Changes of gait pattern after ACL reconstruction are the topics for many studies that analyse different surgical procedures and demonstrate that are a lot of chenas that involved joint extensor/flexor torques, step length and walking base, joint excursions and muscle activity [17].

These patterns could be developed after a process of neuromuscular adaptation like response for pain, instability and the main role is preventing the reinjury [18].

It is a consensus regarding this aspect but are not enough studies that could explain compensatory mechanism and how the tibia displacement could reduce the intraarticular stress. Also, other studies demonstrate some dynamic adjusts phenomena of lower limb after ACL reconstruction and the conclusions are that the lower limb impairments are the result of neuromuscular adaptation process to a new condition [18–20].

4 The Aim of the Study

The aim of this study is to make a comparative analyze of lower limb by gait analysis and identify the lower limbs behaviors after ACL reconstruction. The study includes gait parameters analysis.

5 Method

Our study aims to analyze the variability of gait parameters (angular amplitudes at the hip, knee and ankle), comparison between the healthy lower limb and the surgical lower limb, for seven people that suffered ACL reconstruction. The gait analysis was performed after 1 month from ACL reconstruction and the evaluation included: the range of motion values that define gait symmetry and gait pattern identification, but also step length, cadence. The average age is 30years old, average high 155cm, average weight 79kg.

6 Equipment and Software

In the following section we present three case studies. Kinematic analysis of gait parameters, has been made using the VICON system for movement capture, from Bioengineering Laboratory (www.incesa.ro). The system included 14 infrared cameras; the frequency is 200 Hz (frame/s).

For recording the movement, the system uses software NEXUS, and a special skeleton model named Plug-in–Gait is associated with each subject. The subject wears a black suit which has reflective markers, 14mm diameter (Fig. 1). Markers position are in according to the protocol described by Davis et al. [21] and Oxford foot model.

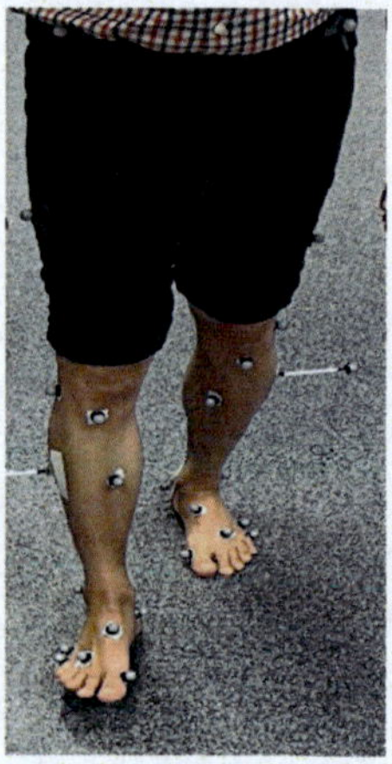

Fig. 1. Markers positions on lower limb respected Oxford foot model.

Using the software we made the movement analysis of lower limb during the gait on a plane surface, at comfortable speed, and follow the trajectories of the main important points on the lower limb like (knee and malleolus) and also variation of angular amplitude for hip, knee and ankle joints.

Participants walked at a self-selected speed in the most natural manner possible on a 10 m walkway at least 3 times, interspersed with suitable rest times.

The values of flexion-extension angles are compared with reference values proposed by Perry in his protocol [22]. In our study the recorded values have been used for evaluation the symmetry of the kinematic parameters of lower limb.

The symmetry has been demonstrated by qualitative shape and for this we propose the following indexes:

Symmetry ratio (R):

$$R = \frac{Xs}{Xd} \tag{1}$$

The factor indicates which of the variables has the highest value, and as such creates asymmetries. The value of $RI = 0$ indicates full symmetry, while $RI \geq 100\%$ indicates asymmetry. Andres and Stimmel [23] used this factor effectively in their study of gait asymmetry in people with disabilities.

Symmetry index (SI):

$$\text{SI (Symetry Index)} = 100\frac{2(\text{Xl} - \text{Xd})}{(\text{Xd} + \text{xl})}[\%\,] \tag{2}$$

The SI factor is a method of percentage assessment of the differences between the kinematic and kinetic parameters for both lower limbs during walking.

The value of $\text{SI} = 0$ indicates full symmetry, while $\text{SI} \geq 100\%$ indicates its asymmetry [24]. The SI index is the method most commonly used and cited in publications on gait symmetry.

Gait asymmetry (GA):

$$\text{GA} = 100\ln\frac{\text{Xs}}{\text{Xd}}[\%] \tag{3}$$

This equation is a logarithmic transform of the RI factor. Plotnik et al. [25], used it to calculate asymmetry on the basis of the duration of the swing phase.

$\text{GA} = 0$ and $\text{GA} \geq 100\%$ denote symmetry and asymmetry, respectively.

Several kinematic and kinetic parameters, such as walking speed, stride length, foot rotation angle, maximum joint range of motion, duration of stance, and swing phases of gait, are frequently used to assess and monitor correctness of gait. We underline that we describe the gait phases like: stance phase (including double support 1-normally 10%, single support-normally 40%, double support 2–10%), swing phase 40%, from gait cycle.

All results are analyzed according with the results of Perry gait values [22].

7 Results

Table 1. Gait phases.

Limb	Stance phase (% from gait phases)	Swing phase (% from gait phases)
Right	65.29	34.71
Left	67.86	32.14

We present the graphics representation of each average joint pattern, during gait and compare with Perry references values (black line). The next graphics will present the hip (Figs. 2), knee (Figs. 3) and ankle (Figs. 4) average joint pattern for operated lower limb (red line) and for healthy lower limb (green line) (Table 1 and 2).

The average hip pattern of operated lower limb is represented in Fig. 2 with the red line. We observe in that at the initial contact the hip flexion is minimal, associated with incoordination and lack of motor control. During stance phase is an important limitation

Table 2. Gait parameters.

	Right limb	Left limb	RI	SI	GA	SA
Gait speed (m/s)	0.51	0.58	−13.99	0.13	13.04	49.20
Cadence (steps/min)	48.17	44.44	6.36	−0.07	−7.32	49.09
Single support (% gait cycle)	80.05	48.62	39.27	−0.49	−50.64	48.86
Swing (% gait cycle)	34.71	32.14	9.78	−0.11	−10.74	49.07
Double support (% gait cycle)	34.95	34.30	1.70	−0.02	−1.75	49.12

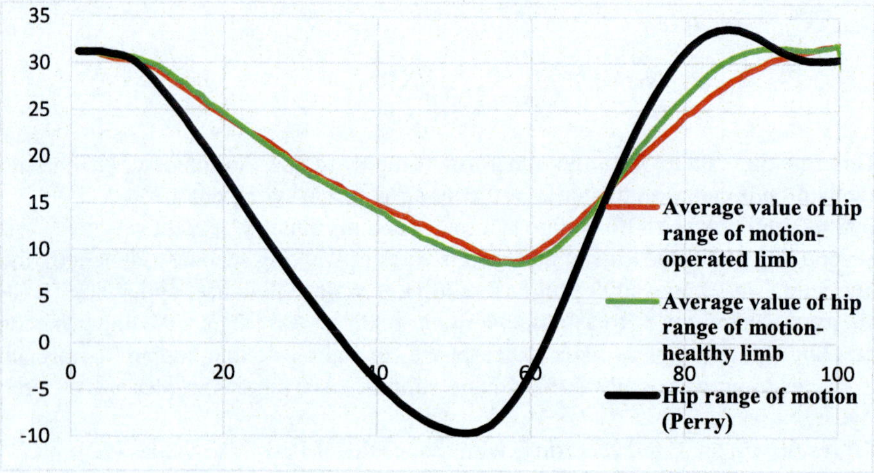

Fig. 2. Hip pattern during gait cycle.

of hip extension around 14°-27°, less then Perry value 42°. In pre swing and swing phases the hip flexion is also limitate and the hip instability in the terminal phase of balance, increase when the lower limb is prepared for landing and support.

During all gait phases we observe a great instability of hip joint.

The average hip pattern of healthy lower limb is represented in Fig. 2 with the green line. The hip pattern has the close pattern like contralateral hip, limits of hip extension during stance phase, but flexion close to reference value and also hip instability could be observed.

In Fig. 3 we observe the knee pattern. The average knee pattern of operated lower limb, represented with the red line, which at the initial contact moment has a decrease of knee flexion and prepare for single stance of lower limb. All patients have a knee flexum position in pre swing and swing phases but the values are less then Perry values. Some of patients have a great knee flexion which is correlated with hip flexion and this could be explain by the development of intrasegmentar compensatory mechanism. In the terminal swing phase, we observe a reduce of knee extension.

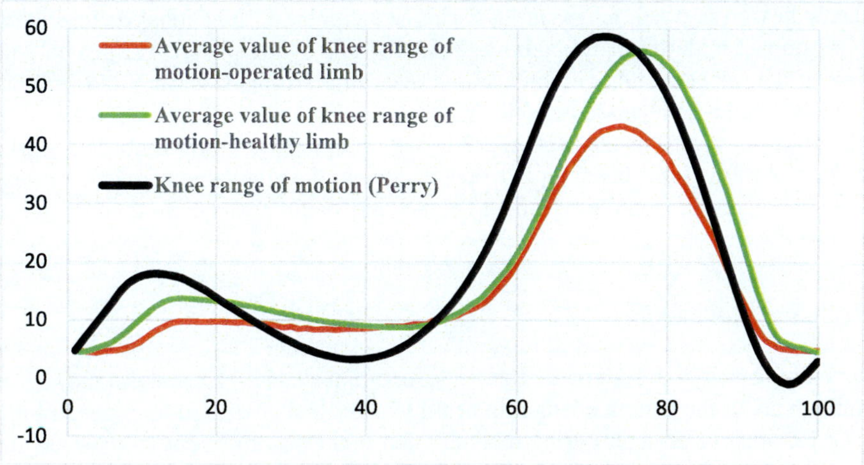

Fig. 3. Knee pattern during gait cycle.

The average knee pattern of healthy lower limb is represented in Fig. 3 with green line. We observe a limitation of knee flexion at initial contact followed by decrease of extension. This means that a compensatory mechanism is developed for maintain the body stability and balance. During pre swing and swing phases knee flexion is closed to reference value.

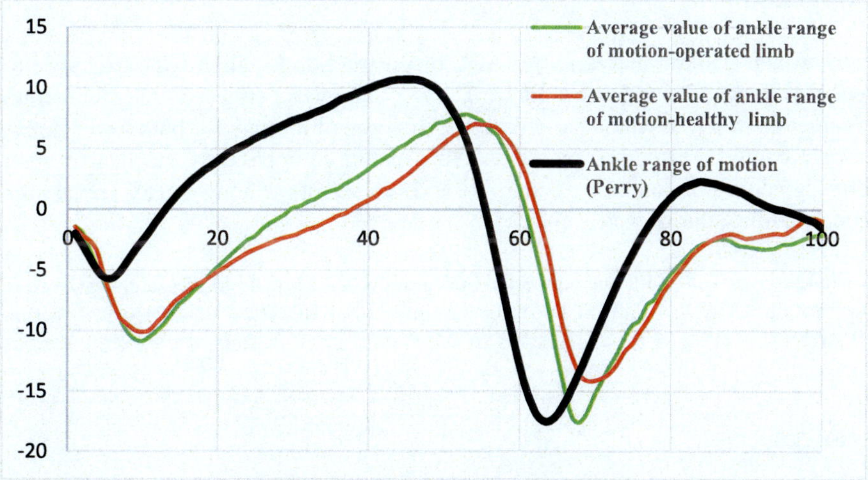

Fig. 4. Ankle pattern during gait cycle.

Figure 4 represents the average pattern of ankle operated lower limb (red line). This pattern consists in development of compensatory mechanism due to the decrease of knee flexion and extension, and the results are increase of dorsiflexion followed by decrease of plantar flexion and neutral position, during stance phase. Functional deficiency of knee has impact under the ankle during pre swing and swing phases and generate an increase of dorsiflexion and contribute to the lower limb lifting. Like for all lower limb joints is observed a great ankle instability.

The green line presents the average ankle pattern of healthy lower limb. The results show that almost the same behavior like operated lower limb, with increase of dorsiflexion and also plantarflexion during initial contact and swing phase more then reference value.

8 Further Research

The subject of lower limb pattern is a challenge for biomechanics gait analysis and al give information about the pattern changes in healthy lower limb. Much more is need future research for analyse the gait during rehabilitation process at different moment and to adapt the rehabilitation program according to the results of gait pattern and compensatory mechanism which is developed.

Identify the symmetry for each gait phases in mandatory for develop the mechanical assistive devices and design the rehabilitation protocols. In the same is useful to understand how is developed the compensatory mechanism and which are the mechanism that involved approximate the same pattern to healthy lower limb. Future research is need for make a link between surgery procedures and gait pattern developed after ACL reconstruction.

9 Conclusions

The present gait pattern analysis after ACL reconstruction highlights the existence of each pattern changes for both lower limbs. The most important effect of ACL reconstruction is under the hip join which has a decrease of range of motion, for both lower limbs. This aspect could be explained by the development of compensatory mechanism inter and intrasegmentar for maintain the stability and balance of the body and also obtain the functional stability during gait.

Acknowledgment. This work was supported by a grant of the Ministry of Research, Innovation and Digitization, CCCDI – UEFISCDI, project number PN-III-P2-2.1-PED-2021-1917, within PNCDI III.

References

1. Hasegawa, S., Kobayashi, M., Arai, R., Tamaki, A., Nakamura, T., Moritani, T.: Effect of early implementation of electrical muscle stimulation to prevent muscle atrophy and weakness in patients after anterior cruciate ligament reconstruction. J Electromyogr Kinesiol **21**, 622–630 (2011)
2. De Valk, E.J., Moen, M.H., Winters, M., Bakker, E.W., Tamminga, R.: Preoperative patient and injury factors of successful rehabilitation after anterior cruciate ligament reconstruction with single-bundle techniques. Art Ther. **29**, 1879–1895 (2013)

3. Ericsson, Y.B., Roos, E.M., Frobell, R.B.: Lower extremity performance following ACL rehabilitation in the KANON-trial: impact of reconstruction and predictive value at 2 and 5 years. Br. J. Sports Med. **47**, 980–985 (2013)
4. Logerstedt, D., Lynch, A., Axe, M.J., Snyder-Mackler, L.: Pre-operative quadriceps strength predicts IKDC2000 scores 6 months after anterior cruciate ligament reconstruction. Knee **20**, 208–212 (2013)
5. Babadi, N., Roostayi, M.M., Rahimi, A., Baghban, A.A., Sarmadi, A., Roostaei, H.: The effect of different hip rotation angles on electromyography activity of the quadriceps muscle during closed kinetic chain tasks in healthy females. J. Phys. Ther. Sci. **29**(30), 1112–1116 (2018)
6. Mikaili, S., Khademi-Kalantari, K., Rezasoltani, A., Arzani, P., Baghban, A.A.: Quadriceps force production during straight leg raising at different hip positions with and without concomitant ankle dorsiflexion. J. Bodyw. Mov. Ther. **22**, 904–908 (2018)
7. Li, W., et al.: Biomechanical evaluation of preoperative rehabilitation in patients of anterior cruciate ligament injury. Orthop Surg. **12**(2), 421–428 (2020). https://doi.org/10.1111/os.12607. Epub 2020 Mar 8
8. Sun, J., Liu, Y., Yan, S., et al.: Clinical gait evaluation of patients with knee osteoarthritis. Gait Posture **58**, 319–324 (2017)
9. Sharafoddin-Shirazi, F., Letafatkar, A., Hogg, J., Saatchian, V.: Biomechanical asymmetries persist after ACL reconstruction: results of a 2-year study. Journal of Experimental Orthopaedics **7**(1), 1 (2020). https://doi.org/10.1186/s40634-020-00301-2
10. Gokeler, A., Seil, R., Kerkhoffs, G., Verhagen, E.: A novel approach to enhance ACL injury prevention programs. J. Exp. Orthop. **5**(1), 1–6 (2018). https://doi.org/10.1186/s40634-018-0137-5
11. Paterno, M.V., Schmitt, L.C., Ford, K.R., et al.: Biomechanical measures during landing and postural stability predict second anterior cruciate ligament injury after anterior cruciate ligament reconstruction and return to sport. Am. J. Sports Med. **38**(10), 1968–1978 (2010). https://doi.org/10.1177/0363546510376053
12. Mueske, N.M., VandenBerg, C.D., Pace, J.L., et al: Comparison of drop jump landing biomechanics and asymmetry among adolescents with hamstring, patellar and quadriceps tendon autografts for anterior cruciate ligament reconstruction. Knee **25**(6), 1065–1073 (2018). https://doi.org/10.1016/j.knee.2018.09.005
13. Mantashloo, Z., Letafatkar, A., Moradi, M.: Vertical ground reaction force and knee muscle activation asymmetries in patients with ACL reconstruction compared to healthy individuals. Knee Surg. Sports Traumatol. Arthrosc. **28**(6), 2009–2014 (2019). https://doi.org/10.1007/s00167-019-05743-5
14. King, E., Richter, C., Franklyn-Miller, A., Wadey, R., Moran, R., Strike, S.: Back to normal symmetry? Biomechanical variables remain more asymmetrical than normal during jump and change-of-direction testing 9 months after anterior cruciate ligament reconstruction. Am. J. Sports Med. **47**(5), 1175–1185 (2019). https://doi.org/10.1177/0363546519830656
15. Lin, P.E., Sigward, S.M.: Contributors to knee loading deficits during gait in individuals following anterior cruciate ligament reconstruction. Gait Posture **66**, 83–87 (2018). https://doi.org/10.1016/j.gaitpost.2018.08.018
16. Dai, B., Butler, R.J., Garrett, W.E., Queen, R.M.: Anterior cruciate ligament reconstruction in adolescent patients: limb asymmetry and functional knee bracing. Am. J. Sports Med. **40**(12), 2756–2763 (2012). https://doi.org/10.1177/0363546512460837
17. Hart, J., Ko, J.W., Konold, T., Pietrosimone, B.: Sagittal plane knee joint moments following anterior cruciate ligament injury and reconstruction: a systematic review. Clin. Biomech. **25**(4), 277–283 (2010)

18. Ferber, R., Osternig, L.R., Woollacott, M.H., Wasielewski, N.J., Lee, J.H.: Gait mechanics in chronic ACL deficiency and subsequent repair. Clin. Biomech. (Bristol, Avon) **17**(4), 274–285 (2002). https://doi.org/10.1016/s0268-0033(02)00016-5
19. Kurz, M.J., Stergiou, N., Buzzi, U.H., Georgoulias, A.D.: The effect of anterior cruciate ligament recontruction on lower extremity relative phase dynamics during walking and running. Knee Surg. Sports Traumatol. Arthrosc. **13**(2), 107–115 (2005)
20. Gao, B., Cordova, M.L., Zheng, N.N.: Three-dimensional joint kinematics of ACL-deficient and ACL-reconstructed knees during stair ascent and descent. Hum. Mov. Sci. **31**(1), 222–235 (2012). https://doi.org/10.1016/j.humov.2011.04.009. Epub 2011 Jul 27 PMID: 21798608
21. Davis, R.B., Õunpuu, S., Tyburski, D.: A gait analysis data collection and reduction technique. Hum. Mov. Sci. **10**, 575–587 (1991)
22. Seliktar, R., Mizrahi, J.: Some gait characteristics of below-knee amputees andtheir reflection on the ground reaction forces. Eng. Med. **15**, 27–34 (1986). https://doi.org/10.1243/EMEDJOUR1986,015(009),pp.02
23. Andres, R., Stimmel, S.: Prosthetic alignment effects on gait symmetry, a case study. Clin. Biomech. **5**(2), 88–96 (1990)
24. Sadeghi, H., Allard, P., Prince, F., Labelle, H.: Symmetry and limb dominance in able-bodied gait: a review. Gait Posture **12**(1), 34–45 (2000)
25. Plotnik, M., Giladi, N., Hausdorff, J.: A new measure for quantifying the bilateral coordination of human gait, effects of aging and Parkinson's disease. Exp. Brain. Res. **181**(4), 561–570 (2007)

The Use of Accelerometers to Track Changes in Cobb Angles During Scoliosis Rehabilitation Exercises

A.-M. Vutan[1], C. M. Gruescu[2(✉)], Carmen Sticlaru[2], and Erwin-Christian Lovasz[2]

[1] West University of Timisoara, Timişoara, România
ana.vutam@e-uvt.ro
[2] Politehnica University of Timisoara, Timişoara, România
{corina.gruescu,carmen.sticlaru,erwin.lovasz}@upt.ro

Abstract. The effectiveness of specific physical exercises for the scoliosis rehabilitation is a topic that is still being discussed in the medical world and orthopedic doctors and physiotherapists have not reached a consensus. Mild and moderate scoliosis benefits from exercise treatment from the moment the deficiency is detected. The value of the Cobb angle is taken into consideration to observe the evolution of a scoliosis and the effectiveness of the treatment carried out, but this is generally done by taking repeated x-rays every 6 months. The study follows the changes that the Cobb angle undergoes during physical exercises specific to scoliosis in the case of a group of 9 subjects diagnosed with mild and moderate scoliosis. The possibility of tracking changes of this angle is given by the use of an equipment made up of accelerometric sensors attached to the skin, just below the spine. Cobb angle values are calculated mathematically by using approximation polynomials. The conclusions of the study are useful for the therapist, who can plan personalized exercise programs adequate to each patient.

Keywords: Scoliosis · Mathematical modelling · Efficiency of exercises · Clinical study

1 Introduction

According to SOSORT (Society of Scoliosis Orthopaedic and Rehabilitation Treatment), scoliosis is a general term comprising a heterogeneous group of conditions consisting in changes in the shape and position of the spine, thorax and trunk [1]. Vertebral disorders are very common in recent years among children and adults, due to lack of physical activity [2] and long-term prolonged sitting position [3].

Approximately 80% of the cases are idiopathic. Adolescent idiopathic scoliosis occurs in the general population in a wide range of prevalence from 1% to 12% [4], depending on the location where the study is conducted.

The treatment of scoliosis is standardized according to the magnitude of curvature measured on frontal radiography [5–7], as follows:

D. Tarnita et al. (Eds.): MESROB 2023, MMS 133, pp. 279–286, 2023.
https://doi.org/10.1007/978-3-031-32446-8_30

- for values of the Cobb angle between 10° and 25°, it is indicated to perform physiotherapeutic scoliosis-specific exercises.
- for values of the Cobb angle between 25° and 50°, orthopedic treatment (brace) and physical exercises specific to scoliosis are indicated.
- for values of the Cobb angle above 50°, surgery is the recommendation.

In 1948 Cobb proposed determining the angle of a vertebral curvature by drawing a line tangent to the upper plateau of the upper neutral vertebra and another tangent line to the lower plateau of the lower neutral vertebra of the same curves. A perpendicular is drawn on each tangent, and the complementary angle of these perpendiculars represents the value of the spine deviation (Fig. 1).

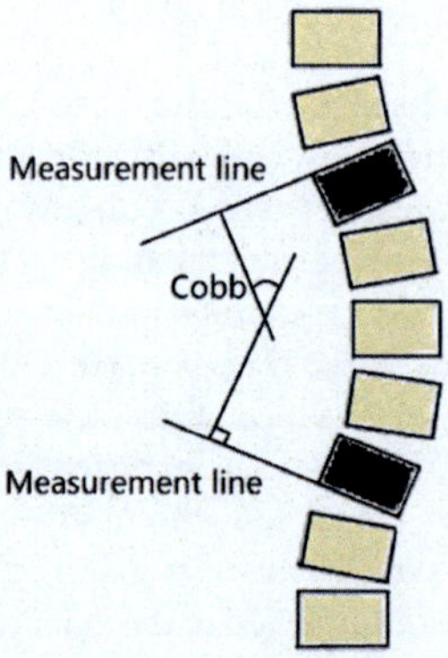

Fig. 1. Computation of the Cobb angle [8]

Physiotherapy for scoliosis consists in carrying out specific physical exercise programs, performed daily by the patient either under the supervision of therapists or independently at home. Physical exercises must always take into account the location of the curves, the magnitude of the Cobb angle, the rotation of the vertebral bodies, the patient's age, the effort capacity and other particularities (the patient's motor skills, the degree of collaboration and involvement of the patient, but also the degree of understanding).

There are several protocols standardized worldwide for physiotherapy programs.

The present study addresses to the classical physiotherapy exercises and exercises from Schroth and Méziéres methods.

The goals of physiotherapy are:

- slowing down the rate of evolution of scoliosis or, if possible, stopping the evolution of scoliosis and reducing the Cobb angle.
- erasing wrong postural reflexes and forming new habits regarding the correct position of the body in space, both statically and dynamically.
- increasing of the respiratory capacity.
- increasing the quality of life of people with scoliosis.

In practices, the physiotherapist performs exercise programs one of the methods and assesses the evolution of the patient through periodical radiographies. The purpose of this paper is to establish the efficiency of the exercises during the development of the program, so that the physiotherapist may decide if the exercises are appropriate for the patient and create personalized programs. The literature does not provide mathematical approaches regarding the efficiency of physical therapy. The authors propose a mathematical modelling of the spine and computation of the Cobb angle [9–12], which are used to assess the efficiency of the exercises for a lot of adolescent patients with scoliosis.

2 Mathematical Modelling of the Spine and Computation of the Cobb Angle

Modelling of the spine is possible only if numerical data, namely coordinates of several significant points on the column is available. Therefore, most of the investigation methods, including radiography, which is currently used, do not allow numerical processing. However, different data acquisition systems can be designed to this purpose. The authors designed and assembled a system consisting of eight accelerometers, attached on the skin of the patient, along the domain of interest of the spine (Fig. 2). The sensors [13] provide the rotation angles in the frontal plane. The microcontroller reads all 8 IMU raw accelerometer values in a continuous loop, computes the angles and sends the values to the connected PC with a frequency of 5 Hz.

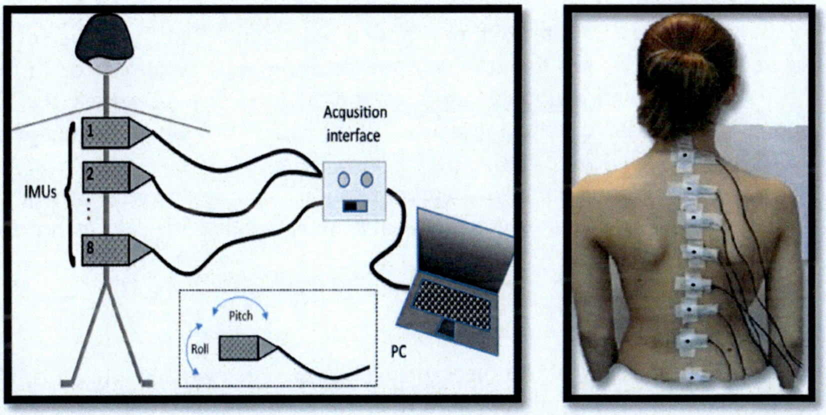

Fig. 2. Scheme of the equipment (left) and positioning of the sensors on the vertebral spinous processes (right) [9]

Knowing the distance between the sensors and the angles in the frontal plane, it is possible to compute the coordinates of eight points. The lowest point may be considered the origin of the reference system, with coordinates (0, 0). The column is modelled by the set of nine points (Fig. 3), which may be used as precision points for an approximation function.

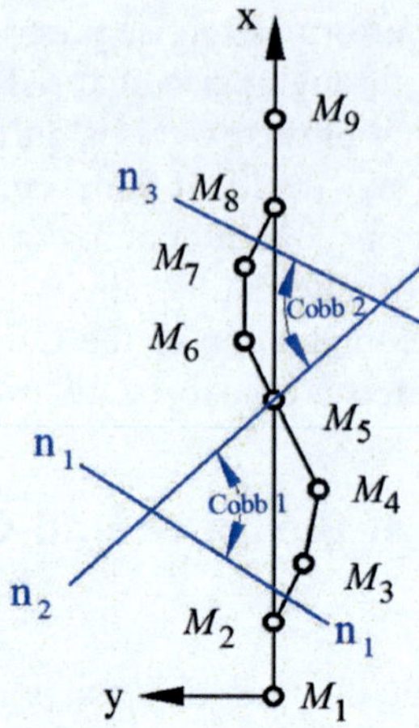

Fig. 3. Nine precision points used for the modelling and Cobb angles [8]

The coordinates of points $M_1 \ldots M_9$ are:

$$\begin{cases} x_{M1} = 0 \\ y_{M1} = 0 \\ x_{Mi+1} = x_{Mi} + l_i \cos\phi_i \quad i = \overline{1,8} \\ y_{Mi+1} = y_{Mi} + l_i \sin\phi_i \quad i = \overline{1,8} \end{cases} \tag{1}$$

For the approximation function, the authors chose a polynomial. For the choice of the polynomial degree, the shape of the graphic representation must be observed. To render the shape of the column and calculate the Cobb angle(s), it is necessary that the graph shows at least two/three inflection points, which indicates a higher degree of the polynomial (fourth or fifth degree).

To determine the inflection points, the approximation function f(x) must be analytically established and the roots of its second derivative must be calculated. Let us consider the function:

$$f''(x) = 0 \tag{2}$$

and its roots, which provide the inflection points $I_1(x_1, y_1)$, $I_2(x_2, y_2)$ and $I_3(x_3, y_3)$. The slope of the normal to the curve in these points is:

$$m_1 = -\frac{1}{f'(x_1)}, \quad m_2 = -\frac{1}{f'(x_2)}, \quad m_3 = -\frac{1}{f'(x_3)}, \tag{3}$$

where f'(x) is the first derivative of the approximation function.

Cobb angles are:

$$Cobb1 = \arctan\left|\frac{m_1 - m_2}{1 - m_1 m_2}\right|, \quad Cobb2 = \arctan\left|\frac{m_2 - m_3}{1 - m_2 m_3}\right|. \tag{4}$$

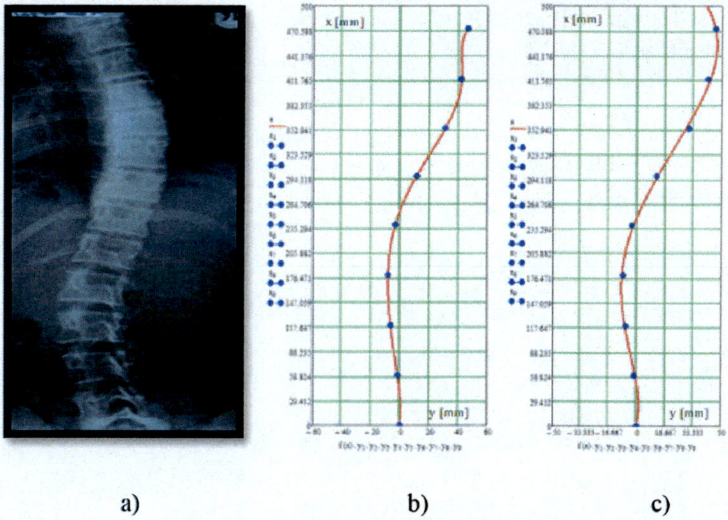

Fig. 4. Radiography (a), model with eighth degree polynomial (b) and model with fifth degree polynomial (c)

Figure 4 illustrates the mathematical procedure. The radiography (Fig. 4.a) may be compared with the model generated with an eighth polynomial (Fig. 4.b) and with a fourth polynomial (Fig. 4.c).

The mathematical modelling and analytical calculus of Cobb angles were used in assessing the efficiency of the physical exercises in the clinical study described below.

3 Clinical Study Regarding the Efficiency of the Physical Exercises

Three exercises belonging to different treatment methods and often used in rehabilitation were taken into analysis: an exercise from Schroth method (performed in the upright position), an exercise from Mezieres method (performed in a seated position) and an exercise from classical physiotherapy (performed in the hanging position). These 3 different types of exercises were performed by 9 subjects with scoliosis, to which Cobb angles are known from radiographs. During the exercises, the sensors of the equipment with accelerometers were positioned on the backs of the subjects participating in the study and the distances between them were noted. The first sensor was positioned at the level of the last lumbar vertebra L1 and the last sensor at the level of the cervical vertebra C7. After positioning the equipment on the back of the subjects, a first data acquisition was carried out in the orthostatic position as the radiographic image acquisition was carried out. Thus, Cobb angles were first calculated for this position for all subjects, considered as the reference position. Afterwards, each subject performed the 3 exercises and data acquisition from the accelerometers was performed for each individual exercise. The Cobb angle values calculated in different exercise sequences were compared with the Cobb angle value obtained on X-ray for each individual subject. The Cobb angles calculated in the positions in which the spine is placed during the 3 exercises taken in the study, decreased compared to the reference value on the radiograph. The results obtained are presented in Table 1.

Tabel 1. Cobb angle values calculated on radiographs and using the mathematical method during exercises from Schroth, Mezieres, and classic rehabilitation exercises (from hanging position) for the 9 subjects in the study

Method	Subj.1	Subj.2	Subj.3	Sub.4	Sub.5	Subj.6	Subj.7	Subj.8	Sub.9
X ray Cobb angle	15°L 17°T	10°L 16°T	13°T 10°L	16L	12°T 16°L	16°T 10°L	12°T-L	13°L 19°T	22°L 23° T
Standing Cobb angle	14.8°L 18.77°T	11.53°L 16,76T	14.33°T 10.56°L	16.48°L 6.50°T	11.72°T 16.72	16,66°T 11.73°L	13.17°L	11.48°L 16.61°T	18.46°L 19.50°T
Schroth Cobb angle	11.18°L 12.77°T	9,15°L 13,29°T	9.75°T 0.00°L	1.82°L 1.59°T	10,84°T 8.06°L	11.45°T 3.69°L	9.54°L	8.51°L 11.35° T	15.11°L 15.46°T
Mezieres Cobb angle	10.30°L 11.38T	8,27°L 11,23°T	9,38°T 0.33°L	2.07°L 2.02°T	10.84°T 8.06°L	9.82°T 1.61°L	8.70°L	9.02°L 10.18°T	14.45°L 15.13°T
Hanging position Cobb angle	14.06°L 5.28°T	10,24°L 11,85°T	4.62°T 11.18°L	14.13°L 11.62°T	11.72°T 9.13°L	11,90°T 1.58°L	11.12°L	21.44°L 3.8°T	16.80°L 17.75°T

For each individual case, mathematical models of the spine were operated for each exercise sequence analyzed. Figure 5 shows an example of modeling.

Analyzing the results obtained from the mathematical calculations on the entire study group, it was found:

- during rehabilitation exercises the Cobb angles change their value depending on the movement chosen to be performed.
- the data taken from the accelerometric sensors can be used to observe the changes undergone by the spine during physical therapy exercises.
- hanging exercises cause an alignment of the vertebral bodies mainly in the thoracic area. Thus, the thoracic Cobb angle can be reduced by hanging on the fixed ladder, but in the lumbar region there was no corresponding correction, probably as a consequence of the difficult muscle control to maintain in this position. There were subjects to whom the Cobb angle in the lumbar region increased during exercise as a compensation for the decrease in the angle in the thoracic region.
- in the case of the specific exercise of the Mézières method, corrections were recorded in the case of the main curvature and less in the case of compensatory curves. Also, the thoracic area seems to correct better compared to the lumbar area.
- in the exercise of the Schroth method, a more efficient approach of the vertebral bodies to the midline is observed. In subjects with two curves, both of them had a decrease in Cobb angle.

The use of the equipment with accelerometric sensors makes possible to follow the changes in the Cobb angles during the exercises and thus the therapist can perform

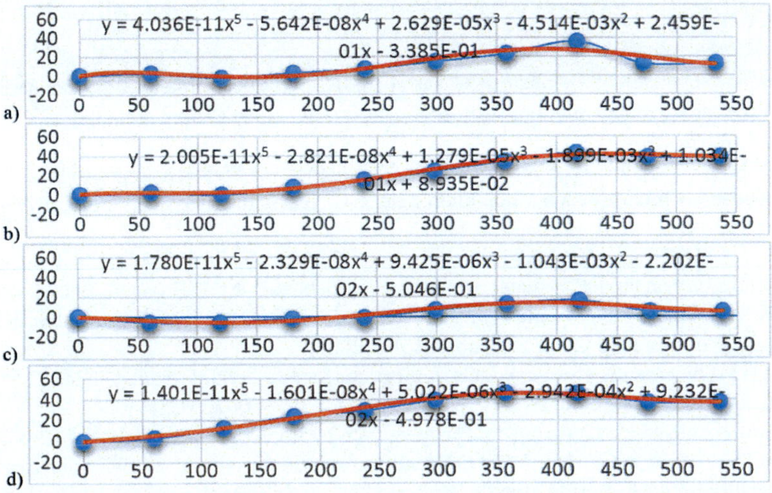

Fig. 5. The model of the column in orthostatism (a), Mezieres (b), Schroth (c) and hanging position (d) – for patient 1 (blue points – coordinates acquired with the equipment, red line – approximation polynomial)

the analysis of the changes that the spinal segments undergo between the first and the last sensor positioned on the skin. By following the evolution of the Cobb angles in certain exercise sequences, the therapist can correct and optimize the exercise program. Recording data during exercise execution helps the therapist determine if the exercise is appropriate for the patient and choose the most effective exercises for each individual patient.

4 Conclusions

In the present research, it was proposed an equipment that can be used to calculate by mathematical approach the Cobb angles in the case of mild and moderate scoliosis. The developed equipment composed by accelerometer makes possible a much easier following of the evolution of a scoliosis, both by the doctor and by the physiotherapist, in the framework of periodic evaluations but also of the therapy sessions in which it is desired to assess the effectiveness of the indicated exercises.

Three exercises that are currently used in rehabilitation clinics were tested, with the aim of observing the changes that Cobb angles undergo in different exercise sequences. Centralizing the data collected during the experiments, it was observed that the specific exercise of the Schroth method, through the three-dimensional corrections, achieves the most effective alignment of the vertebral bodies in the frontal plane, reducing the Cobb angles. The exercise of the Mézières method produces a decrease in the Cobb angle, mainly in the primary curvature and in the case of the exercise performed from the hanging position (from the classic rehabilitation program), a decrease in the Cobb angles were recorded in the thoracic area, while in the lumbar area the changes were minimal.

References

1. Negrini, S., Donzelli, S., Aulisa, A.G., et al.: 2016 SOSORT guidelines: orthopaedic and rehabilitation treatment of idiopathic scoliosis during growth. Scoliosis Spinal Disorders **13**(1), 3 (2018)
2. Juskelene, V., Magnus, P., Bakketeig, L.S., Dailidiene, N.: Prevalence and risk factors for asymmetric posturein preschool children aged 6–7 years. Int. J. Epidemiol. **5**, 1053–1059 (1996)
3. Linton, S.J., Hellsing, A.L., Halme, T., Akerstedt, K.: The effects of ergonomically designed school furniture on pupils' attitudes, symptoms and behavior. Appl. Ergon. **5**, 299–304 (1994)
4. Grivas, T.B., Wade, M.H., Negrini, S., et al.: SOSORT consensus paper: school screening for scoliosis. Where are we today?. Scoliosis **2**, 17 (2007)
5. Weiss, H.R., Negrini, S., et al.: Landauer, Indications for conservative management of scoliosis (SOSORT guidelines). Stud. Health Technol. Inf. **135**, 164–170 (2008)
6. ***. Tratament scolioza. https://scoliosistexas.com/treatment/traditional-scoliosis.html
7. Negrini, S., Aulisa, A.G., et al.: SOSORT guidelines: orthopaedic and rehabilitation treatment of idiopathic scoliosis during growth. Scoliosis **7**(1), 1–35 (2012)
8. Huo, X., et al.: An integrative framework for 3D cobb angle measurement on CT images. Comput. Biol. Med. **82**, 111–118 (2017)
9. Vutan, A.M., Davidescu, A., et al.: A new method of assessing the evolution of scoliosis. In: Proceedings of the 4th International Conference of the Universitaria Consortium (ICU 2018): the Impact of Sport and Physical Education Science on Today's Society, pp. 395–400 (2018)
10. Vutan, A.-M., Ciupe, V., Gruescu, C.M., Lovasz, E.-C.: Experimental method for dynamic evaluation of spinal column deformation exercises. In: Doroftei, I., Oprisan, C., Pisla, D., Lovasz, E.C. (eds.) New Advances in Mechanism and Machine Science. MMS, vol. 57, pp. 137–146. Springer, Cham (2018). https://doi.org/10.1007/978-3-319-79111-1_13
11. Vutan, A.M., Gruescu, C.M., Lovasz, E.C., Ciupe, V.: Discussion on Cobb angle variation during progressive lateral flexion of the trunk. IOP Conf. Ser. Mater. Sci. Eng. **444**, 052020 (2018)
12. Vutan, A.M., Gruescu, C.M., Lovasz, E.C., Ciupe, V.: Method to model the spinal column shape. IOP Conf. Ser. Mater. Sci. Eng. **514**(1), 012046 (2019)
13. MinIMU-9 v5 Gyro, Accelerometer, and Compass (LSM6DS33 and LIS3MDL Carrier) – Product information and resources webpage. https://www.pololu.com/product/2738

Kinematics and Dynamics for Medical Robotics

Forward Kinematic Model Resolution of a Hybrid Haptic Device Using an Inertial Measurement Unit

Majdi Meskini[1,3], Houssem Saafi[1,2], Abdelfattah Mlika[1], Marc Arsicault[3], Juan Sandoval[3], Said Zeghloul[3], and Med Amine Laribi[3(✉)]

[1] Mechanical Laboratory of Sousse (LMS), National Engineering School of Sousse, University of Sousse, 4000 Sousse, Tunisia

[2] Preparatory Institute for Engineering Studies of Gafsa, University of Gafsa, 2000 Gafsa, Tunisia

[3] Department of GMSC, Pprime Institute, CNRS - University of Poitiers, ENSMA - UPR 3346, Poitiers, France

med.amine.laribi@univ-poitiers.fr

Abstract. This paper deals with the experimental validation of a novel hybrid haptic device (nHH) intended to be used in a robotic teleoperation platform for laparoscopic surgery. The contribution of this work is to cope with the complexity of the Forward Kinematic Model (FKM) of the nHH and to validate its resolution experimentally through the use of an additional sensor: an IMU attached to its end-effector (serial part). Thus, this sensor allows to measure the orientation of the end-effector, allowing to solve the forward model of the parallel part of the nHH. Experiments have been conducted on the prototype of the hybrid device and, as expected, the FKM computation time is reduced. The proposed approach is validated and the obtained results demonstrate the significance of placing an IMU sensor on the serial part of the device, which makes the nHH suitable for real-time applications.

Keywords: Hybrid robot · Haptic device · Forward kinematic model · IMU sensor · Real-time application

1 Introduction

In a wide range of fields, human-robot collaboration is crucial. In this context, haptic devices have been created to allow their users to interact with a computer program or a virtual object by providing force and torque feedback. They are employed to enhance immersive solutions in areas like gaming [1], virtual training [2] and augmented reality [3]. One real-world instance where haptic feedback might be extremely helpful is in medical applications, more specifically the minimally invasive surgery (MIS).

A spherical parallel manipulator (SPM) architecture with a center of rotation (CoR) was proposed by several authors and used as a haptic device for MIS [4]. The actuators of the SPM are located on the base as opposed to the serial master haptic device, which

D. Tarnita et al. (Eds.): MESROB 2023, MMS 133, pp. 289–297, 2023.
https://doi.org/10.1007/978-3-031-32446-8_31

cope with the system's inertia problem. However, this parallel-architected haptic device suffers from singularities in its workspace, which amplifies kinematic transformation errors [5].

The complexity of solving the Forward Kinematic Model (FKM) for parallel manipulators has been widely proven [6–8]. When dealing with the Kinematic Model (KM) for these robots, a number of practical issues arise. According to [9], the FKM of a parallel manipulator is actually challenging to solve, and this is due to two main issues: (1) the determination of the admissible solutions, and (2) how to identify the best solution among all the others, which describes the actual posture based on the joint values. Different approaches have been proposed in order to solve the FKM. A solution that involves the resolution of an eight-degree polynomial has been proposed by Gosselin et al. [10]. Nevertheless, given the length of the calculations required in this situation, it is difficult to use this method. The Newton iterative method, which is used by Bai et al. in [11], may be the best numerical method for solving this problem because it only yields one solution. Unlike the least squares method, this approach has the drawback of not guaranteeing that the solution found is the most likely to be effective. These two approaches still have a significant shortcoming because they rely on an estimation of the initial posture, which increases the convergence speed while reducing the computation time. Furthermore, singularities in the workspace of parallel manipulators degrade the FKM's accuracy. The serial method proposed by Meskini et al. [12, 13], where sensors were mounted on a leg, is one of the most recent methods for solving the FKM of parallel manipulators.

Based on the methodology described in [14], this paper presents a pilot study to address the issue of the FKM of a novel hybrid haptic device (nHH) with four possible degrees of freedom (DoF). The proposed architecture is composed of a serial and a parallel kinematic chain. The purposes of the proposed solving method are to reduce the computation time and to choose an exact solution. It is based on the placement of an additional sensor, i.e. an IMU attached to the end-effector (serial chain) of the nHH, indicating its orientation.

This paper is organized as follows. In Sect. 2, the architecture of the novel hybrid haptic device is presented. Sections 3 is devoted to the description of the analytic and the improved method for the resolution of the FKM and the description of experiments. The results of the experiments are presented in Sect. 4. The last section concludes this paper.

2 Architecture of the nHH Device

The nHH device, a newly suggested 4-DoF design, i.e. three rotations around a fixed CoR and one translation, is shown in Fig. 1. The nHH is an association of a parallel kinematic chain and a serial kinematic chain. The parallel chain, defined by a 3-RRR planar manipulator with 3-DoF, manage both the tilt and the self-rotation. The prismatic and spherical joints that make up the serial chain provide control of the translation along an axis passing through a fixed CoR. A universal joint, as shown in Fig. 1, is used to connect the parallel and serial chains. This association overcomes the disadvantages of serial architectures which suffers from the moving masses due to the actuators located in the joints. Further, the nHH has the parallel structures advantage in terms of rigidity and accuracy.

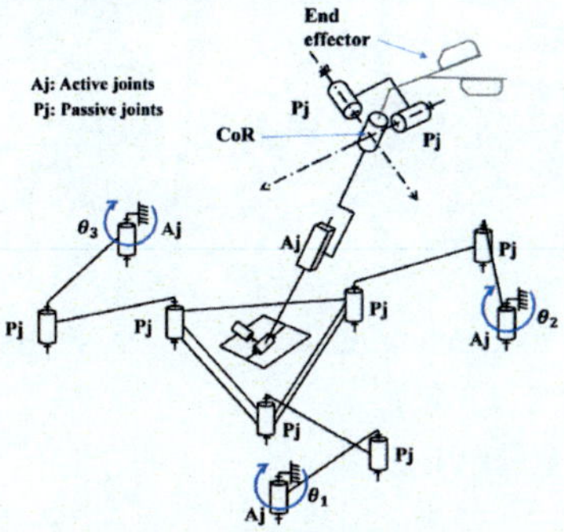

Fig. 1. Hybrid haptic device architecture.

In order to identify the best design parameters of the nHH device leading to the best kinematic performance, an optimization process based on an optimal dimensional synthesis was conducted. The proposed optimization problem is formulated as the minimization of an objective function that reflects the overall performance of the manipulator and is solved using a Genetic Algorithm (GA). The design parameters are presented in Fig. 2.

Where,

$$\mathrm{V} = \left[L_1 \; L_2 \; L_3 \; a \; H \right]^T$$

V: Design vector with the length L_i; $i \in \{1,2,3\}$, the distance a representing the dimension of the base and the distance H between the parallel chain plane and the CoR.

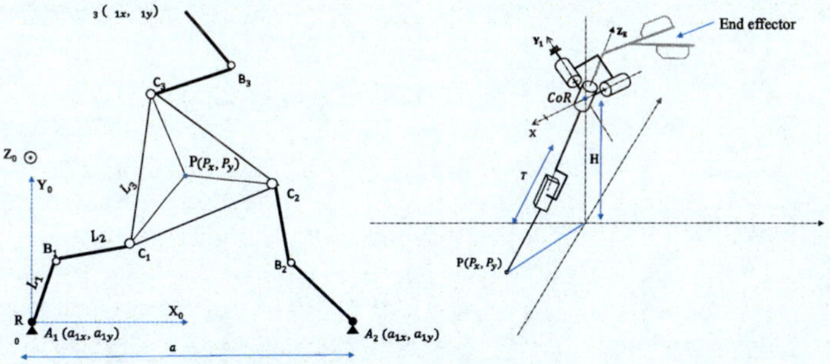

Fig. 2. nHH design parameters.

The CAD model of the nHH device and its manufactured prototype are presented in Fig. 2a. and Fig. 2b, respectively. The prototype given in Fig. 2b includes four actuators located on the active joints, A_j, which handle the four allowed DoF and the expected haptic feedback.

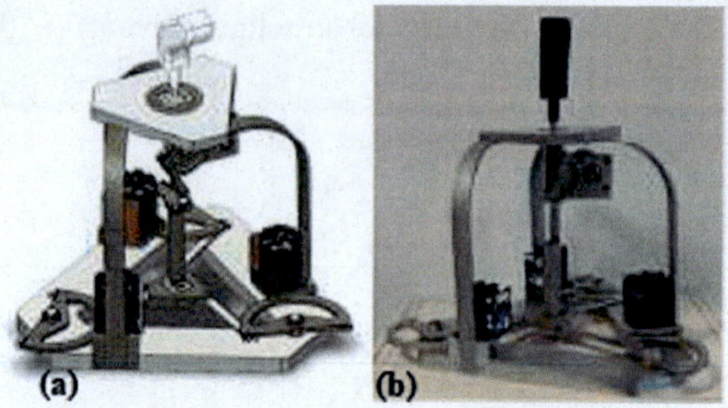

Fig. 3. (a) CAO model of the nHH manipulator and (b) Prototype of the nHH manipulator.

3 The Developed nHH Device

3.1 Direct Kinematic Model of the nHH Device

The direct model is defined by the orientation of the end-effector, (ψ, θ, φ), connected to the serial chain for a given configuration of the actuated joints $(\theta_{1j}, \theta_{2j}, \theta_{3j})$ and the translation, d, along the prismatic joint for a given actuated joint, θ_{4j}. In this paper, experimentations are focused on the experimental validation the FKM. Each motor of the manipulator is equipped with an encoder that calculates the position values for each active joint. Knowing these values, we allow to analytically calculate the position and the orientation of the mobile platform of the parallel chain using a code implemented in MATLAB. Figure 3 provides a visual representation of the solutions obtained after solving the FKM of the parallel chain. As shown, one of the major drawbacks of this method is that we obtain six solutions, then we have to identify the best one that describes the reel configuration.

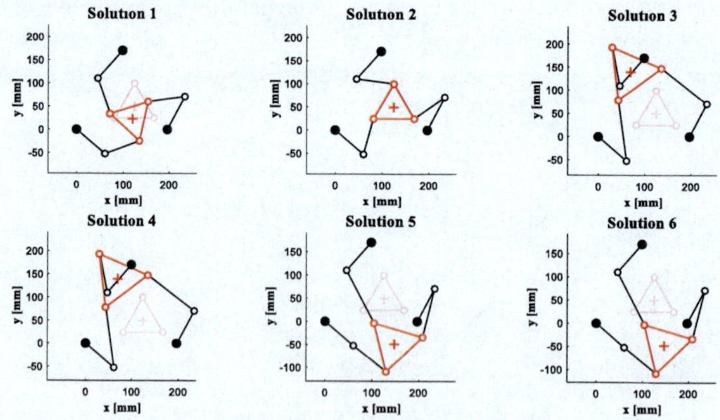

Fig. 4. Different solutions given by the analytic FKM.

The location and orientation of the moving platform of the parallel chain are linked to the orientation of the serial chain. Thus, the relationships between the cartesian coordinates of the point P designing the center of the mobile platform of the parallel chain, the orientation of the moving platform φ_z and the end-effector orientation (ψ, θ, φ) are defined in Eq. (1). Figure 4c illustrates how these relations are established.

$$\begin{cases} P_x = -H\tan\theta\cos\psi \\ P_y = -H\tan\theta\sin\psi \\ \varphi_z = \varphi \end{cases} \tag{1}$$

where, H is the distance between the CoR and the plane of the moving platform plane.

After choosing the reel configuration and after using the equation above, we manage to determine analytically the FKM of the nHH that relates the active joints $(\theta_{1j}, \theta_{2j}, \theta_{3j})$ to the end-effector orientation denoted by $(\psi_a, \theta_a, \varphi_a)$.

For the improved method of calculating the FKM using an additional sensor in the first instance, the sensor is calibrated using a static mechanical device, as shown in Fig. 4a. For this specific position imposed by the static mechanical device, the active angle values are known. Once the IMU sensors is calibrated, the end-effector is placed in different configurations.

Knowing the values of the active joints using the encoders placed in the motors and the information about the orientation of the end-effector given by the IMU, we are able to determine the FKM of the device. In fact, with this method, we have only one unique solution of the FKM. The correct choice solution is based on the comparison between the self-rotation of the mobile platform defined by φ_e and φ_a given by the IMU and the FKM, respectively.

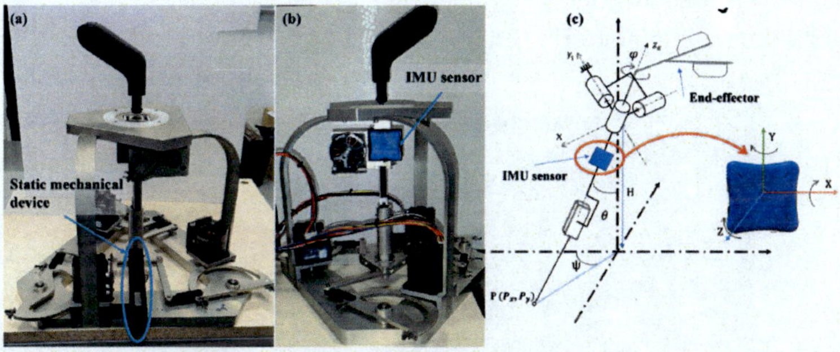

Fig. 5. The nHH device: (a) Calibration of the sensors (b) IMU sensor placement (c) serial chain with the additional sensor (IMU).

In order to verify the feasibility of this method, based on the use of the IMU sensor placed on the serial chain, we carried out several experimentations. In fact, the described algorithm allows the calculation of the error between the pose of the mobile platform, position and orientation, denoted by $(P_{x_e}, P_{y_e}, \varphi_e)$, calculated using the IMU and the one through the analytic model $(P_{x_a}, P_{y_a}, \varphi_a)$. The computation algorithm is presented as follows:

1. Read the IMU quaternion $(\phi_{1i}, \phi_{2i}, \phi_{3i}, \phi_{4i})$ for different orientations of the end effector.

2. Transform the IMU quaternion to Euler angles $(\psi_e, \theta_e, \varphi_e)$.
3. Compute $(P_{xe}, P_{y_e}, \varphi_e)$ using Eq. (1).
4. Read the angular values of the active joints.
5. Compute the mobile platform position and orientation $(P_{x_a}, P_{y_a}, \varphi_a)$ using the analytic model of the FKM.
6. Determining the FKM of the nHH.

The Euler angles can be obtained from the quaternion provided by the IMU, by using the following equations:

$$\begin{cases} \psi_e = atan2(\phi_3, \phi_4) - atan2(\phi_4, \phi_4) \\ \theta_e = \mathrm{acos}\left(2\left(\phi_4^2 + \phi_3^2\right) - 1\right) \\ \varphi_e = atan2(\phi_3, \phi_4) + atan2(-\phi_1, \phi_2) \end{cases} \tag{2}$$

3.2 Experimental Setup and Protocol

The test bench for validation of the FKM using an additional sensor, as presented in Fig. 5, is composed of the nHH device equipped with 4 brushless motors (Simplex Motion SC040), each one coupled to a capstan (10:1 ratio) in the purpose to reduce the speed and multiply the torque. All the motors are connected to a power card, which is connected to a laptop in order to read the angular position values of the motors. The IMU (LPMS-B2 from LP-Research) is linked to the laptop directly using Bluetooth. Once the calibration sensor is done using the static mechanical device, the end-effector pose can be followed by the mobile platform (Fig. 6).

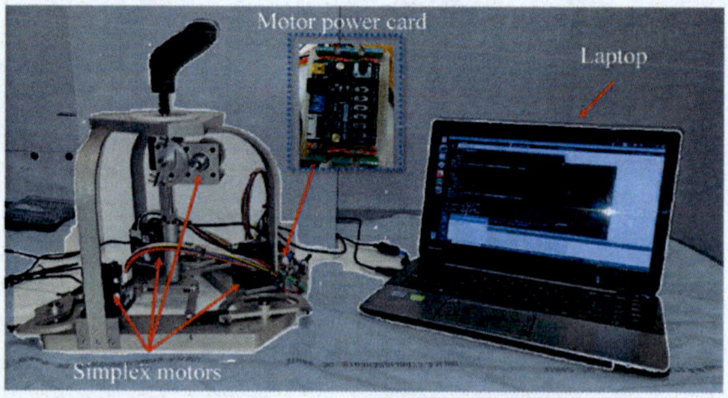

Fig. 6. Test bench for FKM validation.

Several steps have been followed during the experimentations, going from the sensor calibration to the selection of the right configuration of the nHH. These steps can be resumed as given:

(1) Calibrate the sensor in a position with known angle values.
(2) Move the end-effector in a random orientation.
(3) Read the angle encoder values and use them in the analytic FKM calculation.

(4) Read the quaternion provided by the IMU and compute the position and the orientation of the mobile platform of the nHH.
(5) Select the appropriate solution between the six given by the analytic FKM.

Four random poses have been selected in the next section to verify the feasibility of the use of IMU to cope with the complexity of the FKM of the nHH and its multiple solutions.

4 Experimental Results

For four different poses inside the workspace leading to several locations and orientation of the mobile platform of nHH and after calibration, the previous steps from 2 to 5 are performed. Table 1 illustrates the graphic construction of the analytical solution of the FKM with the corresponding values of the self-rotation φ_a. It's important to mention here that only one solution is constructed from the six possible ones. For each pose, the corresponding angle orientation value, φ_e, is given by the IMU. Based on this orientation the correct assembly mode, a solution of FKM, from the six possible modes and happen on the prototype is selected.

Table 1. Experimentation results for FKM resolution using analytic and extra sensor method.

	Pose 1	*Pose 2*	*Pose 3*	*Pose 4*
IMU φ_e	*0.255°*	*-10.31°*	*20.22°*	*30.81°*
Analytic FKM	**Solution 1** 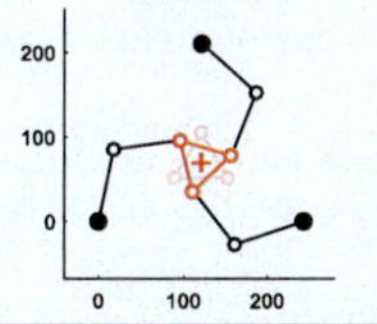	**Solution 5** 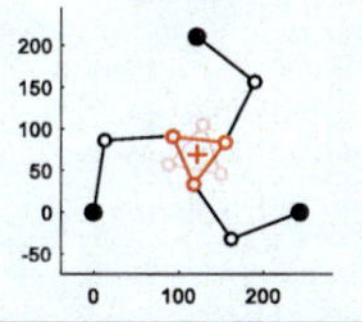	**Solution 1** 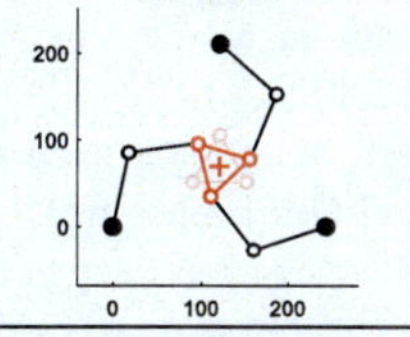	**Solution 4** 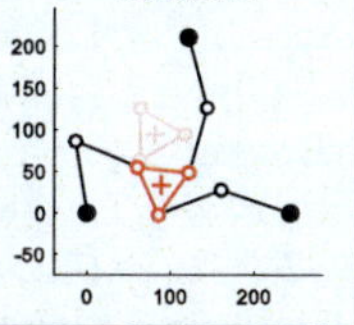
	$\varphi_{a1} = -73.5°$	$\varphi_{a5} = -65.53°$	$\varphi_{a1} = -90.24°$	$\varphi_{a4} = -100.8°$
	Solution 6 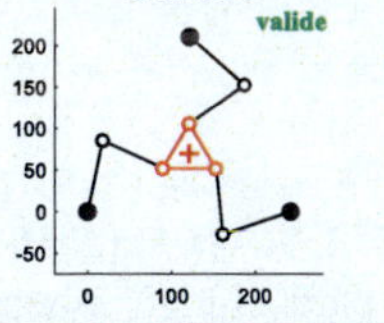	**Solution 6** 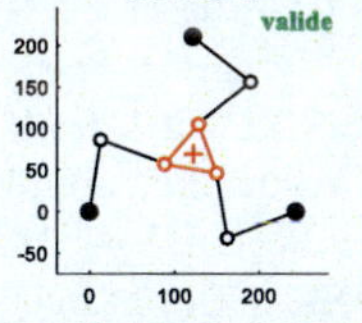	**Solution 2** 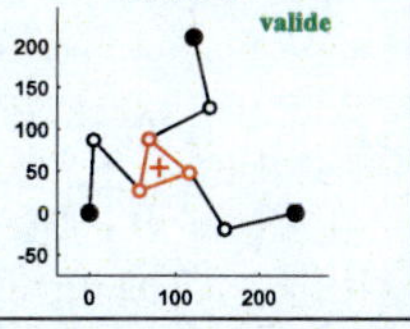	**Solution 1** 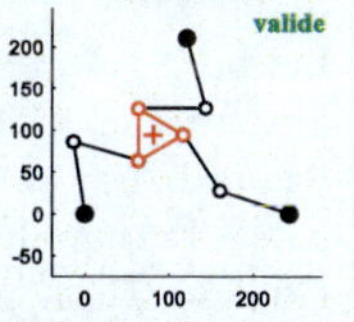
	$\varphi_{a1} = 0.29°$	$\varphi_{a2} = -11.12°$	$\varphi_{a3} = 19.44°$	$\varphi_{a4} = 29.36°$

One of the big advantages for solving the FKM using an extra sensor (IMU) is that it speeds up the computation time and even makes it possible the application of this method in real-time. Table 2 shows the computing time using the two methods implemented on an INTEL i5 processor up to 2.4 GHz.

According to the obtained results, by knowing the orientation of the mobile platform given by the IMU, we manage to resolve the FKM of the nHH and select the right

Table 2. FKM computing time.

Method	Analytic	Using extra sensor
Computation time	1.6s	0.0058s

assembly mode using the extra sensor for any pose inside the workspace of the hybrid device.

5 Conclusion

In this paper, a real-time approach to solve the Forward Kinematic Model of a novel hybrid haptic device is developed using an extra sensor, i.e. an IMU, attached to its end-effector (serial part). Experimentations were performed and the obtained results show the efficiency of the proposed method. The use of an extra sensor improved the resolution of the FKM of the hybrid haptic device, especially of its parallel chain. By this approach, we manage to choose the correct assembly mode among the six possible ones of the direct model, speeding up the computation time, as desired for a real-time use.

References

1. Park, W., Kim, L., Cho, H., Park, S.: Design of haptic interface for brickout game. In: Proceedings of 2009 International Workshop on Haptic Audio Visual Environments. Games, HAVE 2009, pp. 64–68 (2009)
2. Broeren, J., Rydmark, M., Sunnerhagen, K.S.: Virtual reality and haptics as a training device for movement rehabilitation after stroke: a single-case study. Arch. Phys. Med. Rehabil. **85**(8), 1247–1250 (2004)
3. Gosselin, F., Jouan, T., Brisset, J., Andriot, C.: Design of a wearable haptic interface for precise finger interactions in large virtual environments. In: Proceedings of Eurohaptics Conference Symposium Teleoperator Syst. World Haptics Conference WHC 2005, pp. 202–207 (2005)
4. Laribi, A., Romdhane, L., Zeghloul, S.: Synthesis of spherical parallel manipulator for dexterous medical task. Front. Mech. Eng. **7**(2), 150–162 (2012)
5. Saafi, H., Laribi, M.A., Zeghloul, S.: Optimal haptic control of a redundant 3-RRR spherical parallel manipulator. IEEE Int. Conf. Intell. Robot. Syst. **2015**, 2591–2596 (2015)
6. Gosselin, C.M., Merlet, J.-P.: The direct kinematics of planar parallel manipulators: Special architectures and number of solutions. Mech. Mach. Theory **29**(8), 1083–1097 (1994). https://doi.org/10.1016/0094-114X(94)90001-9
7. Baron, L., Angeles, J.: The direct kinematics of parallel manipulators under joint-sensor redundancy. IEEE Trans. Robot. Autom. **16**(1), 12–19 (2000)
8. Merlet, J.P.: Direct kinematics of planar parallel manipulators. In: Proceedings of IEEE International Conference on Robotics and Automation, vol. 4, no. 9212595, pp. 3744–3749 (1996)
9. Tancredi, L., Teillaud, M.: Application de la géométrie synthétique au problème de modélisation géométrique directe des robots parallèles. Mech. Mach. Theory **34**(2), 255–269 (1999). https://doi.org/10.1016/S0094-114X(97)00108-0

10. Gosselin, C.M., Sefrioui, J., Richard, M.J.: On the direct kinematics of spherical three-degree-of-freedom parallel manipulators of general architecture. J. Mech. Des. Trans. ASME **116**(2), 594–598 (1994)
11. Bai, S., Hansen, M.R., Angeles, J.: A robust forward-displacement analysis of spherical parallel robots. Mech. Mach. Theory **44**(12), 2204–2216 (2009)
12. Meskini, M., Saafi, H., Laribi, M.A., Mlika, A., Arsicault, M., Zegloul, S.: Serial approach for solving the forward kinematic model of the DELTA robot. In: Zeghloul, S., Laribi, M.A., Arsicault, M. (eds.) Mechanism Design for Robotics. MMS, vol. 103, pp. 305–312. Springer, Cham (2021). https://doi.org/10.1007/978-3-030-75271-2_32
13. Meskini, M., Saafi, H., Mlika, A., Arsicault, M., Zeghloul, S., Laribi, M.A.: Improved resolution of a forward kinematic model of parallel manipulators using a serial approach. In: CISM International Centre for Mechanical Sciences: Courses and Lectures, vol. 606, pp. 292–300 (2022)
14. Saafi, H., Laribi, M.A., Zeghloul, S.: Improvement of the direct kinematic model of a haptic device for medical application in real time using an extra sensor. In: International Conference on Intelligent Robots and Systems IROS, pp. 1697–1702 (2014)

Influence on the Visual Feedback on Several Balance Assessment Indicators Measured in a Balance Rehabilitation Machine

R. Valenzuela(✉), J. Corral, M. Diez, F. J. Campa, S. Herrero, E. Macho, and Ch. Pinto

University of the Basque Country UPV/EHU, Escuela de Ingeniería de Bilbao, Plaza Ingeniero Torres Quevedo 1, 48013 Bilbao, Spain
ruben.valenzuela@ehu.eus

Abstract. In this paper, a novel parallel platform for balance testing called OREKA is used to analyze the Centre of Pressure movement of several subjects during tilting motions. The platform, based on the 3PRS architecture, is capable of rotations around both horizontal axes and a vertical translation. Several subjects have performed different exercises to validate the capabilities of the platform and the influence of the visual feedback on the COP motion and several balance indicators. The obtained results are promising since the platform presents a higher resolution than the actual scales used in balance assessment and indicate how much the presence of feedback can influence the user behaviour.

Keywords: Balance assessment · force plate · post urography · centre of pressure

1 Introduction

The ability to maintain the body balance depends on the combination of input systems, muscular actions and reactions and neural feedback [1]. Signals are collected and then transmitted to the central nervous system (CNS) which is responsible for processing them to determine the necessary steps to keep the body standing still or walk. When a person is affected by a stroke it affects the motor neurons which then leads to spasticity, this affects daily life and wellbeing of individuals severely limiting the autonomy and therefore, quality of life. In clinical medicine there are several scales for this purpose, such as the Berg Balance Scale (BBS), Timed-Up and Go (TUG), The Short Physical Performance Battery (SPPB), among others. However, the disadvantage is that the assessments made are subjective; for that reason, several studies have been carried out to determine indicators that allow an objective balance evaluation of a person, among which the behavior of the center of pressure (COP) stands out, this is, the point of application of the ground reaction forces resultant under the feet.

The objective of this paper is to explain the use of a dynamometric platform that generates motions to force people to remain in balance and, at the same time, acquire the COP signals for later post-processing and calculating indicators to identify possible irregularities in users.

D. Tarnita et al. (Eds.): MESROB 2023, MMS 133, pp. 298–305, 2023.
https://doi.org/10.1007/978-3-031-32446-8_32

2 Description of the Balance Rehabilitation Device

OREKA is a dynamic platform based on the 3PRS parallel manipulator where the prismatic joints are actuated to allow two rotations around both horizontal axes as well as a vertical displacement. The movement ranges are ± 15° for rotations and a displacement of 250 mm. A screen in front of the user is used as a feedback system, where the medio-lateral (ML) and antero-posterior (AP) displacements of the COP are displayed while the exercise is being performed.

The mobile platform consists of two 800x800 mm aluminium plates with a minimum thickness of 12 mm and reinforcement ribs with a maximum thickness of 20 mm. The user is positioned on the upper platform and the spherical joints are located on the lower platform.

For the signal acquisition system, the lower platform has four INTERFACE GWMC uniaxial force sensors with a measuring range of 2000 N. The force signals are acquired with a sampling frequency of 50 Hz, and a 4th order zero-phase Butterworth filter and a cut-off frequency of 10 Hz is applied prior to any calculation (Fig. 1).

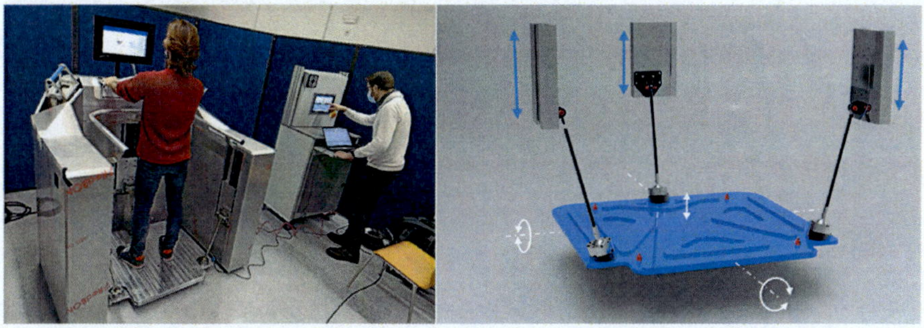

Fig. 1. Left) OREKA balance rehabilitation machine. Right) Diagram of the tilting mechanism.

3 Experimental Methodology

3.1 Subjects

Ten young healthy adults were enrolled. They were teachers and/or students from within the University of the Basque Country UPV/EHU. As a mean ± SD, age was 36.5 ± 7.96 years (range 24 – 43) weight was 74.1 ± 12.5 kg (range 64 – 85), height was 1.76 ± 0.08 m (range 1.67 – 1.85). No subjects reported any discomfort throughout the duration of the test. All gave their informed consent. Ten users performed the tests with the feedback and six participants were asked to return for a second round of tests without the feedback screen.

3.2 Experimental Protocol

OREKA has five types of platform movements programmed, three rotations around the X axis (“anterior-posterior AP”) with different amplitudes and two rotations around the Y axis (“ medio-lateral ML”) with different amplitudes. Each movement can be performed in five different speeds, resulting in twenty-five possible exercises.

Participants were asked to place their feet within an area corresponding to the average foot measurement ($b = 10$ cm $h = 40$ cm) whose centre is located at the midpoint between the sensors of the platform in such a way that the COP reference was as uniform as possible among participants.

Once on the platform, the participant was instructed to keep a straight posture, arms in a natural position and the eyes fixed on the feedback screen or on a marker, both placed 1.5 m away.

When the feedback tests (Fig. 2) were performed, the participants were requested to keep the COP markers as still as possible at its initial position. In the tests without feedback, they were asked to maintain their balance by exerting the required reaction to do so.

Every test had a 60 s duration per exercise resulting in approximately a 30-min session per participant. A sample of 30 s was used to compute the indices, avoiding initial and final transitory phases.

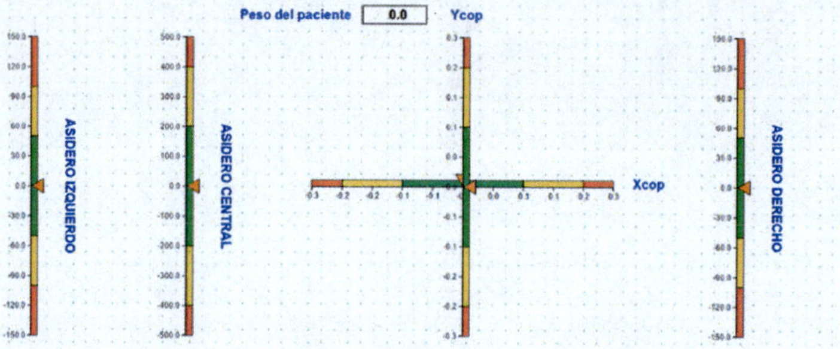

Fig. 2. Visual feedback screen, the yellow markers in the middle cross move accordingly to the COP sway, the rest of the vertical feedback corresponds to the handles.

4 Results

The reaction forces were acquired by the platform sensors and used to compute various indicators to evaluate the behaviour of a person’s equilibrium responding to the movements performed by the platform. These indicators are: average distance ML and AP, maximum distance ML and AP (Fig. 3), minimum distance ML and AP, area of the 95% confidence ellipse of the statokinesigram (SKG) (Fig. 3.), minor axis of the Poincare diagram (SD1) and major axis of the Poincare diagram (SD2) (Fig. 3).

4.1 Measurements of COP Patterns

Figure 3 shows the pattern of the ML and AP displacements, the minimum and maximum distances of the entire sample as well as the mean values for a given test.

Figure 4, left, shows the representation of the COP behaviour in the plane for the same test, where the X axis corresponds to the ML displacements and the Y axis to the AP displacements. It is important to be able to identify its evolution in time to identify the time when the excursions occur outside the 95% confidence ellipse. To this end, colour format was given, which changes from cold to warm colours to represent the beginning and end of the sample respectively.

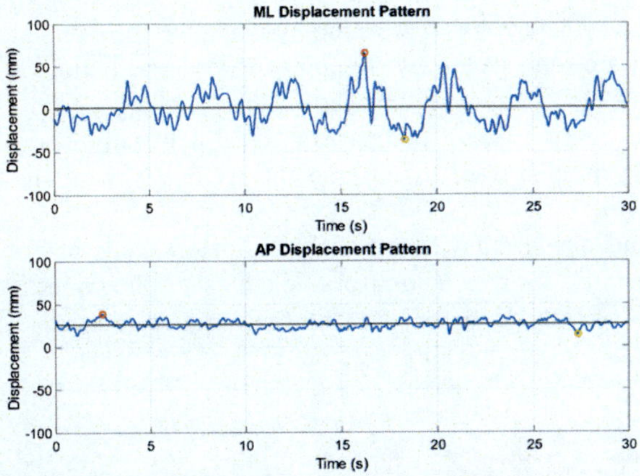

Fig. 3. Example of COP patterns (Statokinesigram, COP-ML, COP-AP) for one subject for a 8° ML rotation at 10 deg./s.

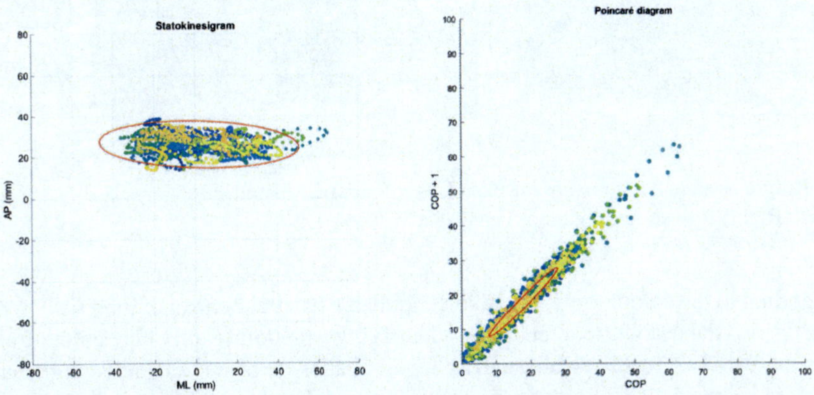

Fig. 4. Left) Statokinesigram for an 8° ML platform rotation at 10 deg./s. Right) Poincaré Diagram for an 8° ML platform rotation at 10 deg./s.

The area of an ellipse is defined as:

$$A_E = \pi ab$$

By using Principal Component Analysis, which states that the first principal component, which is a line that represents the maximum variance direction, and then the second principal component is orthogonal to the first PC. When seeking to calculate a 95% confidence ellipse a constant corresponding to a Chi-square distribution with two degrees of freedom $\chi^2_{0.95,2} = 5.99146$ is used in the following formula to calculate the area:

$$Elipsearea = \pi * PCA_1 * PCA_2 * \sqrt{\chi^2_{0.95,2}}$$

The Poincaré diagram in Fig. 4, right, is a technique that compares a data vector x_i with itself but lag, in this case $m = 1$ $(y = x_{i+m})$. . By using this diagram, one can identify body sway behaviour of a person by using the local and global adjustment of a person, which are represented by the minor (SD1) and major (SD2) axes of the confidence ellipse of the generated point scatter.

In this instance, being a vector comparison, the Euclidean distance from the centre of the trajectory is also used to observe the COP behaviour in both directions simultaneously.

The averages and standard deviations of the indicators were then obtained for each of the platform exercises, for which comparative tables are shown in Tables 1, 2, and 3.

In order to observe the trends between all the exercises and all the speeds of the platform, a 2D colour plot graph is presented in Fig. 5.

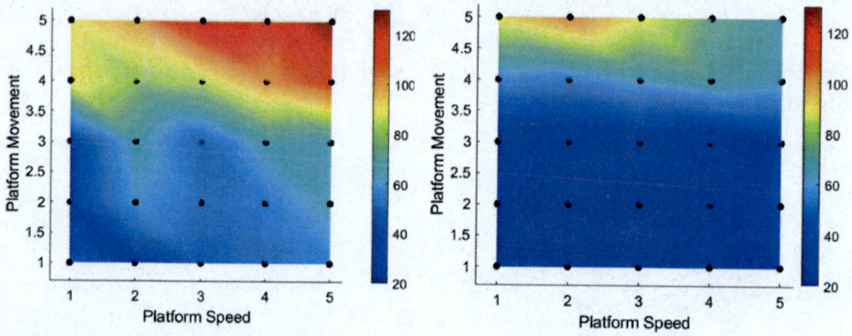

Fig. 5. Ellipse Area as a function of the exercise type (ordinates) and speed (abscissa): Left) with Feedback. Right) Ellipse Area without Feedback.

Attending to the colour plots, users, in general, have better control of their COP when they performed the test without feedback, identifying a predominantly blue colour trend, while in the tests with feedback blue and light blue shades are observed, indicating greater difficulty in keeping the COP static, possibly because they tend to overreact against the COP movement that they see in the feedback screen. The numerical values are shown in Table 1.

Of particular interest is the distribution of the larger areas in the ML direction, Exercises 4 and 5, corresponding to the red shades. When the participants performed the exercise at low speeds without feedback a larger area of the confidence ellipse is presented, while in the tests with feedback such a distribution is presented in the high-speed exercises. It is expected that in future tests this behaviour can be corroborated.

Table 1. Confidence ellipse area in cm^2 with and without feedback.

Feed back	ω (deg./s)	2	5	10	15	20
w	5°A 3°P	36.97 ± 16.79	36.79 ± 16.97	51.89 ± 26.23	54.97 ± 23.78	50.58 ± 24.64
	8°A 4°P	40.48 ± 22.36	57.51 ± 29.16	50.90 ± 32.81	59.17 ± 26.33	64.88 ± 28.09
	13°A 6°P	40.76 ± 21.37	76.88 ± 38.78	57.96 ± 32.75	76.40 ± 36.26	71.00 ± 30.98
	4° ML	92.46 ± 55.21	81.01 ± 33.01	93.13 ± 38.45	85.15 ± 41.13	114.93 ± 42.16
	8° ML	90.87 ± 39.82	99.77 ± 44.94	127.76 ± 46.34	116.50 ± 50.32	129.22 ± 59.21
w/o	5°A 3°P	17.98 ± 11.92	16.20 ± 7.55	16.75 ± 4.38	26.34 ± 12.47	22.34 ± 7.92
	8°A 4°P	16.82 ± 9.81	20.19 ± 8.35	21.55 ± 6.88	20.80 ± 6.66	38.32 ± 15.68
	13°A 6°P	26.98 ± 4.74	24.92 ± 7.36	28.71 ± 10.86	25.51 ± 7.14	31.51 ± 6.38
	4° ML	56.65 ± 20.41	54.76 ± 18.97	62.69 ± 25.93	68.5 ± 31.83	64.26 ± 20.75
	8° ML	92.94 ± 32.53	104.95 ± 36.08	91.18 ± 30.38	73.81 ± 33.59	66.1 ± 20.02

The use of the Poincaré diagram would make it possible to identify different behaviours depending on the shape of the point spread. Figure 3 shows how certain points completely leave the central cloud; however, in other users a more compact figure is observed.

One unexpected behaviour is that the SD1 indicator in the Poincaré diagram remains the same independently of the amplitude and type of the exercises, AP or ML. It increases with the velocity just as the confidence ellipse area, though, and it is also generally higher in the exercises with feedback.

Regarding the SD2 indicator in the Poincaré diagram, it clearly increases with the amplitude of motion of the exercises, but it does not always increase with the velocity, which is something that will require further studies, and maybe increasing the number of tests. Again, as a general trend, SD2 is higher when visual feedback was used.

Table 2. Minor axis (SD1) of the Poincaré plot in cm with and without feedback.

Feed back	ω (deg./s)	2	5	10	15	20
w	5°A 3°P	0.05 ± 0.02	0.07 ± 0.019	0.105 ± 0.023	0.13 ± 0.033	0.16 ± 0.066
	8°A 4°P	0.053 ± 0.01	0.066 ± 0.015	0.11 ± 0.02	0.11 ± 0.02	0.14 ± 0.04
	13°A 6°P	0.05 ± 0.01	0.07 ± 0.02	0.10 ± 0.02	0.11 ± 0.03	0.12 ± 0.03
	4° ML	0.06 ± 0.01	0.07 ± 0.01	0.095 ± 0.027	0.14 ± 0.04	0.19 ± 0.06
	8° ML	0.05 ± 0.02	0.07 ± 0.02	0.10 ± 0.017	0.15 ± 0.03	0.12 ± 0.04
w/o	5°A 3°P	0.03 ± 0.01	0.04 ± 0.01	0.07 ± 0.01	0.08 ± 0.01	0.11 ± 0.02
	8°A 4°P	0.03 ± 0.01	0.04 ± 0.01	0.07 ± 0.01	0.07 ± 0.01	0.08 ± 0.02
	13°A 6°P	0.04 ± 0.01	0.05 ± 0.01	0.08 ± 0.03	0.08 ± 0.03	0.08 ± 0.02
	4° ML	0.04 ± 0.01	0.06 ± 0.01	0.075 ± 0.02	0.12 ± 0.03	0.125 ± 0.03
	8° ML	0.04 ± 0.01	0.06 ± 0.02	0.07 ± 0.02	0.1 ± 0.02	0.11 ± 0.02

Table 3. Major axis (SD2) of the Poincaré plot in cm with and without feedback.

Feed back	ω (deg./s)	2	5	10	15	20
w	5°A 3°P	0.86 ± 0.33	1.02 ± 0.265	1.08 ± 0.33	1.18 ± 0.30	1.16 ± 0.332
	8°A 4°P	1.14 ± 0.44	1.351 ± 0.26	1.235 ± 0.24	1.235 ± 0.265	1.395 ± 0.52
	13°A 6°P	1.10 ± 0.44	1.61 ± 0.56	1.40 ± 0.39	1.44 ± 0.49	1.46 ± 0.53
	4° ML	1.32 ± 0.31	1.20 ± 0.36	1.20 ± 0.48	1.24 ± 0.44	1.53 ± 0.52
	8° ML	1.11 ± 0.33	1.35 ± 0.42	1.68 ± 0.355	1.54 ± 0.49	1.54 ± 0.72
w/o	5°A 3°P	0.65 ± 0.08	0.69 ± 0.11	0.75 ± 0.17	0.84 ± 0.14	0.72 ± 1.30
	8°A 4°P	0.74 ± 0.17	0.74 ± 0.11	0.84 ± 0.20	0.70 ± 0.08	0.95 ± 0.34
	13°A 6°P	1.02 ± 0.29	1.15 ± 0.46	1.01 ± 0.20	0.84 ± 0.16	0.94 ± 0.13
	4° ML	0.89 ± 0.33	0.95 ± 0.28	1.00 ± 0.27	1.05 ± 0.35	1.02 ± 0.19
	8° ML	1.33 ± 0.395	1.44 ± 0.32	1.26 ± 0.32	0.99 ± 0.23	1.07 ± 0.24

5 Conclusions

In this paper, an experimental protocol was carried out to test the OREKA platform capabilities using healthy subjects with different conditions: with and without visual feedback, and with different amplitudes and speeds. With these tests, by means of a dynamometric platform, several indicators are obtained to characterize the equilibrium of a person: the average, maximum and minimum distance in the AP and ML directions, the area of the 95% confidence ellipse and the SD1 and SD2 values of the Poincaré diagram.

As a general trend, all the indicators suggest that the COP motion is higher when the users were asked to react to the visual feedback to keep the COP steady, than when they were told to just stay in a standing pose without visual feedback of the COP motion.

Finally, it is worth highlighting that the prototype has enough resolution to find differences not only between tests with and without visual feedback, but also between individual participants who, if evaluated by traditional clinical methods, would have obtained same balance score. With these results, more detailed analysis is needed to explore the possibilities in terms of diagnosis and rehabilitation of people with balance problems. We look forward to carrying out another experimental protocol to identify the differences between healthy and non-healthy subjects.

Acknowledgements. Authors would like to thank for the funds received for the project PID2019-105262RB-I00 funded by MCIN/ AEI /https://doi.org/10.13039/501100011033, for the project PDC2022–133787-I00 funded by MCIN/AEI /https://doi.org/10.13039/501100011033 and by the European Union Next Generation EU/ PRTR, and for the project 2018222013 funded by the Basque Government. Thanks are also addressed for the funds received of the predoctoral grant PRE2020–092455 funded by MCIN/AEI/https://doi.org/10.13039/501100011033 and by 'FSE invierte en tu futuro'.

References

1. Quijoux, F., et al.: A review of center of pressure (COP) variables to quantify standing balance in elderly people: algorithms and open-access code. Physiol Rep. **9**(22), e15067 (2021)
2. Schubert, P., Kirchner, M.: Ellipse area calculations and their applicability in posturography. Gait Posture **39**(1), 518–522 (2014)
3. Crenna, F., Rossi, G.B., Berardengo, M.: Filtering biomechanical signals in movement analysis. Sensors **21**(13), 4580 (2021)
4. Zhang, S., et al.: Measuring the local and global variabilities in body sway by nonlinear Poincaré technology. IEEE Trans. Instrum. Meas. **68**(12), 4817–4824 (2019)

Kinematic and Dynamic Analysis of a New Mechanism for Assisting Human Locomotion

Ionut Geonea[1(✉)], Nicolae Dumitru[1], Marco Ceccarelli[2], and Daniela Tarnita[1]

[1] Faculty of Mechanics, University of Craiova, Craiova, Romania
{ionut.geonea,nicolae.dumitru,daniela.tarnita}@edu.ucv.ro
[2] University of Rome Tor Vergata, Rome, Lazio, Italy
marco.ceccarelli@uniroma2.it

Abstract. In this paper, an improved solution of a mechanism model used as a design solution for the legs of an exoskeleton intended to assist human walking is analysed from a kinematic and dynamic point of view. It is an improvement that is based on a previous developed solution. A kinematic model is presented, by which we have determined the variation of angles in the joints of the mechanical system. We are particularly interested in the variation of angles in the knee and hip joints, when compared with those made by a human subject in normal walking. Another category of results presented and analysed in the paper are the connecting forces in the kinematic joints of the mechanism. The dynamic study is carried out by dynamic modelling with the help of ADAMS, a software for dynamic analysis of multibody systems. This dynamic study is useful for the design calculation of the mechanical structure of the exoskeleton to ensure structural strength.

Keywords: Medical Robotics · Exoskeletons · Biomechanics · Rehabilitation · Performance Analysis

1 Introduction

As pointed out in [1], the subject of rehabilitation robotics has made significant progress. This is due to the progress in the field of IT technology, which has led to the development of advanced components such as programmable logic controllers, microcontrollers, servomotors and stepper motors. These achievements have been implemented in the field of robotics, leading to high-performance, reliable models and even intelligent autonomous systems [2, 3].

Another development in this direction has been that of exoskeleton robots, which are capable of climbing stairs, providing locomotor assistance to people climbing stairs [4, 5]. They are needed in locomotor rehabilitation clinics, as they supplement the work of the physiotherapist, but not only that, they are also needed to provide locomotor assistance to people with locomotor disabilities in everyday life. This assistance is necessary because there are a very large number of people who following strokes as well as spinal cord injury need locomotor assistance for rehabilitation purposes [6]. The development of robotic

D. Tarnita et al. (Eds.): MESROB 2023, MMS 133, pp. 306–316, 2023.
https://doi.org/10.1007/978-3-031-32446-8_33

rehabilitation systems has undergone two approaches [7]. The first one, where robotic systems in which the structure of the foot is an open kinematic chain. These solutions have driving motors placed in joints (generally in all three joints of the foot, i.e., hip, knee and ankle), faithfully reproducing the structure of the human foot. The disadvantage of this solution is that the drive motors need to be high-performance, powerful and equipped with command-and-control sensors, meaning they are expensive. The second direction is of robotic systems based on the implementation of a closed kinematic chain, desmodromic, i.e., a mechanism, in the exoskeleton leg structure. In general, this type of solution provides assistance only for the knee and hip joints, but this is sufficient to achieve the goal of locomotor assistance. As an advantage, only one driving motor is required. Another advantage is that the mechanism is designed to provide a certain movement with the desired angular amplitude, and in this way the solution is very safe in operation, and cannot cause injury to the patient due to malfunction. In case of failure of the mechanical structure, the movement is no longer transmitted, so the patient cannot be injured. But these solutions can also be equipped with torque sensors to provide controlled locomotor assistance and force feedback from the patient.

This paper presents a new proposed solution of an exoskeleton robotic system which assists human walking. The proposed design solution is studied starting from the results of numerical simulation developed in ADAMS. A kinematic and dynamic analysis of the proposed structural solution is performed.

2 Human Gait Experimental Study

Experimental analysis of human gait is necessary to obtain the laws of variation for flexion-extension angles in the leg joints corresponding to normal gait [8]. The obtained laws of motion are used to obtain the average cycle, corresponding to one step. Wearable goniometer-type sensors are used as equipment to obtain the joint motion laws. Twin-Axis Goniometers simultaneously measure angles in up to two planes of movement. The sensors are connected to a DataLog device, which is attached to the patient and connected to the PC via the Bluetooth interface. The acquired data is saved on the computer's HDD. The assistive system is designed to support flexion-extension movements of the joints, which are performed in the sagittal plane, so we will acquire experimental data for the angles of the leg joints in sagittal plane. In this research we present the results obtained for the average cycle related to normal gait, for a subject: a healthy male of 1.68 m height, 68 kg, and age 35.

In Fig. 1 are plotted the ankle joints angles recorded variation (for the right and left leg) for a complete gait cycle which corresponds to a complete step of human normal gait. The time period of a single step is 1.56 s. In Figs. 2 and 3 are plotted the knee and hip joints angles variation, corresponding to a walking step. The goniometers recorded the variation of flexion-extension angles in the joints of the human leg during normal walking over a period of time. These angles have a certain repeatability, corresponding to one step. We sequenced these angles, corresponding to one step, and by processing successive cycles in Simi Motion, we obtained the average cycle.

Using the Biometrics equipment equipped with electro-goniometers sensors and Biometrics Ltd software, the angular variation laws of all three human leg joint are

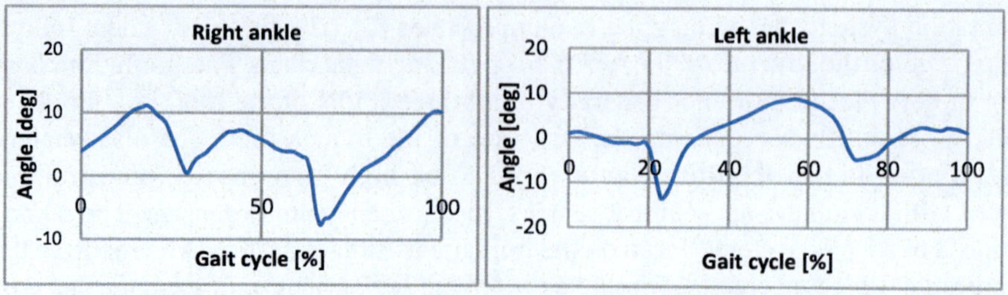

Fig. 1. Acquired ankle joints angles during human walking.

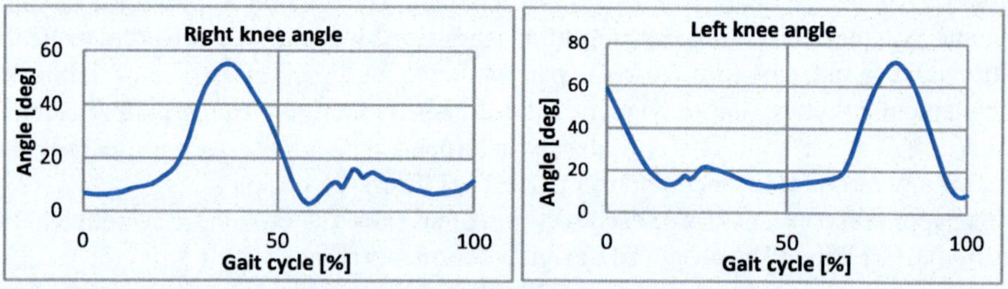

Fig. 2. Acquired knee joints angles during human walking.

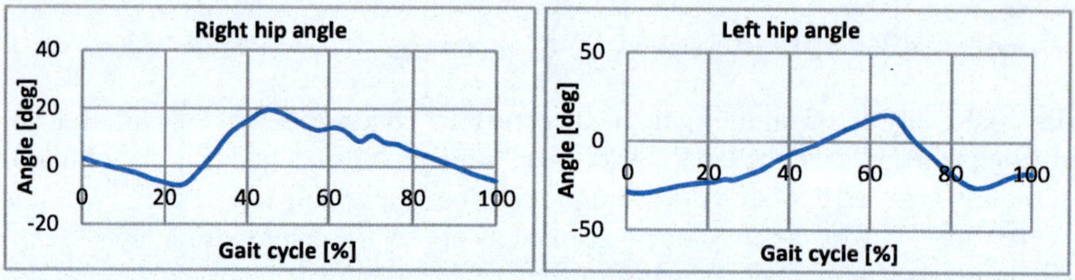

Fig. 3. Acquired hip joints angles during human walking.

acquired in sagittal plane and plotted, in Figs. 1, 2 and 3. The ankle joint flexion extension angle reaches 18°, as is plotted in Fig. 1. The knee joint measured angular maximum value reaches 65°, as is plotted in Fig. 2, and the hip joint measured angle maximum value reaches 30°, as is presented with plots in Fig. 3. These results will help us make a comparison with the motion in the joints of the designed exoskeleton robot.

3 Structure and Design of the Foot Exoskeleton Mechanism

The paper starts from a previously developed solution [9], which we will optimize structurally and kinematically. The objective function of the optimisation is to maximise the rotation angles in the hip and knee joints, to reach values as close as possible to those achieved by humans in normal walking. The mechanism developed previously and implemented as a structural solution for the legs of an exoskeleton robot is shown in Fig. 4, a. According to the kinematic scheme in Fig. 4, a, it can be seen that its structure is based on a quadrilateral kinematic chain, which is driven by a Chebyshev Lambda mechanism. In order to obtain different amplitudes of variation angles in the hip (30°) and knee (65°) joints, this structure is completed with a second quadrilateral kinematic chain, as shown in Fig. 4, b, where we can have two structural variants, because there are two possibilities of connecting link 4 with 7. The introduction of a second kinematic chain of the articulated quadrilateral type in the structure of the mechanism allows different angular amplitudes to be obtained in the hip and knee joints, which leads to an increase in the exoskeleton's performance, i.e., the movement achieved is comparable to that achieved by humans in normal walking.

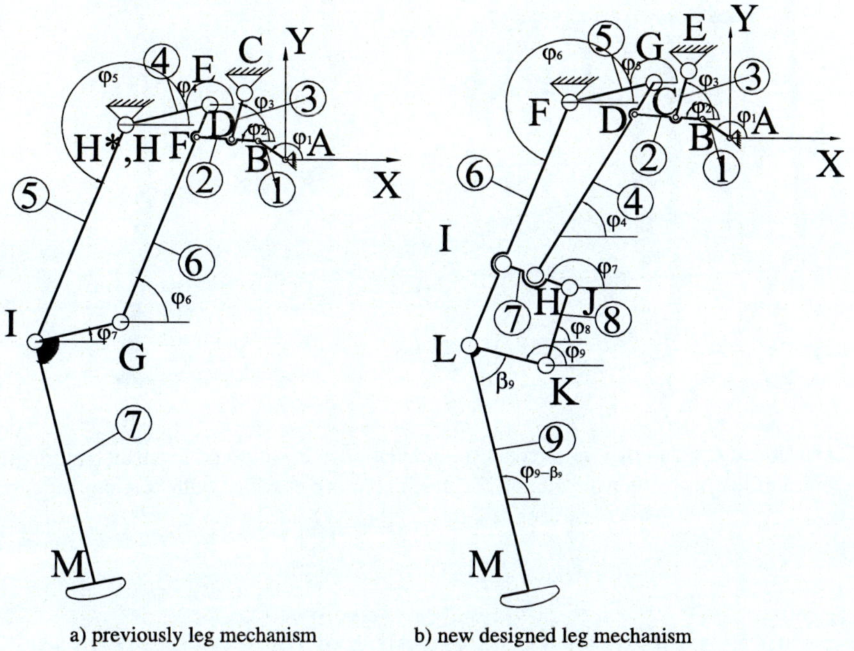

Fig. 4. Kinematic solutions for exoskeleton leg mechanism.

In order to verify and validate the functionality of the robotic system, the kinematic links of the exoskeleton leg are modelled in the first phase with bars (links). After validation of the solution, by kinematic and dynamic simulation in the ADAMS virtual simulation environment, the links will be realized with an optimized design, which will take into account the possibility of modifying the length of the segments that materialize the tibia and femur and the mounting of the bearings in the kinematic joints. Thus, the resulting connection forces in the kinematic joints, obtained from the dynamic modelling, will be a starting point for the dimensioning of the links.

Accordingly, a first design solution, realized in SolidWorks, is shown in Fig. 5. Based on this solution, a kinematic and dynamic study will be performed in ADAMS. As can be seen, the two legs are assembled on an upper frame, the two-driving links, numbered (1) being assembled with an angular offset of 180 degrees. The kinematic joints E and F are connected by means of bolts also on this upper frame. For the optimal manufacturing of the exoskeleton, we propose 3D printing fabrication technology, where the assembling of the links will be done as in Fig. 5.

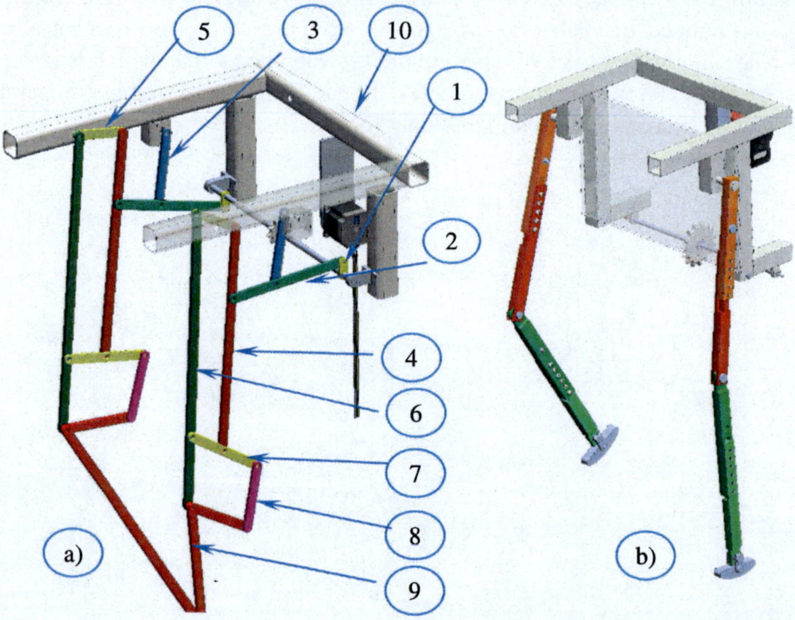

Fig. 5. Developed CAD design as a model for simulation and prototype for manufacturing: a) design with links; b) constructive solution for manufacturing provided with bearings mounting brackets.

4 Kinematic Analysis of the Mechanism of the Exoskeleton Leg

The original kinematic solution that is proposed for the construction of an exoskeleton type robotic system for rehabilitation has the kinematic scheme presented in Fig. 4, b. In this figure, Y axis is vertical, X axis is horizontal and the origin of the coordinate system is placed in the joint A. The lengths of the links and the coordinates of the rotation joints A, E and F are known. Since the solution is patent pending, these data will not be provided. According to the kinematic scheme, the structure of the mechanism has a driving link, which is denoted by (1), and 4 dyad-type structural groups, namely: ECB, DGF, FIH and JKL. The following system of equations can be written:

$$\text{for the ECB dyad}: \begin{cases} l_{BC}\,cos\varphi_2 = (x_E - x_B) + l_{CE}\,cos\varphi_3 \\ l_{BC}\,sin\varphi_2 = (y_E - y_B) + l_{CE}\,sin\varphi_3 \end{cases} \quad (1)$$

$$\text{for the DCF dyad}: \begin{cases} l_{FG}\,cos\varphi_5 = (x_D - x_F) + l_{DG}\,cos\varphi_4 \\ l_{FG}\,sin\varphi_5 = (y_D - y_F) + l_{DG}\,sin\varphi_4 \end{cases} \quad (2)$$

$$\text{for the FIH dyad}: \begin{cases} l_{FI}\, cos\varphi_6 = (x_H - x_F) + l_{HI}\, cos\varphi_7 \\ l_{FI}\, sin\varphi_6 = (y_H - y_F) + l_{HI}\, sin\varphi_7 \end{cases} \quad (3)$$

$$\text{for the JKL dyad}: \begin{cases} l_{JK}\, cos\varphi_8 = (x_L - x_J) + l_{LK}\, cos\varphi_9 \\ l_{JK}\, sin\varphi_8 = (y_L - y_J) + l_{LK}\, sin\varphi_9 \end{cases} \quad (4)$$

In the systems of Eqs. (1) - (4) the following mathematical operations are performed. For each system, square up and add the two equations in the system. We obtain the equations of degree two with trigonometric function as coefficients, as Eq. 5. To determine the law of variation of the angles phi i ($i = 1..9$), there is solved Eq. (6).

$$l_{BC}^2 - a_1^2 - a_2^2 - l_{CE}^2 - 2a_1 l_{CE} cos\varphi_3 - 2a_2 l_{CE} sin\varphi_3 = 0 \quad (5)$$

where we used the following notations:

$(x_E - x_B) = a_1$, $(y_E - y_B) = a_2$,

The solutions of Eq. (5) are obtained by solving equations of type (6).

$$\varphi_i = 2arctg\frac{A_i^2 \pm \sqrt{A_i^2 + B_i^2 - C_i^2}}{B_i^2 - C_i^2} \quad (6)$$

where we have, $i = 2, 3$. The A_i coefficients have the following relations:

$$A_2 = 2a_2 l_{BC};\ B_2 = 2a_1 l_{BC};\ C_2 = l_{CE}^2 - a_1^2 - a_2^2 - l_{BC}^2 \quad (7)$$

$$A_3 = -2a_2 l_{CE};\ B_3 = -2a_1 l_{CE};\ C_3 = l_{BC}^2 - a_1^2 - a_2^2 - l_{CE}^2 \quad (8)$$

Similar equations and solutions are obtained for the systems (2)..(4).

These equations describe the kinematic model of the exoskeleton robotic system. Their numerical solution is obtained in MATLAB environment and then they will be validated by simulating the motion in the multibody-ADAMS View system. The angle variations in the knee and hip joints are calculated, as shown in Fig. 6

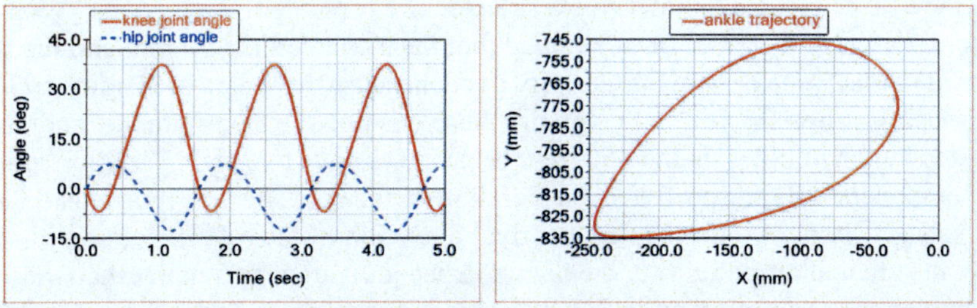

Fig. 6. Knee and hip joints angles variation, and ankle ovoid computed trajectory.

The kinematic model presented in the previous paragraph corresponds to the situation related to the kinematic scheme in Fig. 4, b, namely the kinematic joints of rotation A, F and E are connected to the fixed base. In this situation the mechanism of the exoskeleton leg operates on a supporting frame, and the trajectory described by point M, which corresponds to the ankle joint, must be a closed curve of the ovoid type, as obtained in Fig. 6. To simulate the motion of the exoskeleton, with the help of ADAMS software, we made an assembly of two legs. Aspects of setting up a dynamic simulation model in ADAMS are detailed in previous works [10]. We opted for the constructive solution presented in Fig. 5, which consists of a square tube top frame, joined by welding. Joint A, through which the driving link (1) is connected by the upper frame, is constructed by means of a shaft, on which are assembled at the ends the two cranks (1), positioned at an angle of 180°, to ensure the sequence of steps. For kinematic reasons, we considered the angular velocity of the shaft on which the two-driving links are mounted, of 4 rad/sec. In Fig. 7 it can be observed the trajectory described by the foot, for two simulation cases: - the exoskeleton has the upper frame fixed to the base; - the exoskeleton performs the activity of walking on the floor. For the stationary operation situation, the trajectory described by the ankle is an ovoid one, propitious for the good functioning of the robot, while, on the right side of the figure, the exoskeleton performs the walking on the floor.

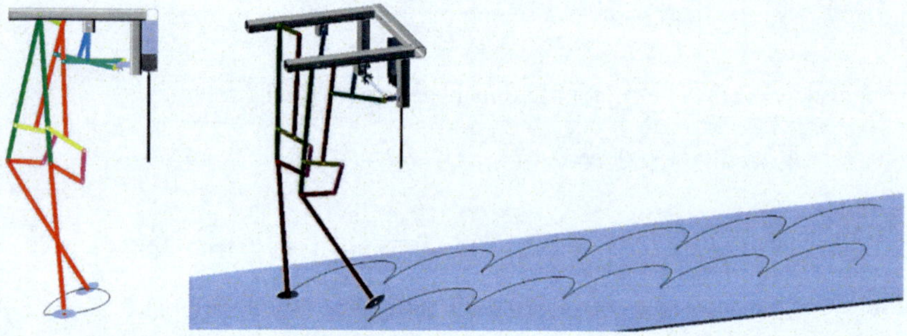

Fig. 7. The path calculated in ADAMS, corresponding to the two operating hypostases.

The simulation output shown in Fig. 7 are displayed in the following. In the Figs. 8, 9 and 10 the laws of variation for the position, velocity and acceleration of the center of mass of the sole of the left foot of the exoskeleton are presented.

According to Fig. 8, it can be concluded that the step height is 90 mm and the step length is 225 mm. These parameters are very good, because the height of 90 mm at which the exoskeleton raises the leg in the swing phase ensures the step without hindrance, and the step length doubles, being 450 mm, because we have two legs. Variation graphs for the components of the speed and acceleration of the sole show a smooth variation, without sudden jumps, which ensures a correct operation of the robot.

Also, the angular amplitudes in the hip and knee joint are a bit smaller than those in normal human gait, as presented in Fig. 11. This is not an obstacle for the exoskeleton to provide locomotion assistance, as we will present below. The results presented in this paragraph are obtained in the case of the first hypothesis, when the joints A, E, F are connected to a fixed base.

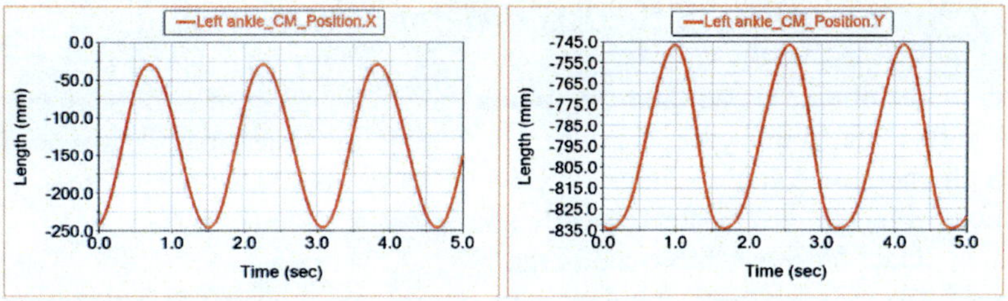

Fig. 8. Variation of the position of the left ankle joint, during the simulation.

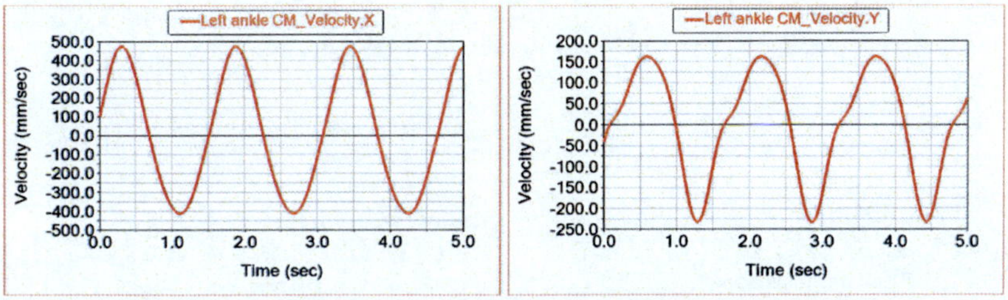

Fig. 9. Time variation for the speed of the centre of mass of the sole of the left foot, during the simulation.

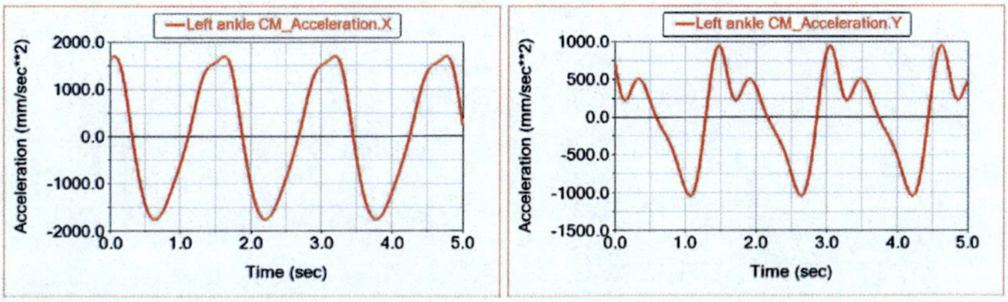

Fig. 10. Time variation for the acceleration of the centre of mass of the left foot sole, during the simulation.

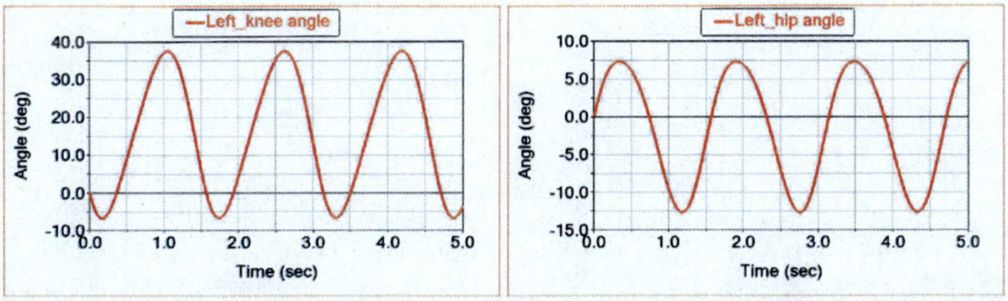

Fig. 11. Graphs of time variation of the angle of the L and F joints (knee and hip), during the simulation.

5 Dynamic Modelling of the Exoskeleton While Walking

For dynamic modelling, we will use the simulation environment of multibody systems, ADAMS View [11]. In this case, we considered the joints previously connected to the fixed base, namely the rotation joints A, E and F to be connected to the upper frame. This frame is allowed to translate vertically and horizontally during the simulation. We defined the contact between the sole and the ground, where we also took into account the friction forces. Under these simulation conditions, the exoskeleton can step on the floor. The graphs in Figs. 12–14, are determined in this case.

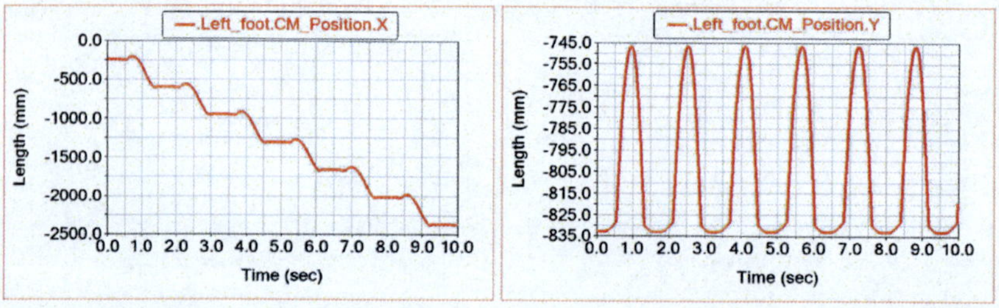

Fig. 12. Graphs of time variation of the position of the centre of mass of the sole, in the case of the stepping activity of the exoskeleton.

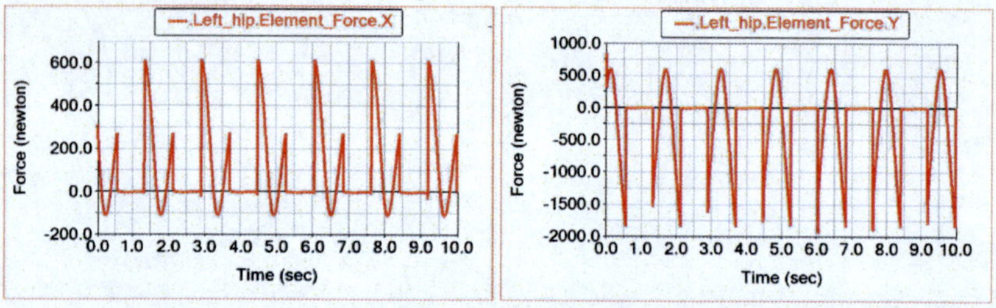

Fig. 13. Graphs of the variation of the components of the connecting forces in the left hip.

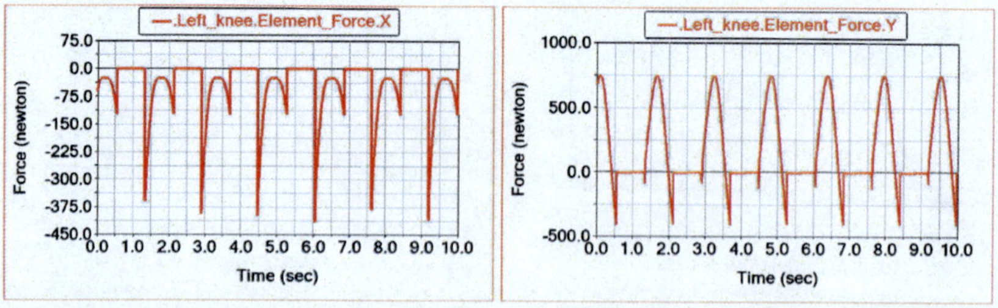

Fig.14. Graphs of the variation of the components of the connecting forces in the left knee.

Thus, in Fig. 12, it can be seen that while walking the height of the exoskeleton step is 90 mm. Also, from this figure you can see that the exoskeleton performs 5 steps and travels a distance of 2250 mm, so the length of a step is 450 mm. Also in the dynamic simulation, we calculated the components of the connecting forces in the hip and knee joints of the exoskeleton, as presented in Figs. 13 and 14. It is observed that higher values are recorded along the vertical Y axis. This mechanism is suitable to be used for rehabilitation, because as shown by the results obtained, it provides similar movement laws in the knee and hip joints as those obtained in normal walking.

6 Conclusion

In this paper, we presented a kinematic and dynamic analysis for an exoskeleton-type robotic system designed to assist human locomotion. The mechanism solution used for the exoskeleton leg is original, being patent pending. The structure of the mechanism comprises a driving link and four RRR type dyads. The kinematics of the proposed mechanism as a constructive solution for the exoskeleton leg are studied by analytical methods and by simulation in ADAMS. The laws of variation of the angles of flexion / extension in the hip and knee joints are suitable for the use of the mechanism as a solution for the assistant exoskeleton of human gait. The dynamic simulation involved the exoskeleton stepping on the floor. The obtained results allow us to validate the proposed solution and move to the next stage of making a physical prototype and experimental testing.

References

1. Chen, B.: Recent developments and challenges of lower extremity exoskeletons. J. Orthop. Transl. **5**, 26–37 (2016)
2. Anama, K., AlJumaily, A.A.: Active exoskeleton control systems: state of the art. Proc. Eng. **41**, 988–994 (2012)
3. Díaz, I., Gil, J.J., Sánchez, E.: Lower-limb robotic rehabilitation: literature review and challenges. J. Robot. **2011**, 1–11 (2011). https://doi.org/10.1155/2011/759764
4. Geonea, I., Tarnita, D.: Motion assistance with an exoskeleton for stair climb. In: 2018 IEEE Int. Conference on Automation, Quality and Testing, Robotics (AQTR) IEEE (2018)
5. Tarnita, D., Geonea, I., Petcu, A., Tarnita, D.-N.: Experimental characterization of human walking on stairs applied to humanoid dynamics. In: Rodic, A., Borangiu, T. (eds.) Advances in Robot Design and Intelligent Control. AISC, vol. 540, pp. 293–301. Springer, Cham (2017). https://doi.org/10.1007/978-3-319-49058-8_32
6. Yan, T.: Review of assistive strategies in powered lower-limb orthoses and exoskeletons. Robot. Auton. Syst. **64**, 120–136 (2015)
7. Huo, W.: Lower limb wearable robots for assistance and rehabilitation: a state of the art. IEEE Syst. J. **10**(3), 1068–1081 (2016)
8. Tarnita, D., Geonea, I., Petcu, A., Tarnita, D.N.: Numerical simulations and experimental human gait analysis using wearable sensors. In: Husty, M., Hofbaur, M. (eds.) New Trends in Medical and Service Robots. MMS, vol. 48, pp. 289–304. Springer, Cham (2016). https://doi.org/10.1007/978-3-319-59972-4_21
9. Geonea, I.: Design and numerical characterization of a leg exoskeleton linkage for motion assistance. In: Proceedings of The World Congress on Engineering and Computer Science 2018, 23–25 October, 2018, San Francisco, USA, pp. 594–599 (2018)

10. Geonea, I., Ceccarelli, M., Carbone, G.: Design and analysis of an exoskeleton for people with motor disabilities. In: The 14th IFToMM World Congress, Taipei, Taiwan (2015)
11. Geonea, I., Dumitru, N., Tarnita, D., Rinderu, P.: Design and kinematics of a new leg exoskeleton for human motion assistance. In: Uhl, T. (ed.) Advance in Mechanisms and Machine Science. MMS, vol. 73, pp. 165–174. Springer, Cham (2019). https://doi.org/10.1007/978-3-030-20131-9_17

The Framework for Mobile Robot Task Planning Based on the Optimal Manufacturing Schedule

Aleksandar Jokić(✉), Milica Petrović, and Zoran Miljković

Faculty of Mechanical Engineering, Department of Production Engineering, University of Belgrade, Kraljice Marije 16, 11120 Belgrade, Serbia
ajokic@mas.bg.ac.rs

Abstract. Integrated process planning and scheduling of manufacturing entities represents one of the most impactful processes for optimizing production systems. The result of integrated process planning and scheduling is visually presented in the form of the Gantt chart that summarizes the timing and order of all manufacturing operations. Moreover, a sequence of actions that needs to be performed by a transportation system to ensure the smooth execution of all manufacturing processes is also incorporated within the Gantt chart. Therefore, in this paper, we develop a framework for mobile robot action planning based on high-level action, e.g., transporting the part from one machine to another. The idea is to automatically plan a sequence of robot-performable actions that, if performed accurately, results in achieving a high-level goal. The framework is developed in the standard Robot Operative System 2 (ROS2) middleware. The system, domain, and essential entities are modeled by using Planning Domain Definition Language (PDDL). The mobile robot actions are modeled by Behavior trees within the PlanSys2 framework. Even though the system for task planning is developed for a manufacturing environment, the framework can be used in various fields such as service or medical mobile robotics applications where scheduling activity is of the essence.

Keywords: Intelligent manufacturing systems · Integrated process planning and scheduling · Mobile robot action planning · ROS2 · PDDL · Behavior trees

1 Introduction

The principles of Industry 4.0 imply high levels of utilization of flexible manufacturing resources. One of the most common frameworks for increasing utilization is thorough optimization of manufacturing schedule. Integrated process planning and scheduling presents one such framework, where individual or multi-objective criteria can be optimized [1]. Depending on the level of flexibility in the manufacturing system and the complexity of the jobs, selecting alternative sequence of operations for all jobs can provide higher levels of utilization while ensuring there are no bottlenecks. After the optimization is performed, the resulting schedule is most commonly presented as a Gantt chart (Fig. 1), where each operation is assigned to a specific machine at a defined moment.

D. Tarnita et al. (Eds.): MESROB 2023, MMS 133, pp. 317–325, 2023.
https://doi.org/10.1007/978-3-031-32446-8_34

Therefore, the Gantt chart represents a high-level plan that needs to be jointly executed by the manufacturing and transportation system. The following three operations that a mobile robot can perform are *loaded/empty trip*, where the robot moves with or without a job to another machine, and *robot waiting* for the processing to finish.

The most reliable, flexible, and efficient transportation system that can be utilized to transport jobs between machines is by employing mobile robots. However, moving from the Gantt chart to the commands modern mobile robotic systems can interpret and perform is not a trivial task. High-level commands, such as carry job 1 from machine 1 to machine 2, assume that the mobile robot can detect job 1, can perform manipulation and unmounting from machine 1, can plan and execute trajectory to machine 2 while avoiding collision with all dynamic obstacles in the environment, and can finally adequately set job 1 to machine 2. Moreover, additional specific tasks, such as visual servoing for fine positioning [2], need to be seamlessly integrated into the overall robot behavior. All the above-mentioned tasks can be even further divided into less complex tasks whose consecutive performance results in achieving a high-level task.

Within the Artificial Intelligence (AI) domain, action planning frameworks have been developed to autonomously plan sequences of low-level actions necessary for the adequate execution of a high-level plan. The analysis of automated planning in the robotic domain is performed in [3]. The most significant difference between action planning systems is in the utilized approaches. AI planning approach can be generally divided into the following two categories – symbolic and model-based planning. Model-based planning uses a model of the problem state, while symbolic-based systems use a set of rules to represent the problem. Model-based planning relies on reasoning about the state of the model to generate a plan, while symbolic-based systems use a set of predefined rules to determine the following action.

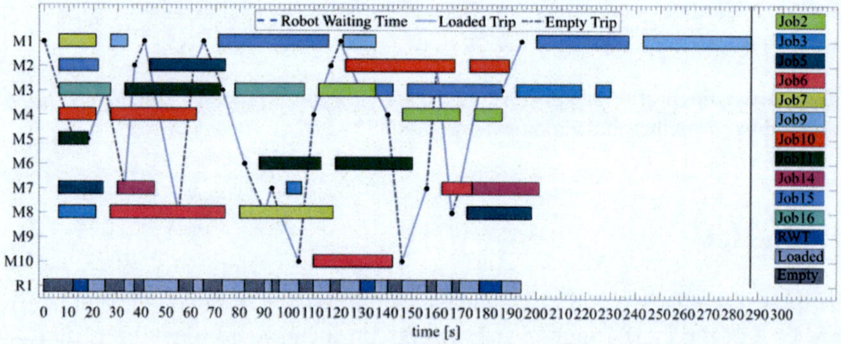

Fig. 1. Example of Gantt chart for a manufacturing system. The duration of mobile robot operations are represented with rectangles beside the R1 column, while operations of the same job are defined with rectangles of the same color and assigned to machines (M1-M10).

2 Literature Review

In work [4], the authors proposed two integrated planning systems, one for each individual robot for low-level tasks, and mission level one for all industrial robots in the manufacturing system. Low-level tasks included sensing operations, motion control, or state update actions performed by an individual robot. World state at the robot level was defined by web ontology language, where the state is defined both by operators and the robot's perception system. Low-level tasks and world state were then utilized to create the PDDL language model and use it to perform planning tasks. The development of a planning system for the industrial robot assembly process was carried out in [5]. The metamodel of the production system was transformed into the PDDL format and utilized in process planning. Multiple variants of the PDDL plan were analyzed depending on the complexity of the model (e.g., with or without durative actions). Fast Downward [6] algorithm with A* heuristic was utilized for solving the problem, and the authors conclude that small and middle-size production line problems can be solved if no durative actions are considered. Some of the state-of-the-art planners that accept input defined in PDDL language are LAMA planner based on A* heuristic [7], Fast Downward Planning System based on causal graph heuristic [6], POPF [8], and [9] TFD planners.

3 Planning System Description

The first requirement for the development of a task planning system was to be useable within Robot Operating System 2 (ROS2) middleware [10, 11]. The robot applications based on the ROS2 system have significant benefits, including modularity, faster integration, and scalability. Moreover, another major advantage includes wide usage in industry and academia, where other researchers can quickly test and adopt the solution. The second requirement included the need to create a robotic application with a flexible and scalable control structure; therefore, the Behavior Trees (BT) are utilized. Behavior trees are a data structure in AI planning used to represent and control the behavior of autonomous agents in simulation or real-world environments [12]. They are used to specify a hierarchy of actions and conditions, with leaves of the tree representing low-level actions and branches representing decision nodes based on conditions. The behavior of the agent is determined by transitioning the tree and executing the action specified by the currently active node. Compared to finite state machines, behavior trees have significant advantages, including a hierarchical design that is reusable, modular, and flexible; they are easier to understand, debug, and scale. Therefore, we have selected PlanSys2 [13] as an adequate framework for implementing our planning system. An added benefit of PlanSys2 is easy integration with the ROS2-based navigation library named Navigation2 [14], utilized for both simulation and real-world control of mobile robots.

3.1 Implementation of Domain and Problem in PDDL

The PlanSys2 framework utilizes PDDL 2.1 with POPF [8] as a planner solver. The implementation includes the definition of the manufacturing system domain and mobile robot durative actions with temporal information. There are four different types of objects, i.e., *robot*, *machine*, *job*, and *operation.* Functions (see Table 1) are utilized to define numerical constraints used to model mobile robot behavior. The transportation of a job cannot start if the machining of the previous operation is not finished, which is defined by the function `start_time`. There are three actions defined in the domain file that the mobile robot can execute, according to the action from the Gantt chart (Fig. 1). Move and wait actions are not presented due to the lack of space; however, the definition of the action `durative-action transport` is given in Table 1. Both predicates, `operation_not_finished` and `operation_finished,` need to be defined due to the lack of possibility to use`not` expression in the goal definition. Moreover, the plan is completed when all transport operations are performed. Since each job has several consecutive manufacturing operations that need to be performed, each transport task (`operation_finished`) is defined with the job that is being transported, the operation that has just finished, and the machine for the next operation. The flexibility of the proposed framework, based on PDDL, provides seamless adaptation for numerous service or medical mobile robot applications, such as [15].

4 Experimental Evaluation

The experiment is performed in a simulated manufacturing environment with 10 machine tools (Fig. 2) and one mobile robot that executes the transportation tasks. Firstly, the entire environment is mapped by utilizing the mobile robot RAICO (Robot with Artificial Intelligence based COgnition); the generated 2D map is shown in Fig. 3.

Secondly, the actions are designed within .xml files as decision trees, where the difference between *transportation* and *move* actions is in the additional time utilized for fine positioning and grasping of a job. Simulation is performed using Gazebo 3D simulation software and the visualization tool RViz for ROS2.

In the PDDL problem file, adequate instances of objects, predicates, and functions are defined (part of the problem file is shown in Table 2). In total, 28 predicates, 26 instances, and 105 functions are defined. All the data utilized in the problem domain is defined according to Fig. 1. (e.g., at which machine is a particular job at the start of the process) and according to the literature [16] (e.g., transportation time between machine tools). Finally, the goal is set to be that all the mobile robot operations are finished. In total, 14 times the mobile robot needs to perform transportation tasks between machines (corresponding to loaded trips of the robot in Fig. 1). Each transportation task is defined by a job number, the number of finished manufacturing operation, and a machine on which the following operation is performed.

Table 1. A part of the PDDL domain definition.

```
(:predicates
(robot_available ?r - robot)
(robot_at ?r - robot ?m - machine)
(job_at ?j - job ?m - machine)
(operation_not_finished ?j - job ?n - operation ?m - machine)
(operation_finished ?j - job ?n - operation ?m - machine)
(ready_to_move ?r - robot)
)
(:functions
    (distance ?m1 - machine ?m2 - machine)
    (curr_time1)
    (start_time ?j - job ?n - operation)
)
(:durative-action transport
    :parameters (?r - robot ?j - job ?n - operation ?m1 ?m2 - machine)
    :duration (= ?duration (distance ?m1 ?m2))
    :condition (and
        (at start(robot_at ?r ?m1))
        (at start(job_at ?j ?m1))
        (at start(robot_available ?r))
        (at start(operation_not_finished ?j ?n ?m2))
        (at start(>= (curr_time1) (start_time ?j ?n)))
    )
    :effect (and
        (at start(not(robot_at ?r ?m1)))
        (at end(robot_at ?r ?m2))
        (at start(not(job_at ?j ?m1)))
        (at end(job_at ?j ?m2))
        (at start(not(robot_available ?r)))
        (at end(robot_available ?r))
        (at end(ready_to_move ?r))
        (at end(not(operation_not_finished ?j ?n ?m2)))
        (at end(operation_finished ?j ?n ?m2))
        (at end(increase (curr_time1) (distance ?m1 ?m2)))))
```

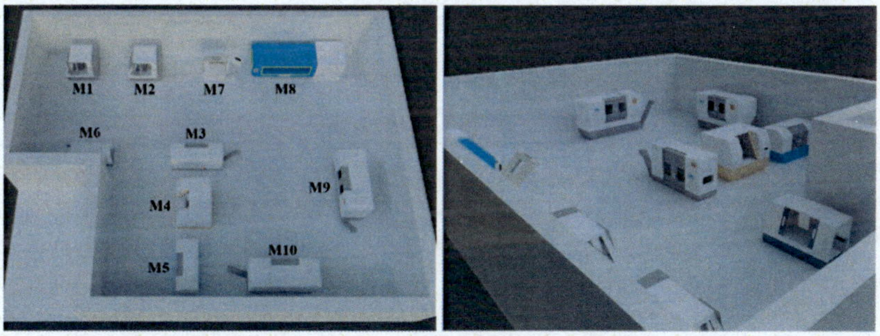

Fig. 2. Manufacturing environment.

The generated mobile robot task plan can be seen in Table 3. The time required for the plan to be generated is around 0.5 s. As can be seen, there are 39 tasks mobile robot needs to perform. Since all actions are durative, each action's duration and starting time are also defined. The mobile robot starts at machine 1, moves to machine 5 (1st task), then waits for the first operation of job 11 to be finished (see Fig. 1), and afterwards transports job 11 from machine 5 to machine 3 (8th task). When both the first and second

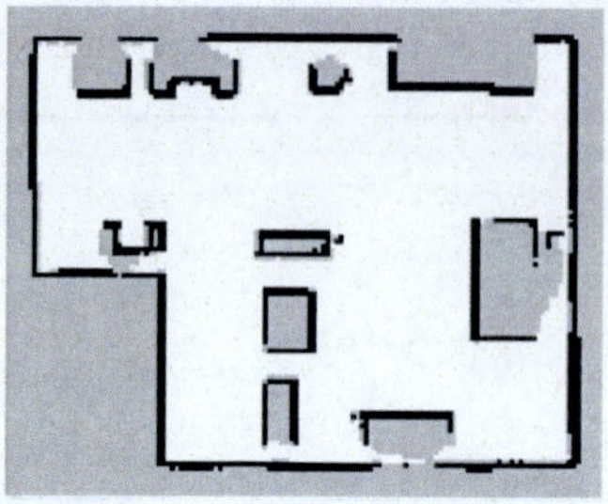

Fig. 3. Manufacturing environment mapped by a mobile robot.

operations of a job are on the same machine, RAICO needs to transport the job only after the second operation is finished (e.g., see 15th action).

Table 2. Examples of instance, predicate, function, and goal definition.

```
1 set instance raico robot
2 set instance m_1 machine
3 set instance job_2 job
4 set instance op_1 operation
5 set predicate (ready_to_move raico)
6 set predicate (robot_available raico)
7 set predicate (robot_at raico m_1)
8 set predicate (job_at job_2 m_3)
9 set function (= (curr_time1) 0)
10 set function (= (distance m_1 m_2) 4)
11 set function (= (start_time job_11 op_1) 18)
12 set predicate (operation_not_finished job_11 op_1 m_3)
13 set goal (and (operation_finished job_11 op_1 m_3)...)
```

As can be observed, the generated plan is not the exact replica of the one defined in Fig. 1. Since the objective was to finish all the operations as fast as possible, with constraints that the job cannot be transported if the previous operation is not finished, the planner has found a plan that is similar but somewhat different. However, since the task timing would slightly vary in the realistic scenario due to the stochastic and unstructured nature of a manufacturing system, the achieved plan is entirely adequate.

After the task planning phase is finished, the generated plan can be executed in the simulation environment. The mobile robot in the 3D environment with the data gathered by a lidar sensor can be seen in Fig. 4. The initial mobile robot pose is predefined, while the map (dark red pixels in the Rviz) and sensor data (blue lines in the Gazebo and pink dots in Rviz) are combined to estimate mobile robot pose during the transportation tasks and avoid any novel obstacle not defined by a map. The generated path mobile robot (see Fig. 4 right) should follow from M5 to M3 is defined according to the known position of each machine tool. Moreover, the coordinate frames of the mobile robot can be seen defined in the global coordinate system. Positions utilized to define where the robot can move in the environment are shown with white pixels, while the shades of red define the confidence in the corresponding pixel position.

Table 3. Generated mobile robot plan.

No.	Time	(Action/Task)	Duration
1	0	(move raico m_1 m_5)	12
2	12.001	(wait raico)	1
3	13.002	(wait raico)	1
4	14.003	(wait raico)	1
5	15.004	(wait raico)	1
6	16.005	(wait raico)	1
7	17.006	(wait raico)	1
8	18.007	(transport raico job_11 op_1 m_5 m_3)	7
9	25.008	(move raico m_3 m_7)	8
10	33.009	(transport raico job_5 op_1 m_7 m_2)	4
11	37.01	(transport raico job_15 op_1 m_2 m_1)	4
12	41.011	(transport raico job_7 op_1 m_1 m_8)	14
13	55.012	(move raico m_8 m_4)	6
14	61.013	(wait raico)	1
15	62.014	(transport raico job_10 op_2 m_4 m_2)	7
16	69.015	(wait raico)	1
17	70.016	(transport raico job_5 op_2 m_2 m_8)	6
18	76.017	(move raico m_8 m_3)	4
19	80.018	(transport raico job_11 op_2 m_3 m_7)	8
20	88.019	(move raico m_7 m_8)	3
21	91.02	(transport raico job_3 op_1 m_8 m_10)	8
22	99.021	(move raico m_10 m_8)	8
23	107.022	(transport raico job_6 op_1 m_8 m_10)	8
24	115.023	(transport raico job_3 op_2 m_10 m_3)	10
25	125.024	(move raico m_3 m_1)	8
26	133.025	(transport raico job_15 op_2 m_1 m_3)	8
27	141.026	(move raico m_3 m_10)	10
28	151.027	(transport raico job_6 op_2 m_10 m_7)	10
29	161.028	(move raico m_7 m_3)	8
30	169.029	(wait raico)	1
31	170.03	(wait raico)	1
32	171.031	(wait raico)	1
33	172.032	(wait raico)	1
34	173.033	(wait raico)	1
35	174.034	(wait raico)	1
36	175.035	(transport raico job_2 op_1 m_3 m_4)	5
37	180.036	(move raico m_4 m_3)	5
38	185.037	(wait raico)	1
39	186.038	(transport raico job_15 op_4 m_3 m_1)	8

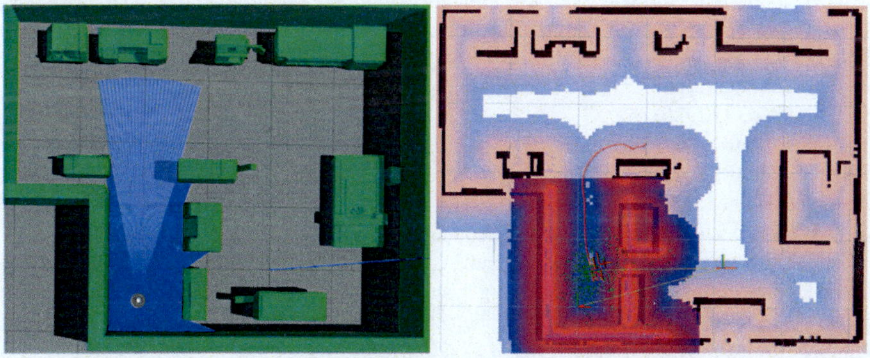

Fig. 4. Mobile robot in the 3D Gazebo (left) and Rviz (right) simulation environment.

5 Conclusion

In this paper, we presented the development and implementation of a mobile robot task planning system based on the optimal manufacturing schedule represented with a Gantt chart. A Gantt chart is utilized to define the initial state of the planning system and the required transportation tasks that need to be completed. The advantage of the proposed approach is its applicability to various tasks where a service mobile robot needs to execute a temporally scheduled plan. To define the logic for the problem domain, PDDL is utilized within the PlanSys2 framework. The entire system is implemented within the ROS2 middleware. All the actions mobile robot performs are defined as behavior trees. Within the experimental evaluation, the temporal plan generated by the proposed planning system is validated and executed by a mobile robot in the Gazebo and Rviz simulation environments. The plan is generated effectively, and the implementation can be used in a real-time application on one of the common development boards, such as Nvidia Jetson Nano. The experimental evaluation shows that a mobile robot can adequately use the generated plan for the transportation of manufacturing jobs. Future research directions include implementing and evaluating the developed system on the own developed mobile robot RAICO in a real laboratory manufacturing environment.

Acknowledgement. This research has been financially supported by the Minister of Science, Technological Development and Innovation of the Serbian Government, through the project "Integrated research in macro, micro, and nano mechanical engineering – Deep learning of intelligent manufacturing systems in production engineering" (contract No. 451–03-47/2023–01/200105).

References

1. Petrović, M., Jokić, A., Miljković, Z., Kulesza, Z.: Multi-objective scheduling of a single mobile robot based on the grey wolf optimization algorithm. Appl. Soft Comput. **131**, 109784 (2022)
2. Jokić, A., Petrović, M., Miljković, Z.: Semantic segmentation based stereo visual servoing of nonholonomic mobile robot in intelligent manufacturing environment. Expert Syst. Appl. **190**, 116203 (2022)
3. Karpas, E., Magazzeni, D.: Automated planning for robotics. Ann. Rev. Control Rob. Auton. Syst. **3**, 417–439 (2020)
4. Crosby, M., Petrick, R., Rovida, F., Krueger, V.: Integrating mission and task planning in an industrial robotics framework. In: Twenty-Seventh International Conference on Automated Planning and Scheduling, pp. 471–479 (2017)
5. Wally, B., Vyskočil, J., Novák, P., et al.: Production planning with IEC 62264 and PDDL. In: IEEE 17th International Conference on Industrial Informatics (INDIN), pp. 492–499 (2019)
6. Helmert, M.: The fast downward planning system. J. Artif. Intell. Res. **26**, 191–246 (2006)
7. Richter, S., Westphal, M.: The LAMA planner: guiding cost-based anytime planning with landmarks. J. Artif. Intell. Res. **39**, 127–177 (2010)
8. Coles, A., Coles, A., Fox, M., Long, D.: Forward-chaining partial-order planning. In: Proceedings of the International Conference on Automated Planning and Scheduling, vol. 20, pp. 42–49 (2010)

9. Eyerich, P., Mattmüller, R., Röger, G.: Using the context-enhanced additive heuristic for temporal and numeric planning. In: Nineteenth International Conference on Automated Planning and Scheduling, pp. 130–137 (2009)
10. Quigley, M., Conley, K., Gerkey, B., et al.: ROS: an open-source robot operating system. In: ICRA Workshop on Open Source Software (2009)
11. Macenski, S., Foote, T., Gerkey, B., Lalancette, C., Woodall, W.: Robot operating system 2: design, architecture, and uses in the wild. Sci. Robot. **7**(66), 6074 (2022)
12. Colledanchise, M., Ögren, P.: Behavior Trees in Robotics and AI: An Introduction. CRC Press, Boca Raton (2018)
13. Martín, F., Clavero, J.G., Matellán, V., Rodríguez, F.J.: Plansys2: a planning system framework for ROS2. In: 2021 IEEE/RSJ International Conference on Intelligent Robots and Systems (IROS), pp. 9742–9749 (2021)
14. Macenski, S., Martín, F., White, R., Clavero, J.G.: The marathon 2: a navigation system. In: 2020 IEEE/RSJ International Conference on Intelligent Robots and Systems (IROS), pp. 2718–2725 (2020)
15. Jeon, S., Lee, J.: Performance analysis of scheduling multiple robots for hospital logistics. In: IEEE 14th International Conference on Ubiquitous Robots and Ambient Intelligence (URAI), pp. 937–940 (2017)
16. Petrović, M., Miljković, Z., Jokić, A.: A novel methodology for optimal single mobile robot scheduling using whale optimization algorithm. Appl. Soft Comput. **81**, 105520 (2019)

Periodic Actuations of Two-Link Planar Robot Arm with Revolute and Prismatic Joints

Jing Zhao[1], Daniela Tarnita[2(✉)], and Dan B. Marghitu[1]

[1] Department of Mechanical Engineering, Auburn University, Auburn, AL 36849, USA
jzz0053@auburn.edu

[2] Faculty of Mechanics, University of Craiova, Craiova, Romania
daniela.tarnita@edu.ucv.ro

Abstract. A two-link planar robotic arm with revolute and prismatic joints is considered. The control torque on the first link and the control force on the second link are periodic functions. The controllers are selected using generalized forces. For the system's dynamics, the phase plane is plotted. The proposed work used entropy as a quantitative measurement of the regularity for the controlled periodic motion which was not investigated in the past. The approximate entropy decreases with the magnitude of the actuation periods.

Keywords: Robotic arm · Prismatic joint · Dynamics

1 Introduction

Robotic manipulators are widely used in a variety of applications, from industrial processes where tedious tasks are involved [1] to space explorations which can pose risks for human operators [2]. The dynamic modeling and control of robotic manipulators have captured a broad interest among researchers in the past forty years. Lagrange's formulation provides an efficient form of expressing the equation of motion of robots [3]. Kane's method can be implemented to study the dynamics of manipulators [4].

The behavior of a robotic system is often nonlinear due to the actuation algorithms and the interaction between the system and the environment. Genta offers a useful introduction to the dynamics and control of robots [5]. Villani and De Schutterm provided a thorough review of the main approaches to force control in robotic systems, including the discussion of the advantages and disadvantages of each method [6]. Brogårdh, Moosavian and Papadopoulos discussed the development of control methods, particularly in industrial robotics [7] and space robots [8]. Zhang et al. summarized the applications of chaos in robotics [9].

Lyapunov methods present a powerful tool for describing stability properties of nonlinear systems [10]. The integration of control Lyapunov functions with other model-based controllers has been employed to achieve long-term optimal behavior without compromising the nonlinearity of the system dynamics [11]. Entropy quantifies the amount of information in terms of uncertainty in a dynamical system [12]. However, accurate calculation of entropy requires a large amount

D. Tarnita et al. (Eds.): MESROB 2023, MMS 133, pp. 326–333, 2023.
https://doi.org/10.1007/978-3-031-32446-8_35

of data, and therefore approximate entropy is used in practical applications [13]. In conjunction with a reinforcement learning algorithm, an entropy function has been used to ensure stable and robust control of a soft mobile robot [14].

To date, most of the studies on modeling and control of robotic manipulators considered manipulators with purely revolute joints. Combining sliding prismatic joints with such systems allows the arms to perform manipulation tasks in a larger space [15]. The aim of this study is to investigate the dynamics of a two-link robotic arm with revolute and prismatic joints. The actuating torque and force are determined using generalized forces with a PD controller. Equations of motion of the system under periodic actuation are derived by using Lagrange's equation. We use the phase plane and the approximate entropy. The approximate entropy quantitatively tells the regularity of the controlled motion, therefore could be used as an indicator of robust control. The approximate entropy can characterize the regularity of the motion of the robot arm.

2 Dynamics of the System

2.1 Kinematics of the Links

The robot arm with a slender rotating link 1, of mass m_1, and a translational joint 2, of mass m_2, is sliding without friction, as shown in Fig. 1. The length of link 1 is L, the mass center of link 1 is C_1, and the mass moment of inertia of link 1 with respect to the pivot point O is I_O. The mass moment of inertia of slider 2 with respect to its mass center point C_2 is I_{C2}. The acceleration due to gravity is g. The kinematic robot has two degrees of freedom and two generalized coordinates. The angle $\theta(t) = q_1(t)$ and the distance $OC_2 = r(t) = q_2(t)$ are selected as the generalized coordinates as shown in Fig. 1.

The position vector of the center of the mass C_1 of link 1 is

$$\mathbf{r}_{C_1} = x_{C_1}\,\mathbf{\imath} + y_{C_1}\,\mathbf{\jmath} = \frac{L}{2}\cos q_1(t)\,\mathbf{\imath} + \frac{L}{2}\sin q_1(t)\,\mathbf{\jmath}. \tag{1}$$

The position vector of the center of the mass C_2 of link 2 is

$$\mathbf{r}_{C_2} = x_{C_2}\,\mathbf{\imath} + y_{C_2}\,\mathbf{\jmath} = q_2(t)\,\cos q_1(t)\,\mathbf{\imath} + q_2(t)\,\sin q_1(t)\,\mathbf{\jmath}. \tag{2}$$

The velocity vectors of C_1 and C_2 are the derivative with respect to time of the position vectors

$$\mathbf{v}_{C_1} = \dot{x}_{C_1}\,\mathbf{\imath} + \dot{y}_{C_1}\,\mathbf{\jmath} \;\text{ and }\; \mathbf{v}_{C_2} = \dot{x}_{C_2}\,\mathbf{\imath} + \dot{y}_{C_2}\,\mathbf{\jmath}. \tag{3}$$

The velocity vector of A is the derivative with respect to time of the position vector of A

$$\mathbf{v}_A = \dot{\mathbf{r}}_A = \dot{x}_A\,\mathbf{\imath} + \dot{y}_A\,\mathbf{\jmath}. \tag{4}$$

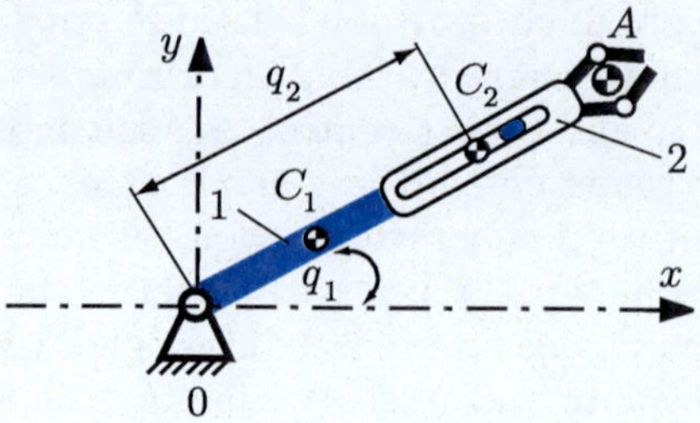

Fig. 1. Two-link planar arm with revolute and prismatic joints.

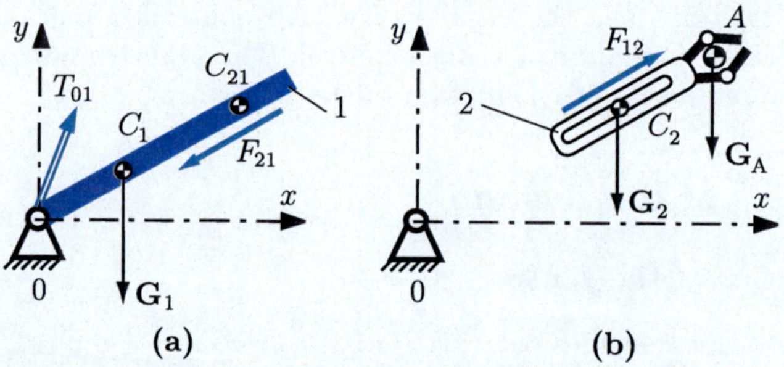

Fig. 2. Active forces: (a) link 1 and (b) slider 2.

2.2 Generalized Active Forces

The active forces on the system are shown in Fig. 2.

The gravity forces on links 1 and 2 at the mass centers C_1 and C_2 are

$$\mathbf{G}_1 = -m_1\, g\, \mathbf{j} \quad \text{and} \quad \mathbf{G}_2 = -m_2\, g\, \mathbf{j}, \tag{5}$$

and the gravity force of the concentrated mass at A is

$$\mathbf{G}_A = -m_A\, g\, \mathbf{j}. \tag{6}$$

The control moment transmitted from 0 on 1 at O is $\mathbf{T}_{01} = T_{01}\,\mathbf{k}$ and the force transmitted from 1 on 2 at C_2 is $\mathbf{F}_{12} = F_{12}\,(\cos q_1(t)\,\mathbf{\imath} + \sin q_1(t)\,\mathbf{\jmath})$. There are two generalized active forces for q_i, $i = 1, 2$

$$\begin{aligned} Q_i = {} & \mathbf{G}_1 \cdot \frac{\partial \mathbf{r}_{C_1}}{\partial q_i} + \mathbf{T}_{01} \cdot \frac{\partial \boldsymbol{\omega}}{\partial \dot{q}_i} - \mathbf{F}_{12} \cdot \frac{\partial \mathbf{v}_{C_2^1}}{\partial q_i} \\ & + \mathbf{F}_{12} \cdot \frac{\partial \mathbf{v}_{C_2}}{\partial q_i} + \mathbf{G}_2 \cdot \frac{\partial \mathbf{r}_{C_2}}{\partial q_i} + \mathbf{G}_A \cdot \frac{\partial \mathbf{r}_A}{\partial q_i}, \end{aligned} \tag{7}$$

where $\mathbf{v}_{C_2^1}$ is the velocity of a point C_2^1 on link 1 that is coincident with C_2: $\mathbf{r}_{C_2^1} = \mathbf{r}_{C_2}$.

2.3 Kinetic Energy

The kinetic energy of the two links and the concentrated mass at A are

$$T_1 = \frac{1}{2} I_O \boldsymbol{\omega} \cdot \boldsymbol{\omega},$$
$$T_2 = \frac{1}{2} m_2 \mathbf{v}_{C_2} \cdot \mathbf{v}_{C_2} + \frac{1}{2} I_{C_2} \boldsymbol{\omega} \cdot \boldsymbol{\omega},$$
$$T_A = \frac{1}{2} m_A \mathbf{v}_A \cdot \mathbf{v}_A, \tag{8}$$

where I_O is the mass moment of inertia of link 1 about O, I_{C_2} is the mass moment inertia of link 2 about C_2. The kinetic energy of the system is

$$T = T_1 + T_2 + T_A \tag{9}$$

Lagrange's equations of motion are

$$\frac{d}{dt}\left(\frac{\partial T}{\partial \dot{q}_i}\right) - \frac{\partial T}{\partial q_i} = Q_i, \;\; i = 1, 2. \tag{10}$$

The Chaucy problem for Eq. (10) is: $t = 0 \Longrightarrow q_1(0) = q_{10}$, $q_2(0) = q_{20}$, $\dot{q}_1(0) = \dot{q}_{10}$, $\dot{q}_2(0) = \dot{q}_{20}$. The direct path of the robot is from q_{10}, q_{20} to q_{1f}, q_{2f}. The controllers for the direct path are selected as

$$T_{01c} = -\beta_{01}\,\dot{q}_1(t) - \gamma_{01}\,(q_1(t) - q_{1f}) - (Q_1(t) - T_{01}),$$
$$F_{12c} = -\beta_{12}\,\dot{q}_2(t) - \gamma_{12}\,(q_2(t) - q_{2f}) - (Q_2(t) - F_{12}). \tag{11}$$

The return path of the robot is from q_{1f}, q_{2f} to q_{10}, q_{20} and the controller are

$$T_{01r} = -\beta_{01}\,\dot{q}_1(t) - \gamma_{01}\,(q_1(t) - q_{10}) - (Q_1(t) - T_{01}),$$
$$F_{12r} = -\beta_{12}\,\dot{q}_2(t) - \gamma_{12}\,(q_2(t) - q_{20}) - (Q_2(t) - F_{12}). \tag{12}$$

The controllers are considered periodic with a period T

$$T_{01c}(t+T),\; F_{12c}(t+T),\; T_{01r}(t+T),\; F_{12r}(t+T). \tag{13}$$

The dynamical equations of motion are solved for the direct and return paths with periodic controllers.

3 Results and Discussion

The physical and control parameters of the robot arm used for the simulation are shown in Table 1. The initial conditions and the target position for the direct path are specified in Table 2. The dynamics of the robots are investigated under three cases: $T = 8$ s, $T = 2.5$ s, and $T = 1$ s. Ten cycles are simulated for each case.

Table 1. Physical and control parameters of the robot arm.

Physical parameters	Value	Control parameters	Value
m_1	1 (kg)	β_{01}	50 (N s)
m_2	1 (kg)	β_{01}	50 (N s)
m_A	5 (kg)	γ_{01}	300 (N)
L	2 (m)	γ_{01}	300 (N)
I_{C_2}	1 (kg m^2)		
g	9.81 (m/s^2)		

Table 2. Initial conditions and target position for the direct path.

Initial conditions	Value	Direct target position	Value
q_{10}	0	q_{1f}	$\pi/4$ (rad)
q_{20}	0.5 (m)	q_{2f}	2 (m)
$\dot{q}_{10}$	0		
$\dot{q}_{20}$	0		

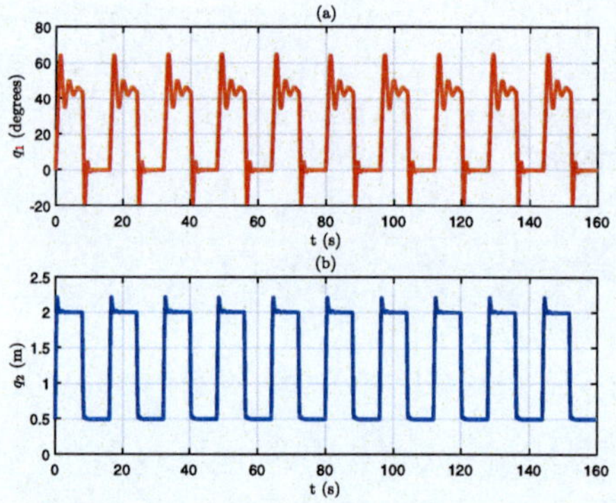

Fig. 3. Control response of the robot arm with $T = 8$ s: (a) $q_1(t)$ and (b) $q_2(t)$.

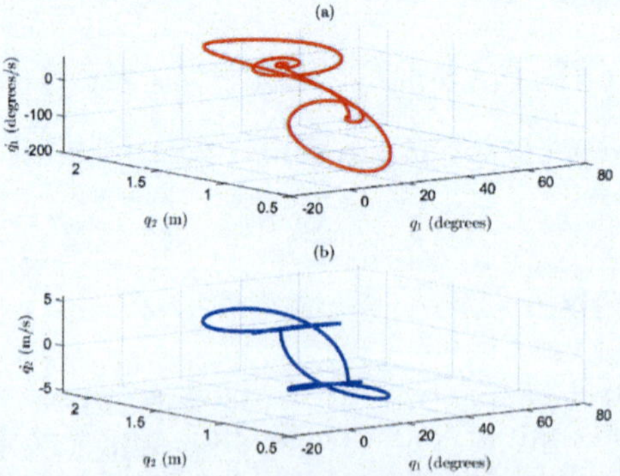

Fig. 4. Phase plane of the robot arm with $T = 8$ s: (a) $\dot{q}_1(q_1, q_2)$ and (b) $\dot{q}_2(q_1, q_2)$.

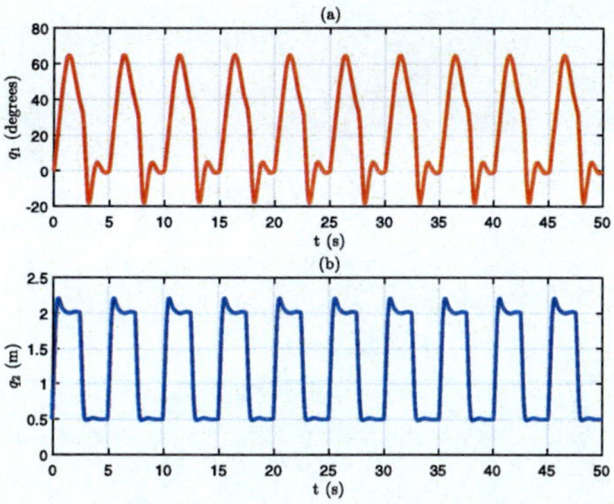

Fig. 5. Control response of the robot arm with $T = 2.5$ s: (a) $q_1(t)$ and (b) $q_2(t)$.

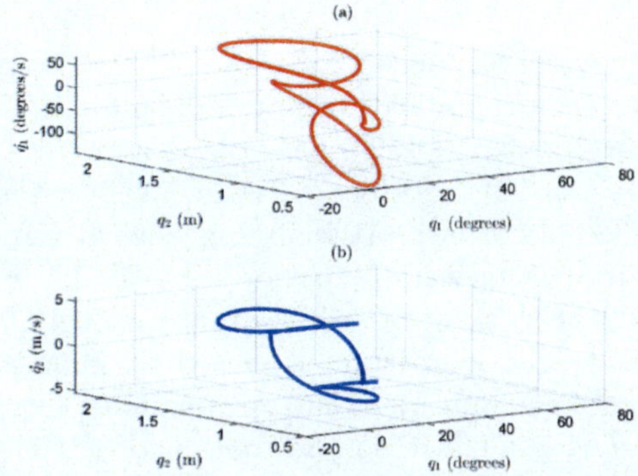

Fig. 6. Phase plane of the robot arm with $T = 2.5$ s: (a) $\dot{q}_1(q_1, q_2)$ and (b) $\dot{q}_2(q_1, q_2)$.

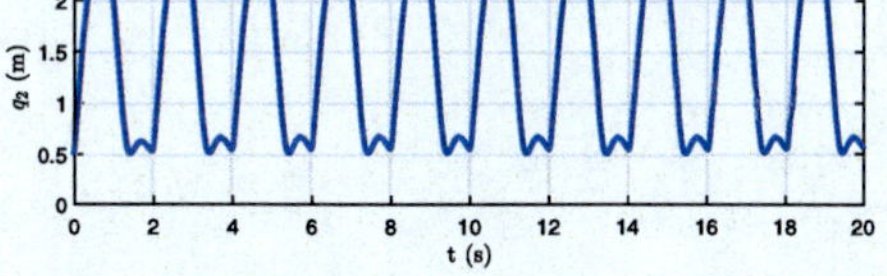

Fig. 7. Control response of the robot arm with $T = 1$ s: (a) $q_1(t)$ and (b) $q_2(t)$.

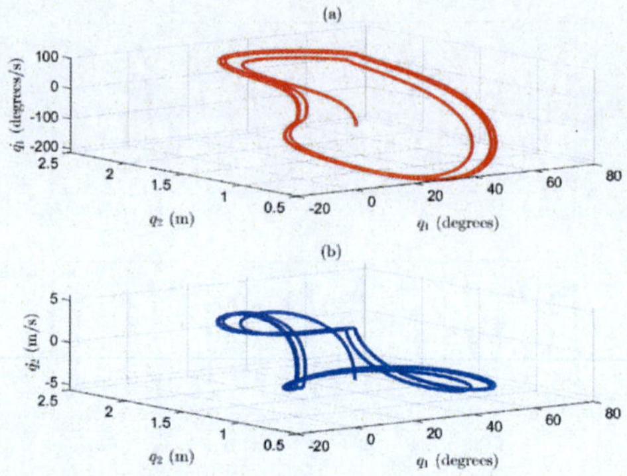

Fig. 8. Phase plane of the robot arm with $T = 1$ s: (a) $\dot{q}_1(q_1, q_2)$ and (b) $\dot{q}_2(q_1, q_2)$.

Figure 3 shows the control response for $T = 8$ s. The phase plane is depicted in Fig. 4 with the closed trajectory indicating a periodic motion. Figure 5 represents the control response for $T = 2.5$ s. The phase plane is plotted in Fig. 6 with the closed orbit implying a periodic motion. Figure 7 shows the control response for $T = 1$ s. The phase plane is plotted in Fig. 8 with limit cycles following the separated trajectories suggesting a periodic motion. Figure 9 shows the approximate entropy of the q_2 position of the robot arm with $T = 1$ s, $T = 2.5$ s, $T = 8$ s, and $T = 15$ s. The algorithm proposed by Pincus [13] was used to compute the approximate entropy. Here the approximate entropy was evaluated for q_2 because it has a larger effect on the motion of the end-effector A. It is shown that for q_2 the approximate entropy decreases with the magnitude of the period T. In other words, with higher magnitudes of the actuation period, the robotic arm system tends to be more regular, and the dynamics are more predictable over fluctuations.

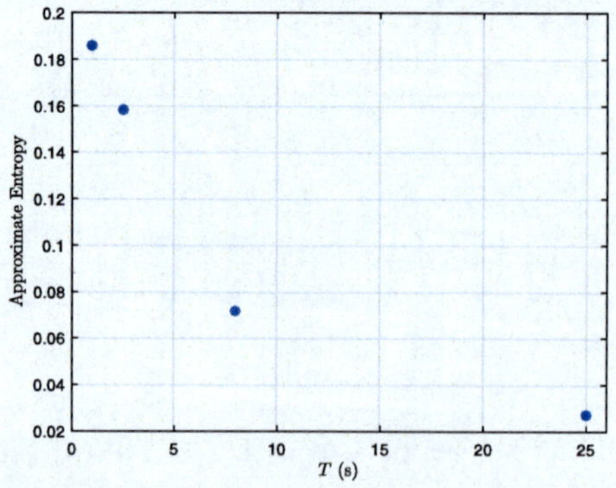

Fig. 9. Approximate entropy of the robot arm with various T.

4 Conclusion

In this study, the dynamics of a two-link planar robotic arm with revolute and prismatic joints under periodic actuations are investigated. The actuators have the form of a PD controller with an additional term calculated from the generalized forces. The performance of this controller has been verified under various magnitudes of the actuation period. The periodic motion was obtained in all the cases, even though a steady state was not reached until several cycles of simulation for the shortest actuation period considered in this study. The approximate entropy is a function of the period of the actuators and is decreasing with the period. The robotic arm system is more regular for higher periods.

References

1. Hashemi, S.M., Abbas, H.S., Werner, H.: Control. Eng. Pract. **20**(3), 248 (2012)
2. Liu, X.F., Li, H.Q., Chen, Y.J., Cai, G.P., Wang, X.: Multibody. Syst. Dyn. **33**(3), 315 (2015)
3. Marghitu, D.B.: Mechanisms and Robots Analysis with MATLAB®. Springer Science & Business Media, London (2009). https://doi.org/10.1007/978-1-84800-391-0
4. Kane, T.R., Levinson, D.A.: Dynamics, Theory and Applications. McGraw Hill, New York (1985)
5. Genta, G.: Introduction to the Mechanics of Space Robots, vol. 26. Springer Science & Business Media, Dordrecht (2011). https://doi.org/10.1007/978-94-007-1796-1
6. Villani, L., De Schutterm, J.: Handbook of Robotics. Springer, New York (2008)
7. Brogårdh, T.: Present and future robot control development: an industrial perspective. Annu. Rev. Control. **31**(1), 69–79 (2007)
8. Moosavian, S.A.A., Papadopoulos, E.: Tutorial review on space manipulators for space debris mitigation. Robotica **25**(5), 537 (2007)
9. Zang, X., Iqbal, S., Zhu, Y., Liu, X., Zhao, J.: Int. J. Adv. Rob. Syst. **13**(2), 60 (2016)
10. Reher, J., Kann, C., Ames, A.D.: 2020 American Control Conference (ACC), pp. 2444–2451. IEEE (2020)
11. Chang, Y.C., Roohi, N., Gao, S.: Neural lyapunov control. Adv. Neural Inf. Process. Syst. **32** (2019)
12. Son, C.: Optimal control planning strategies with fuzzy entropy and sensor fusion for obotic part assembly tasks. Int. J. Mach. Tools Manuf **42**(12), 1335 (2002)
13. Pincus, S.M.: Approximate entropy as a measure of system complexity. Proc. Natl. Acad. Sci. **88**(6), 2297 (1991)
14. Kim, J.I., Hong, M., Lee, K., Kim, D., Park, Y.L., Oh, S.: Learning to walk a tripod mobile robot using nonlinear soft vibration actuators with entropy adaptive reinforcement learning. IEEE Roboti. Autom. Lett. **5**(2), 2317 (2020)
15. Kalyoncu, M.: Mathematical modelling and dynamic response of a multi-straight-line path tracing flexible robot manipulator with rotating-prismatic joint. Appl. Math. Model. **32**(6), 1087 (2008)

Mechanism Design and Inverse Kinematics of a 5-DOF Medical Assistive Manipulator

Anton Antonov and Alexey Fomin(✉)

Mechanical Engineering Research Institute of the Russian Academy of Sciences (IMASH RAN), Moscow 101000, Russia
antonov.av@imash.ru, alexey-nvkz@mail.ru

Abstract. This article presents an inverse kinematic analysis of a medical assistive manipulator, whose output link has three translational and two rotational degrees of freedom (3T2R motion pattern). The manipulator consists of a 2-DOF parallel kinematic part and a 3-DOF serial kinematic part. An original design of the manipulator looks promising for medical applications that require a movable frame above the patient. The article develops an algorithm for calculating displacements in the actuated joints when the desired motion of the output link is prescribed. The suggested algorithm is based on the product-of-exponentials formula. It provides a closed-form solution with no assumptions about the manipulator geometry. A case study demonstrates an example of application and verifies the proposed techniques.

Keywords: parallel-serial manipulator · hybrid manipulator · 3T2R motion pattern · inverse kinematics · PoE formula · screw theory · twist

1 Introduction

The COVID-19 pandemic has caused a lot of dangers for the human society. To deal with these issues, many robotic applications have been proposed since the pandemic emergence [13]. In particular, robotic systems based on parallel mechanisms are widely applied in medicine at the moment. The end-effector of these systems has several degrees of freedom (DOFs), and it is controlled by several kinematic chains. There are devices applied in surgery, e.g., a PARASURG-9M robot for minimally invasive surgery (including abdominal surgery, urology, and thoracic surgery) [8], a robot for cochlear implant surgery [7], and a robot for skull surgery [3]; in rehabilitation procedures, e.g., mechanisms for ankle rehabilitation [9,11] and upper- and lower-limb rehabilitation [4,12]; and in other operations, e.g., a spherical robot for tele-echography applications [1] and a robot for cardiopulmonary resuscitation [5].

The current study considers a medical assistive manipulator, whose output link has five DOFs. Figure 1 illustrates a schematic view of the proposed manipulator, where the moving frame with the end-effector is above the patient.

D. Tarnita et al. (Eds.): MESROB 2023, MMS 133, pp. 334–342, 2023.
https://doi.org/10.1007/978-3-031-32446-8_36

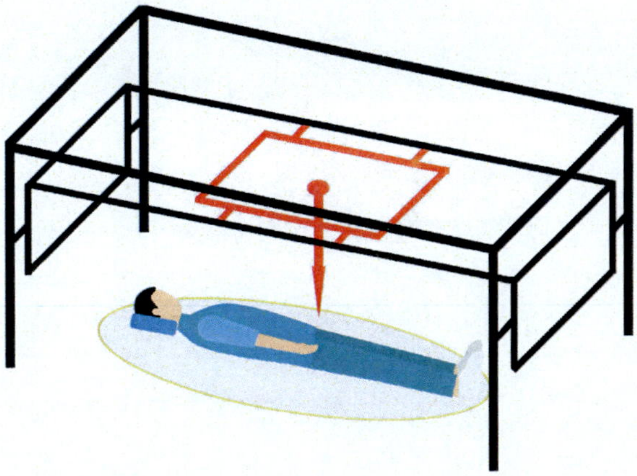

Fig. 1. Schematic view of the proposed system.

Manipulator design corresponds to the novel kinematic scheme introduced recently in paper [2]. In the current work, we will focus on its inverse kinematics, which is the major contribution of the article. This problem is crucial for manipulator control, and its solution forms a basis for solving other problems of kinematic and dynamic analyses.

2 Manipulator Architecture

Figure 2 shows a kinematic scheme of the considered manipulator. It includes a parallel part formed by links 1, ..., 6, and a serial part formed by links 7, 8, and 9. We will call links 1, 6, and 9 the base, the platform, and the output link, respectively. Links 1 and 2 are coupled by prismatic (P) joints; links 4 and 6, 4 and 5, and 5 and 6 are coupled by revolute (R) joints, whose axes are parallel to each other and orthogonal to the P joints above. Thus, there is one PRR kinematic chain and one PR kinematic chain between base 1 and platform 6—the platform has two degrees of freedom in a planar motion. The serial part has a PPR structure and provides output link 9 with three more DOFs. The output link has five DOFs in total, which we can classify as three translational and rotational (a 3T2R motion pattern). The restricted rotation is about the axis orthogonal to the axes of the R joints. The manipulator has five actuated joints, indicated in Fig. 2 by parameters $q_1, \ldots, q_5$.

3 Inverse Kinematics

Inverse kinematics aims to find displacements in the actuated joints when the output link configuration is given. For the considered manipulator, these displacements are $q_1, \ldots, q_5$, as mentioned in the previous section. The output link configuration can be characterized by vector $\mathbf{p}_S \in \mathbb{R}^3$, which describes

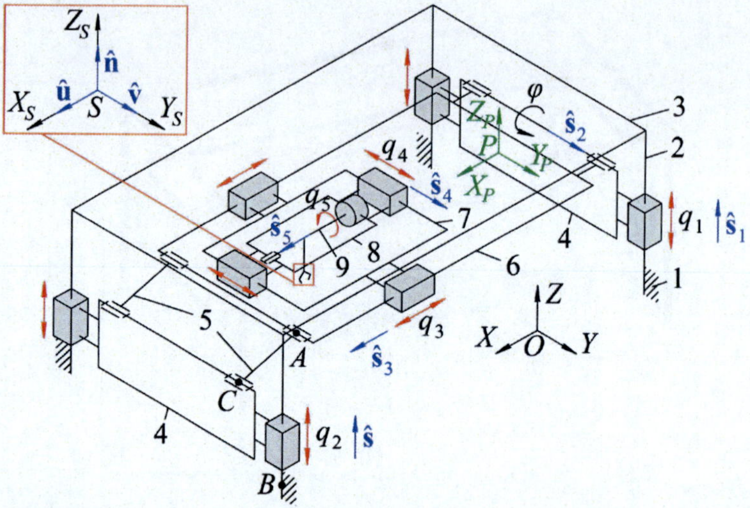

Fig. 2. Considered hybrid manipulator and some kinematic notations. Red arrows indicate the actuated joints.

the position of some point S, and by unit vector $\hat{\mathbf{n}} \in \mathbb{R}^3$, $\|\hat{\mathbf{n}}\|_2 = 1$, which describes the orientation. We set both $\mathbf{p}_S$ and $\hat{\mathbf{n}}$ relative to some stationary reference frame $OXYZ$, placed on the base. Since the output link has only two rotational DOFs, vector $\hat{\mathbf{n}}$ is sufficient to describe its orientation. Let us also attach reference frame $SX_SY_SZ_S$ to the output link and introduce transformation matrix $\mathbf{T}_S \in SE(3)$, which defines the frame configuration relative to $OXYZ$:

$$\mathbf{T}_S = \begin{bmatrix} \hat{\mathbf{u}} \; \hat{\mathbf{v}} \; \hat{\mathbf{n}} \; \mathbf{p}_S \\ 0 \; 0 \; 0 \;\; 1 \end{bmatrix}, \tag{1}$$

where $\hat{\mathbf{u}}$ and $\hat{\mathbf{v}}$ are unit vectors, which constitute the right system with vector $\hat{\mathbf{n}}$. Vectors $\hat{\mathbf{u}}$ and $\hat{\mathbf{v}}$ can have arbitrary directions.

Let us look at the PRPPR serial kinematic chain between the base and the output link, defined by links 1, 4, 6, 7, 8, and 9 (Fig. 2). We can write a product-of-exponentials (PoE) formula for this chain as follows [6, ch. 4]:

$$\mathbf{T}_S = \left(\prod_{i=1}^{5} \exp([\boldsymbol{\xi}_i]\theta_i) \right) \mathbf{M}_S, \tag{2}$$

where $\mathbf{M}_S \in SE(3)$ is a transformation matrix, which corresponds to some initial configuration of the output link; $i = 1, \ldots, 5$ is a joint number, counting from the base; θ_i is a displacement in the i-th joint; $\boldsymbol{\xi}_i \in \mathbb{R}^6$ is a (unit) twist, which corresponds to the i-th joint in the initial configuration; $[\boldsymbol{\xi}_i] \in se(3)$ is a matrix representation of twist $\boldsymbol{\xi}_i$. One can find expanded expressions of $[\boldsymbol{\xi}_i]$ and $\exp([\boldsymbol{\xi}_i]\theta_i)$ in [6, ch. 3].

For the considered PRPPR chain, twists $\boldsymbol{\xi}_i$ and displacements θ_i has the following form:

$$\boldsymbol{\xi}_1 = \begin{bmatrix} \mathbf{0} \\ \hat{\mathbf{s}}_1 \end{bmatrix}, \quad \boldsymbol{\xi}_2 = \begin{bmatrix} \hat{\mathbf{s}}_2 \\ \mathbf{r}_2 \times \hat{\mathbf{s}}_2 \end{bmatrix}, \quad \boldsymbol{\xi}_3 = \begin{bmatrix} \mathbf{0} \\ \hat{\mathbf{s}}_3 \end{bmatrix}, \quad \boldsymbol{\xi}_4 = \begin{bmatrix} \mathbf{0} \\ \hat{\mathbf{s}}_4 \end{bmatrix}, \quad \boldsymbol{\xi}_5 = \begin{bmatrix} \hat{\mathbf{s}}_5 \\ \mathbf{r}_5 \times \hat{\mathbf{s}}_5 \end{bmatrix}, \tag{3}$$

$$\theta_1 = q_1, \qquad \theta_2 = \varphi, \qquad \theta_3 = q_3, \qquad \theta_4 = q_4, \qquad \theta_5 = q_5, \tag{4}$$

where $\hat{\mathbf{s}}_1, \ldots, \hat{\mathbf{s}}_5$ are unit vectors, parallel to the axes of the corresponding joints; $\mathbf{r}_2$ and $\mathbf{r}_5$ are vectors that define position of the axes of the corresponding joints; φ is a platform rotation angle about the axis defined by vector $\hat{\mathbf{s}}_2$.

Parameters $\mathbf{M}_S$, $\hat{\mathbf{s}}_1, \ldots, \hat{\mathbf{s}}_5$, $\mathbf{r}_2$, and $\mathbf{r}_5$ depend on the manipulator design and location of frames $OXYZ$ and $SX_SY_SZ_S$, and they are assumed to be known. Thus, when we are given matrix $\mathbf{T}_S$, Eq. (2) represents a system of equations with respect to variables θ_i, $i = 1, \ldots, 5$, written in Eq. (4). To simplify the equations, we can direct the OZ axis parallel to vector $\hat{\mathbf{s}}_1$ and the OY axis parallel to vector $\hat{\mathbf{s}}_2$ without loss of generality:

$$\hat{\mathbf{s}}_1 = \begin{bmatrix} 0 \; 0 \; 1 \end{bmatrix}^{\mathrm{T}}, \quad \hat{\mathbf{s}}_2 = \begin{bmatrix} 0 \; 1 \; 0 \end{bmatrix}^{\mathrm{T}}. \tag{5}$$

Now, let us substitute Eqs. (1), (3)–(5) into Eq. (2) and consider an equation that corresponds to the second row and the third column in Eq. (2). This equation depends on displacement q_5 as follows:

$$a_1 \cos q_5 + b_1 \sin q_5 + c_1 = 0, \tag{6}$$

where a_1, b_1, and c_1 are known coefficients independent of φ and $q_1, \ldots, q_5$.

The trigonometric equation above gives two different solutions for variable q_5, which can be found using conventional methods [10]. Next, we consider two equations that correspond to the first and the third rows and the third column in Eq. (2). These equations look similar to Eq. (6):

$$\begin{aligned} a_2 \cos\varphi + b_2 \sin\varphi + c_2 = 0, \\ a_3 \cos\varphi + b_3 \sin\varphi + c_3 = 0, \end{aligned} \tag{7}$$

where $a_2, \ldots, c_3$ are known coefficients independent of φ and $q_1, \ldots, q_4$.

The expressions above represent a system of two linear equations with respect to variables $\cos\varphi$ and $\sin\varphi$. In addition, symbolic computations show that $a_2 = b_3$ and $b_2 = -a_3$. When $a_2 b_3 - a_3 b_2 \neq 0$, this system has a unique solution [10], from which we find variable φ using the atan2 function [6, ch. 6]. Each solution of Eq. (6) will define a different solution for variable φ.

Let us next look at two equations that correspond to the first two rows and the fourth column in Eq. (2):

$$\begin{aligned} a_4 q_3 + b_4 q_4 + c_4 = 0, \\ a_5 q_3 + b_5 q_4 + c_5 = 0, \end{aligned} \tag{8}$$

where $a_4, \ldots, c_5$ are known coefficients independent of $q_1, \ldots, q_4$.

When $a_4 b_5 - a_5 b_4 \neq 0$, the system above provides a unique set of solutions for variables q_3 and q_4 (for each solution q_5). Finally, consider an equation that corresponds to the third row and the third column in Eq. (2):

$$a_6 q_1 + b_6 = 0, \tag{9}$$

where a_6 and b_6 are known coefficients independent of q_1 and q_2.

When $a_6 \neq 0$, the above equation gives a unique solution q_1 (for each solution q_5). Thus, we have found all variables θ_i, $i = 1, \ldots, 5$, which include four displacements q_1, q_3, q_4, and q_5 in the actuated joints. To find remaining displacement q_2, we can apply the PoE formula again. First, we attach reference frame $PX_PY_PZ_P$ to the platform. Let transformation matrix $\mathbf{T}_P$ define the frame configuration relative to $OXYZ$ in a general posture, and matrix $\mathbf{M}_P$—in the initial posture. We compute matrix $\mathbf{T}_P$ as follows:

$$\mathbf{T}_P = \exp([\boldsymbol{\xi}_1]\theta_1)\exp([\boldsymbol{\xi}_2]\theta_2)\mathbf{M}_P. \tag{10}$$

Next, we can write expressions for coordinates $\mathbf{p}_A$ and $\mathbf{p}_C$ of points A and C, which correspond to the revolute joints (Fig. 2):

$$\begin{bmatrix} \mathbf{p}_A \\ 1 \end{bmatrix} = \mathbf{T}_P \begin{bmatrix} \mathbf{r}_A \\ 1 \end{bmatrix}, \tag{11}$$

$$\mathbf{p}_C = \mathbf{p}_B + q_2 \hat{\mathbf{s}}, \tag{12}$$

where $\mathbf{r}_A$ are coordinates of point A in frame $PX_PY_PZ_P$; $\mathbf{p}_B$ are coordinates of point B in frame $OXYZ$, with B being some reference point for variable q_2; $\hat{\mathbf{s}}$ is a unit vector parallel to the axis of the actuated joint. These parameters depend on the manipulator geometry, and they are assumed to be known.

To find variable q_2, we write an expression that connects coordinates $\mathbf{p}_A$ and $\mathbf{p}_C$:

$$(\mathbf{p}_A - \mathbf{p}_C)^2 = l_{AC}^2, \tag{13}$$

where l_{AC} is a known and constant distance between points A and C.

If we substitute Eqs. (11) and (12) into Eq. (13), we will get a quadratic equation with respect to variable q_2. This equation gives a set of two different solutions in a general case. Note that there are two different sets of solutions, each of which corresponds to a different value q_5 we found earlier. This completes the solution of the inverse kinematics.

4 Case Study

Let us consider an example of the inverse kinematic analysis for the manipulator with the following geometry (linear parameters are in mm):

$$\hat{\mathbf{s}}_3 = \hat{\mathbf{s}}_5 = \begin{bmatrix} 1 \\ 0 \\ 0 \end{bmatrix}, \hat{\mathbf{s}}_4 = \begin{bmatrix} 0 \\ 1 \\ 0 \end{bmatrix}, \hat{\mathbf{s}} = \begin{bmatrix} 0 \\ 0 \\ 1 \end{bmatrix}, \mathbf{r}_2 = \begin{bmatrix} -300 \\ 0 \\ 0 \end{bmatrix}, \mathbf{r}_5 = \begin{bmatrix} 0 \\ 0 \\ 0 \end{bmatrix}, \mathbf{r}_A = \begin{bmatrix} 250 \\ 150 \\ 0 \end{bmatrix},$$

$$\mathbf{p}_B = \begin{bmatrix} 300 \\ 150 \\ 0 \end{bmatrix}, \quad \mathbf{M}_S = \begin{bmatrix} 1 & 0 & 0 & 0 \\ 0 & 1 & 0 & 0 \\ 0 & 0 & 1 & -100 \\ 0 & 0 & 0 & 1 \end{bmatrix}, \quad \mathbf{M}_P = \begin{bmatrix} 1 & 0 & 0 & 0 \\ 0 & 1 & 0 & 0 \\ 0 & 0 & 1 & 0 \\ 0 & 0 & 0 & 1 \end{bmatrix}, \quad l_{AC} = 75.$$

Suppose the output link has to follow the trajectory depicted in Fig. 3. The trajectory includes two straight-line segments (1–2 and 3–4) and two circular segments (2–3 and 4–1), which are symmetric relative to the OXZ and OYZ planes. Along the entire path, the output link stays parallel to the OYZ plane. The output link maintains its orientation on the straight-line segments and alters it to the opposite one on the circular segments. The motion begins at point 0, which is at the center of circular segment 4–1. Each straight-line segment takes 4 s to move, and each circular segment takes 2 s.

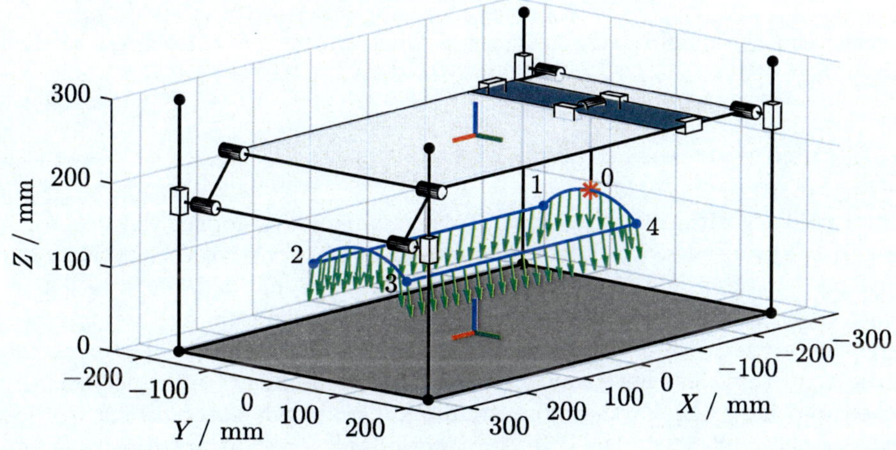

Fig. 3. The reference trajectory and the manipulator at the beginning of its motion. Green arrows correspond to vector $-\hat{\mathbf{n}}$. Two RGB triads correspond to reference frames $OXYZ$ and $PX_PY_PZ_P$. (Color figure online)

Figure 4 illustrates the solution to the inverse kinematics problem[1]. The calculated values of the actuated coordinates and their time behavior match the

[1] MATLAB script that applies the proposed algorithm is available free online at http://dx.doi.org/10.17632/vct5jzkzk6.1.

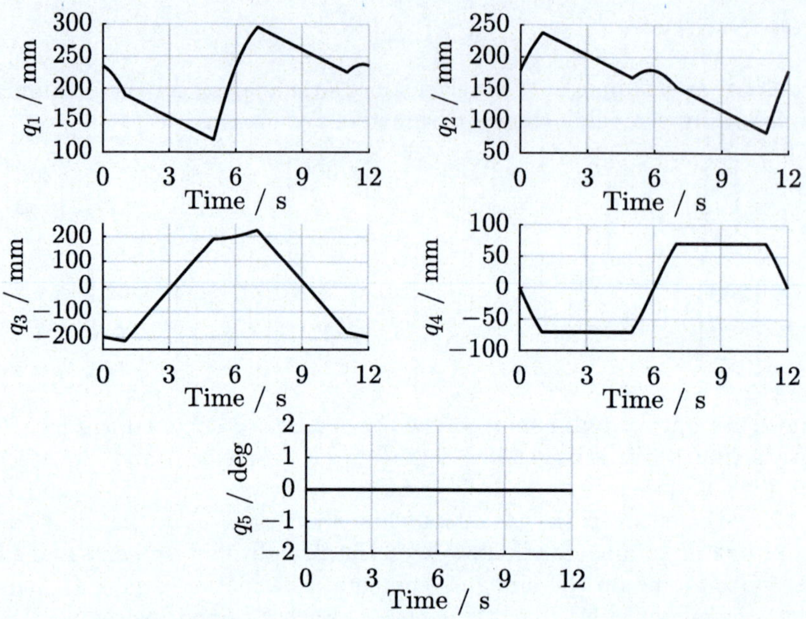

Fig. 4. Solution to the inverse kinematic problem.

trajectory and the manipulator geometry. This confirms the correctness of the proposed algorithm.

5 Discussion

The proposed algorithm for solving the inverse kinematics applies the PoE formula (Eqs. (2) and (10)) to obtain the desired expressions. To solve the problem, we need to describe the initial configuration of the manipulator in terms of parameters $\boldsymbol{\xi}_i$, $i = 1, \ldots, 5$, $\mathbf{M}_S$, and $\mathbf{M}_P$, which depend only on the manipulator geometry and reference frames $OXYZ$, $PX_PY_PZ_P$, and $SX_SY_SZ_S$. Note that the algorithm does not require introducing any auxiliary reference frames attached to other links. Furthermore, we did not make any assumptions on the location of the joint axes—the algorithm works well for arbitrary directions of vectors $\hat{\mathbf{s}}_3$, $\hat{\mathbf{s}}_4$, and $\hat{\mathbf{s}}_5$.

Because of the space limitation, we did not present explicit expressions for coefficients in Eqs. (6)–(9). When solving the inverse kinematics, we should check these coefficients to make sure that the corresponding equations provide real-valued solutions. There can also be situations when the equations have an infinite number of solutions. Such situations are closely related to singular configurations that should be analyzed before the motion planning.

6 Conclusion

This article has considered the inverse kinematics of the 5-DOF hybrid manipulator, which includes the 2-DOF parallel part and the 3-DOF serial part. The proposed algorithm, based on the PoE formula, allows us to get a closed-form solution with no assumptions on the manipulator geometry. The considered case study verifies that the algorithm is correct.

The obtained expressions constitute a basis for subsequent kinematic analysis, which will include direct kinematics and workspace determination. One further development of the performed study is velocity analysis, which can be done using the screw theory approach we considered here. In addition, the presented techniques can also be adapted to other hybrid manipulators.

Acknowledgements. This research was supported by Russian Science Foundation (RSF) under grant No. 22-79-10304, https://rscf.ru/project/22-79-10304/.

References

1. Essomba, T., Laribi, M.A., Zeghloul, S., Poisson, G.: Optimal synthesis of a spherical parallel mechanism for medical application. Robotica **34**(3), 671–686 (2016). https://doi.org/10.1017/S0263574714001805
2. Ganiev, R.F., Glazunov, V.A., Filippov, G.S.: Urgent problems of machine science and ways of solving them: wave and additive technologies, the machine tool industry, and robot surgery. J. Mach. Manuf. Reliab. **47**(5), 399–406 (2018). https://doi.org/10.3103/S1052618818050059
3. Kobler, J.-P., et al.: Configuration optimization and experimental accuracy evaluation of a bone-attached, parallel robot for skull surgery. Int. J. Comput. Assist. Radiol. Surg. **11**(3), 421–436 (2015). https://doi.org/10.1007/s11548-015-1300-4
4. Laribi, M.A., Carbone, G., Zeghloul, S.: On the optimal design of cable driven parallel robot with a prescribed workspace for upper limb rehabilitation tasks. J. Bionic Eng. **16**(3), 503–513 (2019). https://doi.org/10.1007/s42235-019-0041-4
5. Li, Y., Xu, Q.: Design and development of a medical parallel robot for cardiopulmonary resuscitation. IEEE/ASME Trans. Mechatron. **12**(3), 265–273 (2007). https://doi.org/10.1109/TMECH.2007.897257
6. Lynch, K.M., Park, F.C.: Modern Robotics: Mechanics, Planning, and Control. Cambridge University Press, Cambridge (2017). https://doi.org/10.1017/9781316661239
7. Pile, J., Simaan, N.: Modeling, design, and evaluation of a parallel robot for cochlear implant surgery. IEEE/ASME Trans. Mechatron. **19**(6), 1746–1755 (2014). https://doi.org/10.1109/TMECH.2014.2308479
8. Pisla, D., Gherman, B., Vaida, C., Suciu, M., Plitea, N.: An active hybrid parallel robot for minimally invasive surgery. Rob. Comput.-Integr. Manuf. **29**(4), 203–221 (2013). https://doi.org/10.1016/j.rcim.2012.12.004
9. Saglia, J.A., Tsagarakis, N.G., Dai, J.S., Caldwell, D.G.: A high-performance redundantly actuated parallel mechanism for ankle rehabilitation. Int. J. Rob. Res. **28**(9), 1216–1227 (2009). https://doi.org/10.1177/0278364909104221
10. Waldron, K.J., Schmiedeler, J.: Kinematics. In: Siciliano, B., Khatib, O. (eds.) Springer Handbook of Robotics, pp. 11–36. Springer, Cham (2016). https://doi.org/10.1007/978-3-319-32552-1_2

11. Wang, C., Fang, Y., Guo, S., Chen, Y.: Design and kinematical performance analysis of a 3-RUS/RRR redundantly actuated parallel mechanism for ankle rehabilitation. J. Mech. Rob. **5**(4), 041003 (2013). https://doi.org/10.1115/1.4024736
12. Wang, H., Li, W., Liu, H., Zhang, J., Liu, S.: Conceptual design and dimensional synthesis of a novel parallel mechanism for lower-limb rehabilitation. Robotica **37**(3), 469–480 (2019). https://doi.org/10.1017/S0263574718001121
13. Zemmar, A., Lozano, A.M., Nelson, B.J.: The rise of robots in surgical environments during COVID-19. Nat. Mach. Intell. **2**(10), 566–572 (2020). https://doi.org/10.1038/s42256-020-00238-2

Design and Operation of a Robotized Bed for Bedridden COVID Patients

Marco Ceccarelli[1] (✉), Matteo Russo[1], Jorge Araque Isidro[1], Betsy D. M. Chaparro-Rico[2], and Daniele Cafolla[3]

[1] University of Rome Tor Vergata, 00133 Rome, Italy
{marco.ceccarelli,matteo.russo}@uniroma2.it
[2] Independant researcher, Swansea, UK
[3] Faculty of Science and Engineering, Department of Computer Science, Swansea University, Swansea, UK
daniele.cafolla@swansea.ac.uk

Abstract. Improvement of the conditions of bedridden patients is analyzed in terms of the effects of prolonged time or bed rest in order to define a design solution for a bed that can improve comfort and avoid worsening. The structure and functionality of a robotized bed solution is presented with characteristics which can be useful for bedridden patients and for those affected by COVID in intensive care units with the fundamental characteristics that refer to adequate mobility of the patient in the bed itself.

Keywords: Robotic beds · Bedridden conditions · Design · Operation analysis · COVID patients

1 Introduction

Hospital-type beds are important for bedridden patients with difficult health illnesses and for these reasons the development of better beds has increased in recent years. These improvements are focused on different areas, especially to make more comfortable and safer the stay in bedridden conditions. Healthcare workers also need protection to do a better job without health risks from contact with patients with contagious diseases.

Hospital-type beds are specifically designed for the care of people whit health complications. Therefore, they must have medical and biomedical instrumentation that allows health personnel to constantly monitor a patient. Another reason for the use of hospital beds, mainly in Intensive Care Units (ICUs), is that they must facilitate the maneuvers that can be required for the health care of each patient as outlined for example in [1–5].

Therefore, new technological solutions are required to address the issues for better comfort, improvement of bedridden conditions, and avoid complications due to long bedridden status. Furthermore, in order to help the nurses and other health workers to avoid diseases due to patient management like in the fight against COVID-19 it is important to have available suitable solutions. There are already solutions using pneumatic actuators to move patients from side to side facilitating the work of nurses as reported in

D. Tarnita et al. (Eds.): MESROB 2023, MMS 133, pp. 343–350, 2023.
https://doi.org/10.1007/978-3-031-32446-8_37

[1–5]. Remote monitoring can be also used to avoid contagious risk also to the medical operators. A solution for robotized hospital bed control is also possible with a webcam and digital image processing so that mechatronic designs have been also proposed as those presented in [6–10].

The main objective of this paper is to present the design and a controlled operation of a robotized hospital-type bed that performs movements of segments of the bed that allow a patient to move from right to left and from left to right. These movements are carried out in the upper part of a patient's body by means a mechanism that is specifically designed to move each segment of the bed, according to a previous solution presented in [1, 5, 11]. The robotic bed solution is presented with its main characteristic in the mechanical design and controlled operation as function of a proper driving mechanism. This driving mechanism is driven by a dc motor and a control system is designed with feedback sensors that provide the position of the bed segment, pressure sensors monitoring the status of the imbedded patient, and medical sensors monitoring patient's vital sign to be observed by the health sanitary operators.

2 Requirements

The most special hospital beds are in ICU because those patients have complex health situations, and their treatments need special biomedical devices to monitor vital signs and medical devices to help patients with different complications.

Main complications in bedridden patients can be identified in lung secretion stationary and sore source, as summarized in the schemes in Fig. 1. Without a proper mobilization of the patients and with the sedation of the cough reflex due to prolonged bed stay, secretions may accumulate in the lower lobes of the pulmonary complex. This is the reason why prone position has been successfully proposed mainly in treating the COVID patients, [12]. Constant movement of semi-rotation along the patient's axial plane may contrast mucus engorgement and subsequent lung atelectasis.

In addition, pressure ulcers are often source of problems with bedridden patients as areas of damaged skin and adjacent tissues as due to applied pressure, friction, or shear, as pointed out in [4, 13]. Sores can also be a source of infections and other complications putting the patient's life at risk. To avoid the sore problem in patients, nurses are used to turn them from side to side every two hours, and in this procedure, health care workers could suffer medical complications due to repetitive forced movements and the risk of contagion with sick patients [4, 13].

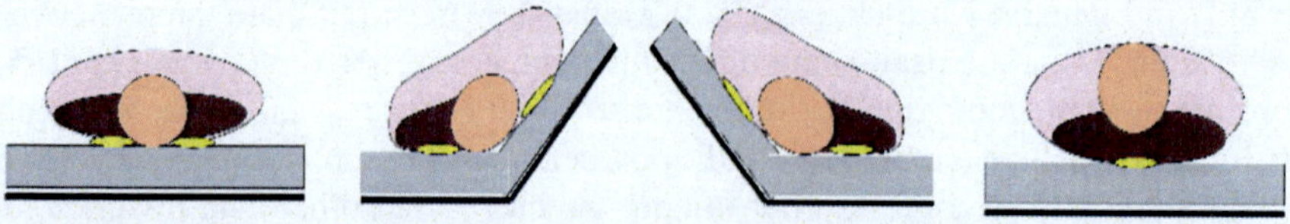

Fig. 1. Effects of prolonged bedridden conditions in terms of location of pulmonary secretions (in brown) and source of decubitus (in yellow)

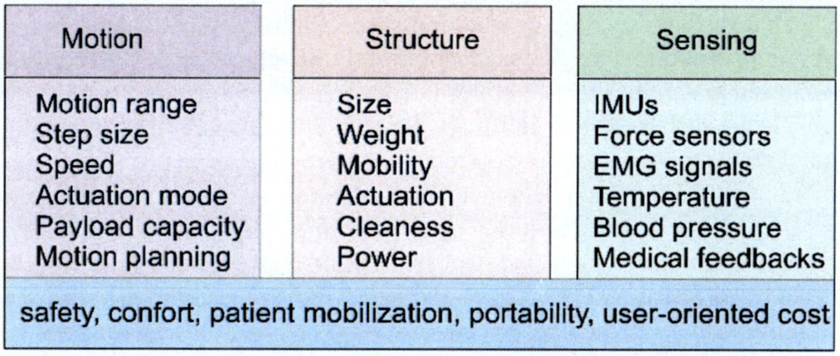

Fig. 2. Requirements for design of beds for bedridden patients

Figure 2 summarizes peculiarities and requirements for the design of a robotic bed solution for bedridden patients with above-mentioned clinical complications, although they can be considered for patients suffering of other pathologies requiring long-term immobilization on a bed. The items in Fig. 2 refer to the main characteristics that may affect the design and functionality of a robotic bed in terms of mobility, structure, and sensorization against the main issues with bedridden patients. As regards the motion, requirements can refer to the range of motion of bed segments with the necessary motion resolutions without excessive speed. This motion capacity is possible with an electric-type servomotor controlled in position even with open-loop algorithms. In addition, it is to consider of equipping the robotic bed with a battery power station (beneath the bed yet) that can allow the use of the bed even in locations far from power sockets at least for a sufficiently long period. The actuation solutions should be equipped with suitable mechanisms that allow to use those light compact servomotors with adequate performance for the bed structure. The load capacity can be defined as the body mass that each segment is expected to move. This load capacity can be sized to values below 30 kg for each segment in lateral movement of the body. The use of position-controlled servomotors makes possible to use programmable motion s that can be defined by medical operators according to the patient's state and required therapy even for remote programming. The ability to move the patient's body in lateral rotation can also be programmed with vibratory movements that allow biomechanical stresses but may increase the efficiency of any drainages on the patient.

Referring to structure design as in Fig. 2, the traditional frame of hospital beds can be adjusted with segmentations that allow patient mobility with solutions that limit dimensions and overall weight. The mechanical design of robotic beds will size also the servo-actuators and the mechanisms that are connected to them in order to determine the movement of the segments with configurations without additional risks for the patient and assisting medical operators. Aspects linked to sanitary cleaning and sanitation of the entire structure are stringent requirements according to medical sanitation protocols. The power consumption for the bed structure with its sensors and interfaces should be limited to respect the interference constraints (such as for example, as of primary interest, in electromagnetic fields) with medical equipment and even on the patient's condition.

As indicated in Fig. 2 particular attention should be addressed to sensors for regulating robotic operation of the bed and monitoring the effects of the bed movements on the patient health condition. Therefore, for the controlled operation typical sensors can be considered such as IMUs and force sensors. Furthermore, on the mobile bed segments and on the mattress sections, medical-type sensors can be installed to monitor the patient's status like for example temperature, blood pressure and any other sensors. EMG sensors can be used for monitoring the benefit of bed movements on the patient's musculoskeletal structure.

The design and functionality of a robotic bed will have also to ensure safety and comfort requirements as prescribed by medical protocols and critical situations as in the case of the COVID-19 pandemic. In addition, to general requirements, it is convenient that a robotic bed should be easily transportable within hospital environments and its functionality can be managed by medical operators and hospital personnel without complications and at limited costs.

3 Design of a Robotized Bed

The proposed design of a robotic bed is reported in the schemes in Figs.3 and 4.

In Fig. 3a), [1, 5, 11], the bed mechanical design is indicated with full bed frame (1), the upper part bed Sect. (2) movable around the joint (6), the bed segments (3) and 4) moveable with respect each other around the joint (5). The movable be segments are equipped with motors with driving mechanism as in the scheme in Fig. 3b).

The primary functionality of lateral rotation as in Fig. 3b) is operated according to the scheme in Fig. 1 so that the patient's torso can be rotated adequately even alternately, with any particular impediment to the patient's immobilization condition. The main design parameters in the driving mechanism are indicated in Fig. 3b) as S linear actuator stroke, F_C linear actuator force, F_{LX} and F_{LY} X and Y components of joint reaction force, T_R joint reaction force with X and Y components, M patient mass.

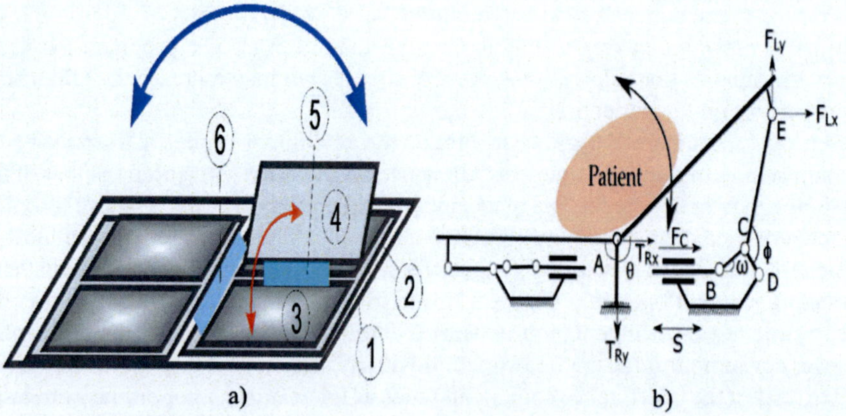

Fig. 3. A conceptual design of a bed structure for bedridden patients: a) the bed structure; b) the driving mechanism of a bed segment

Motor control system can be designed with a proper PI algorithm according to the conceptual design in Fig. 4 using sensors in bed segments and patient body for bed motion and medical monitoring with central role of the control unit. Considering the proposed robotized hospital bed with two upper-part segments, movements can be carried out to allow the mobilization of a bedridden patient as controlled by sensors with data from the patient, the segments of the bed, the mechanism and the actuators. A PI control can be conveniently used to operate the slow motion of a bed segment with its proper positioning.

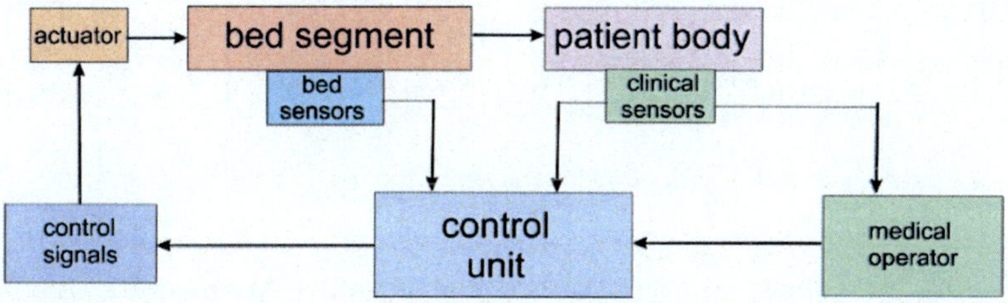

Fig. 4. A conceptual design of a robotic bed design for bedridden patients

4 Operation of a Robotized Bed

Figure 5 summarizes aspects of the functionality of the robotized in terms of operation aims and effects through the motion and force aspects in the bed segment movements with design and operation features matching with requirements as in Fig. 2. Particular attention is focused on the synergic implementation and mechanical design of the structure to ensure motion and load capacity within the expected ranges, considering that the mechanical structure with actuation and medical equipment influence each other.

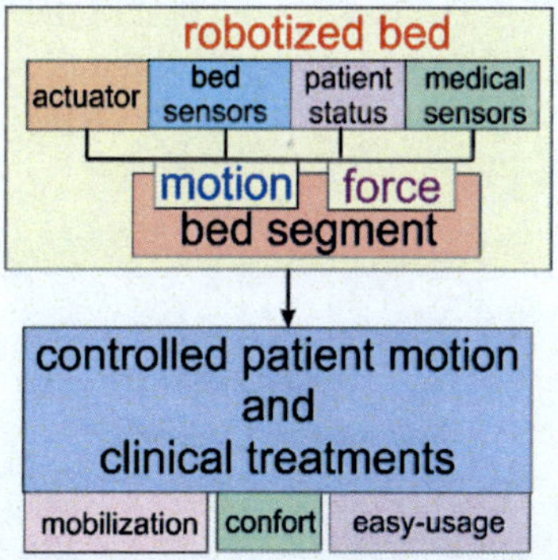

Fig. 5. Operation of the designed robotic bed for bedridden patients

Figure 6 shows the structure of a control unit for the driving mechanism of a bed segment in Fig. 4 when a suitable PI controlled operation is planned in terms of speed and position also considering the medical sensors. The design layout in Fig. 6 is conceived in modular way with components in software and hardware that are designed for an easy installation and maintenance in order to preserve the compact user-oriented design of the segmented hospital bed in Fig. 3 with operation features summarized in Fig. 4.

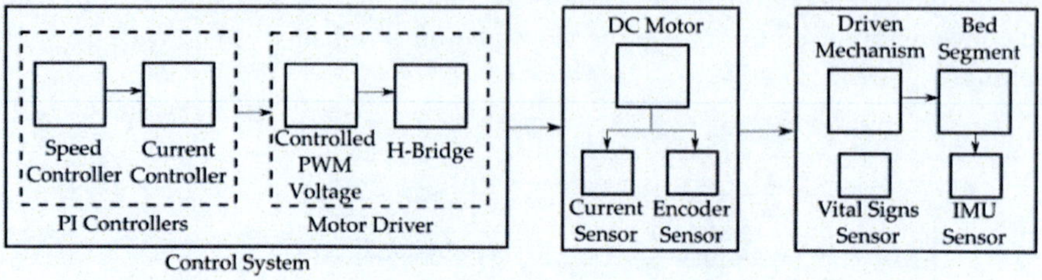

Fig. 6. Control design of the operation of the designed robotic bed

The driving mechanism in Fig. 3 b) is designed in a CAD model as reported in Fig. 7. The performance analysis of the robotized hospital bed has been as reported in the snapshot of Fig. 7 by considering three different modes of functioning, namely without any additional mass (empty bed without a patient); with a limited mass of 10 kg, representing a child or young patient; with a mass of 40 kg, representing an adult. The computed results in Fig. 8 are expressed in terms of motor stroke, Fig. 8a) and angular velocity of the bed segment, Fig. 8 b), as a characterization of the motion operation in numerical and quality aspects as obtained using the PI control in the bed movements for the goals in Figs. 5 and 6. The obtained controlled motion is smooth as per the smooth action of the linear actuator, giving a smooth regular motion of the bed segment, although a small irregularity in the continuity of the angular velocity in correspondence of the inversion of the motion towards the home horizontal position. The motor stroke is limited to 4.1 cm with an angular velocity of the bed segment reaching the maximum of 0.4 deg/s, that can be considered a very comfortable value for the patient in the bed, with an operation duration of 8 s. The motor actuation of the bed segment with no load requires less than 5 A while the case with 40 kg load requires almost 6 A. Considering the case of the simultaneous actuation of the two bed segments, the whole bed system requires 12 A of power supply current.

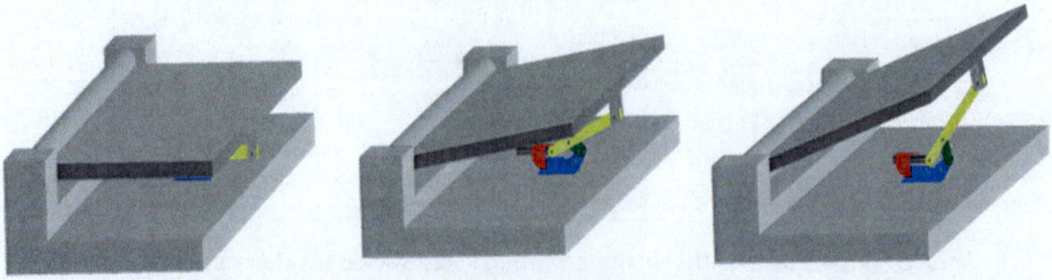

Fig. 7. A simulation of the operation of the designed robotic bed

In summary, the control design with its fairly simple design structure of PI controller cane be considered suitable and well proportionated to the segment bed design with the main aspects in compact fairly easy user-oriented system that permits also the respect of safety and sterilization conditions as in hospital frames.

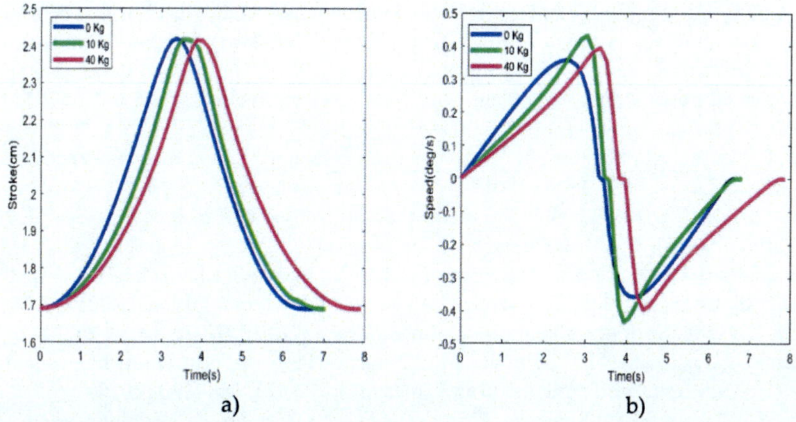

Fig. 8. Computed results of the simulation in Fig. 7 in terms of: a) actuator stroke; b) angular velocity of the segment bed

5 Conclusions

The analysis of the conditions and effects of a long bed rest allows to identify requirements for a fairly easy improvement of current hospital-type beds for patients who may suffer from pulmonary complications and pressure ulcers. Adequate mobility can improve and minimize these effects even to avoid them and therefore a solution has been designed that allows adequate mobility of bedridden patients with a robotic solution that is also designed for a bed control by healthcare professionals in a programmed and remote form. The proposed solution can be particularly convenient in the treatment of COVID patients in intensive care units as outlined by examining the functionality and design characteristics of the proposed robotic bed.

References

1. Ceccarelli, M., Sarmati, L., Ambrogi, V.: A robotized hospital bed for COVID-19 patients in intensive care treatments. In: 2021 IEEE International Conference on Automation/XXIV Congress of the Chilean Association of Automatic Control (ICA-ACCA), pp. 1–6 (2021). https://doi.org/10.1109/ICAACCA51523.2021.9465310
2. Fortney, S.M., Schneider, V.S., Greenleaf, J.E.: The physiology of bed rest. In: Handbook of Physiology. vol. 2, pp. 889-939. Oxford University Press, New York (1996)
3. Moghadam, V.D., Shafiee, H., Ghorbani, M., Heidarifar, R.: Prone positioning in management of COVID-19 hospitalized patients. Braz. J. Anesthesiol. **70**(2), 188–190 (2020)

4. Guérin, C.: Prone Position. Acute Respiratory Distress Syndrome, pp. 73–83. Springer, Cham (2017)
5. Ceccarelli, M.: Bed with moving part, patent nIT102020000014263, Italy (2020)
6. Shih-Wei, P., Feng-Li, L., Li-Chen, F.: Mechanism design and mechatronic control of a multifunctional test bed for bedridden healthcare. IEEE/ASME Trans. Mechatron. **15**, 234–241 (2010)
7. Atasoy, N.A., Çavuşoğlu, A., Atasoy, F.: Real-Time motorized electrical hospital bed control with eye-gaze tracking. Turkish J. Electr. Eng. Comput. Sci. **24**(6), 5162–5172 (2016)
8. Kajol, H., Junaid, S., Jain, S., Chaudhary, A., Prajwal, K.T.: Design and development of a voice actuated hospital bed for patient care. Int. J. Recent Technol. Eng. **8**(4), 1751–1757 (2019)
9. Ghersi, I., Mariño, M., Miralles, M.: Smart medical beds in patient-care environments. BMC Med. Inform. Decis. Mak. **18**, 63 (2018)
10. Rithalia, S., Kenney, L.: Hospital bed mattresses: an overview of technical aspects. J. Med. Eng. Technol. **24**(1), 32–39 (2000)
11. Araque Isidro, J.E., Ceccarelli, M.: Driving mechanism in robotized hospital bed for patients with COVID 19. In: Zeghloul, S., Laribi, M.A., Arsicault, M. (eds.) MEDER 2021. MMS, vol. 103, pp. 179–186. Springer, Cham (2021). https://doi.org/10.1007/978-3-030-75271-2_19
12. Moghadam, V.D., Shafiee, H., Ghorbani, M., Heidarifar, R.: Prone positioning in management of COVID-19 hospitalized patients. Braz J Anesthesiol. **70**(2), 188–190 (2020)
13. Joshua, S., Mervis, M.D., Tania, J., Phillips, M.D.: Pressure ulcers: pathophysiology, epidemiology, risk factors, and presentation. J. Am. Acad. Dermatol. **81**(4), 881–890 (2019). https://doi.org/10.1016/j.jaad.2018.12.069

Design of a Medical Robot with Folding Mechanism Used for Disinfection in the Hard-to-Reach Areas

Elida-Gabriela Tulcan(✉), Carmen Sticlaru, and Erwin-Christian Lovasz

Polytechnic University of Timişoara, 300006 Timişoara, Romania
elida.tulcan@student.upt.ro, {carmen.sticlaru, erwin.lovasz}@upt.ro

Abstract. The paper presents a design of a medical robot used for disinfection in the hard-to-reach areas from the medical environment and other facilities. The robot uses UV light with wavelengths between 200 nm and 280 nm, because of its germicidal properties, to inactivate microorganisms from all kind of surfaces. Its folding mechanism, a four-bar linkage, allows it to be used in different configurations. Its extended position (maximum position) ensures the disinfection of drawers, nightstands, bed rails, bed frames and other small furniture pieces, while its folded position (minimum position) ensures the disinfection of both the hard-to-reach areas, such as the area under the hospital beds and other furniture, and the floors, which cannot be performed with the currently available disinfection robots.

Keywords: medical robots · folding mechanisms · disinfection · mobile robots

1 Introduction

Service robots have been developed with the main purpose of assisting humans in performing tasks that are usually dangerous or repetitive.

They can be classified in three categories [1]:

- Professional robots – used in commercial activities, for example: cleaning robots, delivery robots and medical robots;
- Domestic robots – used in household, for example: robot vacuums, robot lawn mowers, window cleaner robots and pool cleaner robots;
- Personal robots – for personal use, for example: educational robots, entertainment robots and humanoid robots.

Lately, there has been an increasing interest in using disinfection robots by different public institutions, such as hospitals, hotels and airports. This is also because disinfection robots make the disinfection process faster and more efficient [2]. Still, they cannot yet replace manual cleaning, only complement it [3]. Disinfection robots use UV-C light

D. Tarnita et al. (Eds.): MESROB 2023, MMS 133, pp. 351–359, 2023.
https://doi.org/10.1007/978-3-031-32446-8_38

(ultraviolet light with wavelength range from 200nm to 280nm) for its germicidal properties to perform surface, air and water disinfection, mostly in medical facilities. Since the whole process doesn't require the usage of any chemical substances, it's considered to be eco-friendly.

According to the CDC (Centers for Disease Control and Prevention), disinfection describes a process that eliminates many or all pathogenic microorganisms on inanimate objects [4]. Basically, UV-C light destroys cells by damaging their DNA, since the exposure to the radiation at certain wavelengths modifies the genetic material of microorganisms and destroys their ability to reproduce [5]. Each nosocomial pathogen has a different persistence time on surfaces. For example, most gram-positive bacteria survive for months on dry surfaces, most viruses from the respiratory tract survive for days, while herpes viruses persist from only a few hours up to seven days [6].

Air disinfection is performed using UV-C lamps in ceiling fixtures or HVAC systems to clean circulating air continuously. It's important to mention that the lamps have shields so that the radiation is only directed upwards and that they are far enough from the ground, in order not to harm people.

Surface disinfection is performed using UV-C light to kill pathogens on any objects or medical equipment, while no one is in the room. The water disinfection is the simplest process, as a UV-C lighting unit is placed in the water [7].

Some examples of UV-C disinfection robots were presented by Zaman et al. in [8]. The Xenex robot uses pulsed xenon UV light for disinfection and has a size of 760 x 510 x 970 mm, while SIFROBOT is an autonomous robot and has a size of 410 x 410 x 1350 mm, which allows it to operate in tight spaces. Their own design, UVC-PURGE, has a small form factor and real time camera feedback which makes it easy to navigate in congested places. Ruan et al. in [9] designed an autonomous indoor disinfection robot, while they verified the effectiveness of the developed robot in different environments, such as hospitals, hotels, offices, and laboratories. Lastly, an interesting solution was provided in [10], a mobile disinfection robot with folding mechanism, that can also be used in the hard-to-reach areas from the medical facilities (Fig. 1). The seven-bar linkage also has a large height variation, increasing more than three times from the folded position to the extended position and allows the optimal location of four UV-C lighting systems that emit light in all directions in order to ensure the optimal disinfection process.

The state of the art pointed out that the currently available disinfection robots don't have a folding mechanism structure and were not designed to ensure the disinfection of the areas where the space is limited, narrow or tight, but have the advantages of having a compact base size and disinfecting a relatively large area at once. This paper, together with [10], is part of a series of research papers where we study different elementary and simple mechanisms, in order to design a medical disinfection robot with folding mechanism, that has a compact size and a height variation between the folded and the extended position as high as possible, for an overall better disinfection process of the hard-to-reach areas.

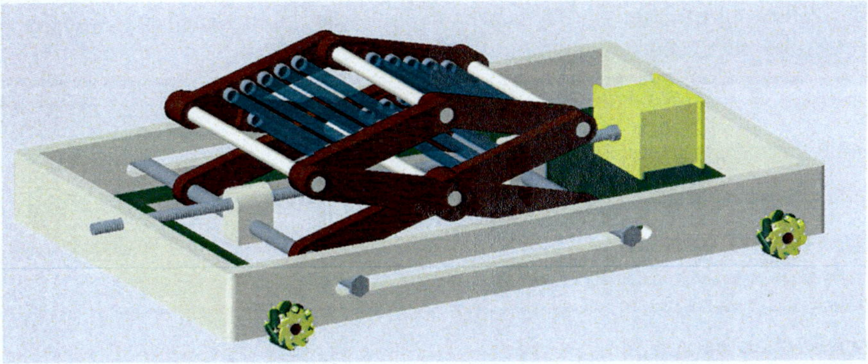

Fig. 1. Disinfection robot with folding mechanism [10]

2 Analysis of the Mechanism

Considering the points previously mentioned, the proposed folding mechanism structure is a four-bar linkage, a modified in-line slider-crank, which is presented in Fig. 2.

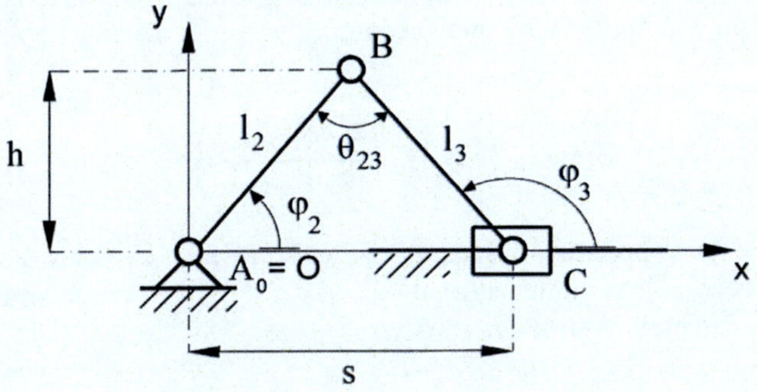

Fig. 2. Kinematic scheme of the mechanism

The height of the robot is represented by h, the drive stroke is represented by s, the lengths of the elements are represented by l, the passive angles are represented by φ_2 and φ_3, while the input transmission angle is represented by θ_{23}.

There are two extreme positions of the folding mechanism:

- extended, where φ_2 and h have the maximum value whereas φ_3, θ_{23} and s have the minimum value;
- folded, where φ_3, θ_{23} and s have the maximum value whereas φ_2 and h have the minimum value.

The following equations were used to compute the input transmission angle, the current stroke and the current height of the mechanism:

$$\theta_{23} = \varphi_3 - \varphi_2 \tag{1}$$

$$s = \sqrt{{l_2}^2 + {l_3}^2 - 2 \cdot l_2 \cdot l_3 \cdot cos(\theta_{23})} \tag{2}$$

$$h(s) = \frac{2 \cdot \sqrt{p(s) \cdot (p(s) - s) \cdot (p(s) - l_2) \cdot (p(s) - l_3)}}{s} \tag{3}$$

where the following notation was used:

$$p(s) = \frac{s + l_2 + l_3}{2} \tag{4}$$

In order to compute the passive angles φ_2 and φ_3, it is necessary to write the vectorial equation for the mechanism, in complex numbers:

$$s = l_2 \cdot e^{i \cdot \varphi_2} - l_3 \cdot e^{i \cdot \varphi_3} \tag{5}$$

By separating the term which contains the angle φ_3 in Eq. (5), writing its complex conjugate equation and multiplying them accordingly results the angle φ_2 as a function of stroke s:

$$\varphi_2(s) = arccos\left(\frac{s^2 + {l_2}^2 - {l_3}^2}{2 \cdot s \cdot l_2}\right) \tag{6}$$

Repeating the same process, by separating the term which contains the angle φ_2 in Eq. (5), writing its complex conjugate equation and multiplying them accordingly results the angle φ_3 as a function of stroke s:

$$\varphi_3(s) = arccos\left(\frac{-s^2 + {l_2}^2 - {l_3}^2}{2 \cdot s \cdot l_3}\right) \tag{7}$$

3 Design of the Robot

Due to functional and design requirements, the lengths of the elements were chosen to be equal $l_2 = l_3 = 300$ mm, while the input transmission angle θ_{23} was chosen to range between 70° and 160° in order to ensure the non-blocking movement of the mechanism.

Figure 3 and Fig. 4 present the variation of the passive angles φ_2 and φ_3 as a dependency of the stroke s. As it can be observed, angle φ_2 decreases while stroke s increases, whereas angle φ_3 increases together with stroke s.

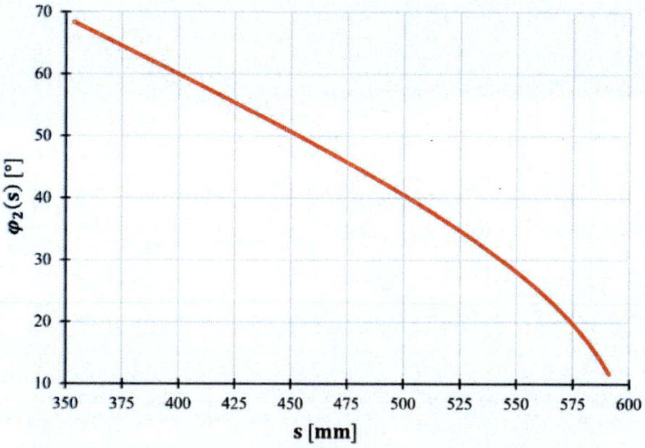

Fig. 3. Variation of the passive angle $\varphi_2(s)$

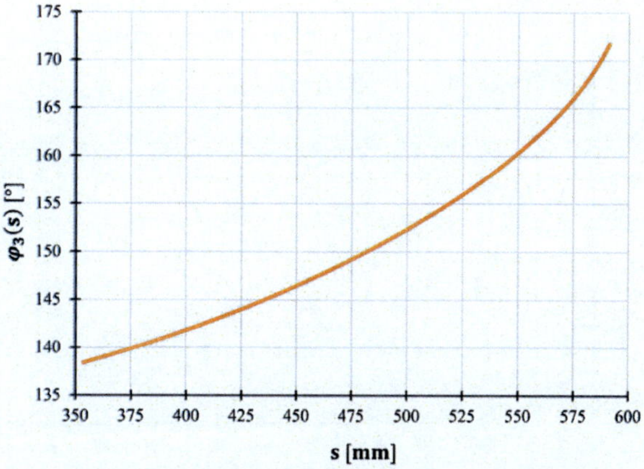

Fig. 4. Variation of the passive angle $\varphi_3(s)$

Figure 5 and Fig. 6 present the variation of angle θ_{23} and height h as a dependency of the stroke s. As it can be seen, angle θ_{23} increases together with stroke s, whereas height h decreases while stroke s increases.

Figure 7 shows the folding mechanism of the robot in the extended position. In this position φ_2 and h have the maximum value, whereas φ_3, θ_{23} and s have the minimum value. This configuration is mainly intended to be used for vertical surfaces and corners, nightstands, drawers, bed rails, bed frames and other small furniture pieces, since the shape of the mechanism's position ensures an optimal disinfection process for the mentioned areas. Values of the parameters related to the extended position of the mechanism are presented in Table 1.

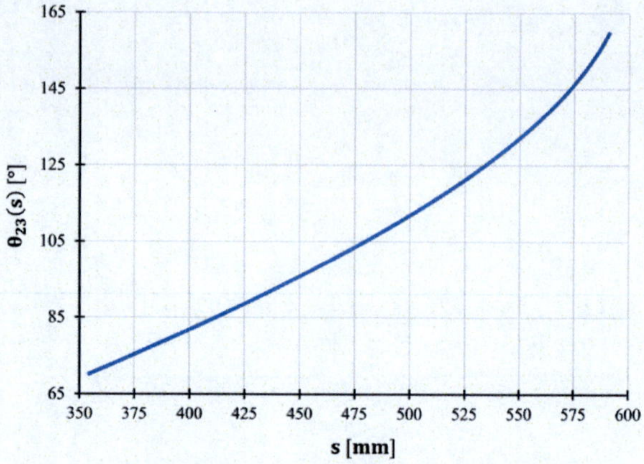

Fig. 5. Variation of the input transmission angle $\theta_{23}(s)$

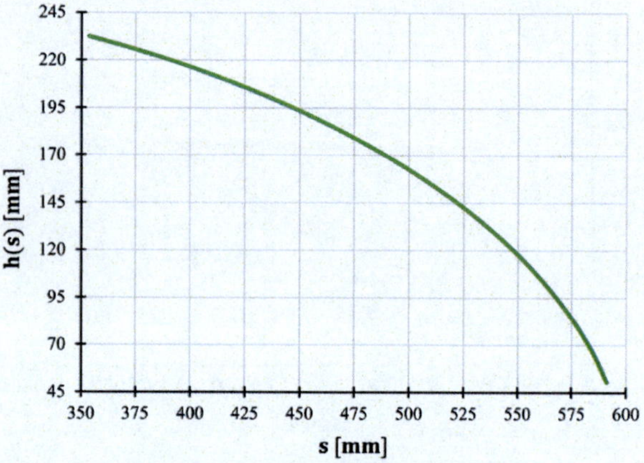

Fig. 6. Variation of the height h(s)

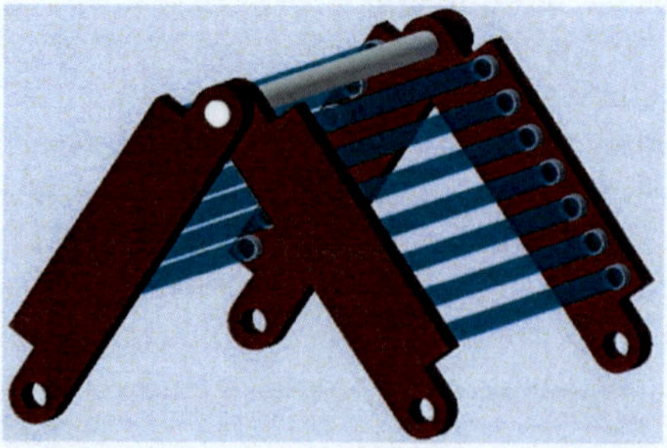

Fig. 7. Robot's mechanism – Extended position

Table 1. Reference values of the parameters – Extended position

Parameter	Value
φ_{2max}	68,3°
φ_{3min}	138,3°
θ_{23min}	70°
h_{max}	232,4 mm
s_{min}	353,7 mm

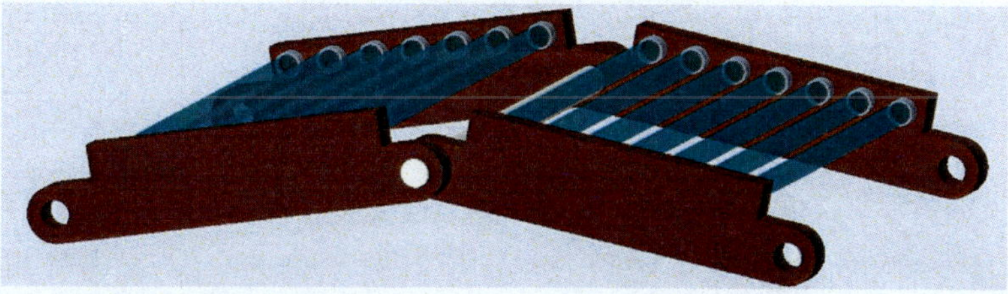

Fig. 8. Robot's mechanism – Folded position

Figure 8 shows the folding mechanism of the robot in the folded position. In this position φ_3, θ_{23} and *s* have the maximum value, while φ_2 and *h* have the minimum value. This configuration is intended to be used in the hard-to-reach areas or areas where the space is small or narrow, such as the areas under the hospital beds and other furniture, which are known as reservoirs of infection. Also, this position is optimal to be used for the floors disinfection, since the maximum stroke s_{max} is almost 600 mm, it can disinfect a large area at a time, therefore maximizing the efficiency of the disinfection process. Values of the parameters related to the folded position of the mechanism are presented in Table 2.

Table 2. Reference values of the parameters – Folded position

Parameter	Value
φ_{2min}	11,6°
φ_{3max}	171,6°
θ_{23max}	160°
h_{min}	50,6 mm
s_{max}	591,1 mm

Figure 9 shows the design of the medical disinfection robot. The disinfection robot uses two UV-C lighting systems, placed on the coupler and the crank of the slider-crank, that emit light in all directions, in order to ensure the optimal disinfection process. The robot is actuated by an electric motor through a ball screw transmission and its mobile platform is equipped with four mecanum wheels, independently actuated by their own motor, thus being separately controlled, in order to allow the omnidirectional movement. The compact size of the mobile platform of 850 × 650 × 60 mm allows the navigation of the robot in small and tight spaces that need to be disinfected, while the two designed guides ensure the stability of the mechanism during the robot's operation. Additionally, a large part of the bottom mobile platform was cut in order to ensure the disinfection of the floor in any current position of the medical robot.

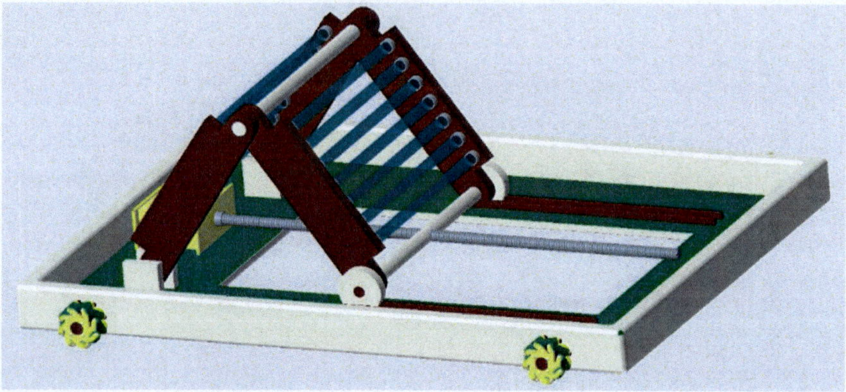

Fig. 9. Design of the medical disinfection robot

4 Conclusions

The presented design of a medical disinfection robot with folding mechanism represents a solution for disinfecting the hard-to-reach areas and floors. Its folding mechanism allows two main configurations, with several in between, for a better disinfection process. The mobile platform has mecanum wheels, for a better maneuverability and navigation in small spaces. The main advantage of this disinfection robot is that it has a simple mechanism and it's easy to maneuver in small and narrow spaces. It also allows a large variation of the folding mechanism's height, with an increase of more than four times from the folded position to the extended position. The height of the robot in the extended position could be increased, but that would also mean increasing its size, since the drive stroke would also then substantially increase.

Further studies will be performed in order to establish the optimal folding mechanism structure for the disinfection robot. We have already designed another disinfection robot with a folding mechanism, a seven-bar linkage known as the scissor jack mechanism [10]. Also, other folding mechanisms structures will be considered for studies and validation purposes and tests will be performed to determine the optimal UV-C dose, exposure time, mechanism position and distance between the robot and the exposed surfaces, in order to ensure the efficiency of the disinfection process.

References

1. Lovasz, E.-C., Rădulescu, C., Moldovan, C.-E.: Roboți de prestări de servicii (Service Robotics), vol. 2, Editura Politehnica, Timişoara (2020)
2. Mehta, I., Hsueh, H-Y., Taghipour, S., Li, W., Saeedi, S.: UV disinfection robots: a review. Robot. Autonom. Syst. **161**, 104332 (2023)
3. Diab-El, S.M., et al.: Ultraviolet disinfection robots to improve hospital cleaning: real promise or just a gimmick? Antimicrob. Resist. Infect. Control **10**, 33 (2021)
4. What is UV-C Disinfection Lighting: The Basics, https://www.stouchlighting.com/faqs-about-uv-disinfection-lighting-the-basics. Accessed 06 Jan 2023
5. Lindblad, M., Tano, E., Lindahl, C., Huss, F.: Ultraviolet-C decontamination of a hospital room: amount of UV light needed. Burns **46**(4), 842–849 (2020)
6. Kramer, A., Schwebke, I., Kampf, G.: How long do nosocomial pathogens persist on inanimate surfaces? A systematic review. BMC Infect. Dis. **6**, 130 (2006)
7. Kesavan, J.S., Sagripanti, J.-L.: Disinfection of airborne organisms by ultraviolet-c radiation and sunlight. In: Aerosol Science: Technology and Applications, pp. 417–439 (2014)
8. Zaman, A., et al.: UVC-PURGE: a novel cost-effective disinfection robot for combating COVID-19 pandemic. IEEE Access **10**, 37613–37634 (2022)
9. Ruan, K., Wu, Z., Xu, Q.: Smart Cleaner: a new autonomous indoor disinfection robot for combating the COVID-19 pandemic. Robotics **10**, 87 (2021)
10. Tulcan, E.-G., Sticlaru, C., Lovasz, E.-C., Gruescu, C.M., Sandu, M.O.: Design of a Folding Mechanism for a Mobile Robot used for Medical Disinfection. Facta Universitatis, Series, Mechanical Engineering (2023). [submitted for publication]

Anthropomorphic Hands

Patient Tailored Hand Exoskeletons - A 3D-Printable Concept for Force Transmission and Feedback

Mateus Enzenberg, Simon Winkler(✉), and Yeongmi Kim

MCI, University of Applied Science, Innsbruck, Austria
{mateus.enzenberg,simon.winkler,yeongmi.kim}@mci.edu

Abstract. A hand exoskeleton can assist motor function of a hand. However, bulky design and misalignment of the hand due to the variation of the hand sizes are the limiting factors. In this paper, we present a printable patient-tailored hand exoskeleton based on parameters derived from 3D scanning the hand. Forces on each link of the finger are measured to detect user intention and allow to trigger extension or flexion motion of the exoskeleton. With the compact design, a range of motion of 90°, 90° and 53° are obtained for Meta Carpophalangeal, Proximal Interphalangeal and Distal Interphalangeal joint respectively. The results showed that the novel linkage design and customization process allows building a hand exoskeleton with individually controllable fingers and sufficient force output while being within the weight requirements.

Keywords: Exoskeleton · rehabilitation · assistance · bio-mechanics · 3D-printing · robotics · activities of daily living

1 Introduction

Impairments of the upper limbs lead to difficulty in performing various activities of daily living (ADL). Motor deficits on the distal arm, such as flexion and extension of the fingers, are found to be more significant than the proximal ones [1]. Without training or assistance, patients may stop using the affected body parts which result in a behaviour referred to as *learned nonuse* [2]. Rehabilitation after stroke is traditionally done in form of guided therapy sessions and by using training devices to perform repetitive exercises [3]. It is therefore required to both train patients effectively and to assist their movements during daily living. While manual therapy and assistance by medical professionals requires substantial time and workload, a wearable robotic device can perform the task in an automated way. The complexity and variability of the human hand render development of such systems difficult, limiting their degrees of freedom (DOF) and range of motion (ROM) in terms of designing wearable hand robotic device [4].

Also, to reduce size, weight, and other design parameters, the number of DOFs of exoskeletons may be limited. This reduces complexity and introduces under-actuated joints, deviating from the original hand functionality. Each active joint requires an individual actuator, adding weight to the system. Some devices

D. Tarnita et al. (Eds.): MESROB 2023, MMS 133, pp. 363–370, 2023.
https://doi.org/10.1007/978-3-031-32446-8_39

found in the literature actuate multiple fingers with one actuator to reduce the number of actuators [5]. Other devices keep the proximal parts of the device lightweight by introducing a secondary part worn on the patient's waist or other remote parts of the body [6]. The distal parts of the hand provide little space for actuator and mechanism placement, requiring a space-efficient way of transmitting the forces to the desired endpoints. There are six commonly used types of mechanical finger linkage designs [7]. Most devices utilize redundant and tendon-driven mechanisms. Both the matched axis as well as the tendon driven mechanism rely on both the inner and the outer side of the hand to function, which is found undesirable for patients [8]. Some devices utilize the back and side parts of the finger while leaving the front surface unobstructed [9,10]. This may interfere with movements of the Meta Carpophalangeal (MCP) joint because it is not possible to get access to the required axis from the side of the fingers [9].

The remote center of motion (RCM) requires the highest number of individual components to function but enables a defined motion without interfering with the front side of the hand. An alternative way of achieving this defined movement is by implementing sliders into the design as it has been implemented in previous work [10,11]. Both base-to-distal, as well as the joint-less structure, provide little guidance to the finger's movements. The joint-less structure is found to be the lightest design on average [7]. A mixture of mechanisms on the same finger to match desired requirements may also be achieved [10]. As the anatomical parameters vary, the device has to be adaptable or customizable to ensure a match between the designed movement axes and the ones that are given [12]. This is increasingly difficult for hand exoskeletons compared to elbow and shoulder exoskeletons, due to the higher DOFs and limited space [13]. In order to overcome the shortcomings of the current designs, we present a novel design of a hand exoskeleton based on a compact variation of the redundant link design and a patient-tailored manufacturing method via 3D scanning of the hand.

2 Methods

2.1 Design Requirements

The design for the active hand exoskeleton is based on both the overall intended use and from data given by expert and patient interviews regarding design requirements [8]. The design shall be used to both assist and train patients suffering from impairments affecting the flexion and extension of the fingers as well as the thumb. It shall be able to actively drive each finger individually. It shall be able to fully open and close the finger. The design should support the fingers in a way that does not obstruct the palm of the hand and remain primarily on the back of the hand. Further, it shall implement sensors to detect the intention of the user for flexion or extension movements. The assembled fingers should not exceed a weight of 300 g combined, with the option to place components on the arm to distribute weight.

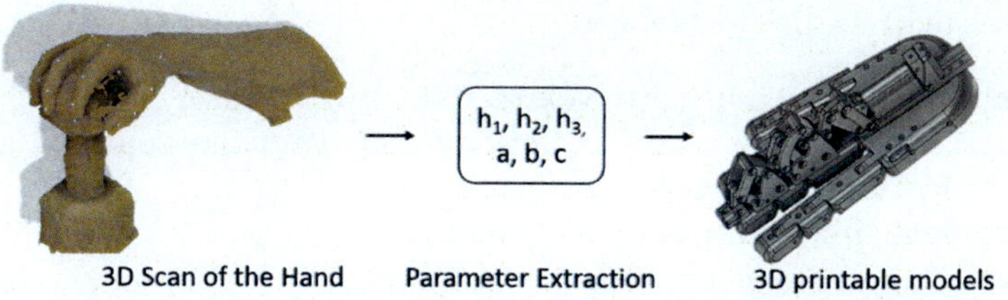

Fig. 1. The customization procedure using a 3D model of the hand with manually set joint surface markers to extract design parameters for the finger links.

2.2 Hand Measurement

To ensure a match between the device and the hand, the first step is to identify lengths and angles of the finger joints with the wrist joint as a common reference. A common way of measuring the ROM of fingers is goniometry [14]. For distances, a linear ruler may be used to measure distances between surface points. This process is rather time intensive. It also relies on the performance of the operator and may be subject to human error. Another way of localizing joints and measuring distances is using 2D imaging of the hand [15]. Using this approach, finger thickness and hand curvature parameters can not be extracted in a single picture. The hand forms a rounded shape during relaxation, which is not the case if it is pushed flat on a surface while taking a picture [16]. The joint markers are set manually by observation of surface features in the picture [15]. In this paper, we utilize photogrammetry to create a 3D model of the hand. This way both depth, as well as curvature and angles of joints, can be extracted by placing markers on the model surface. To minimize marker misplacement, the hand is positioned on a fixed object at a partially closed position to simplify joint location. As shown in Fig. 1, a scan from 200 pictures of the static hand is taken to create the 3D model and extract the design parameters. Using an iPhone 13 pro running *Polycam*, total scanning time is approximately 3 min.

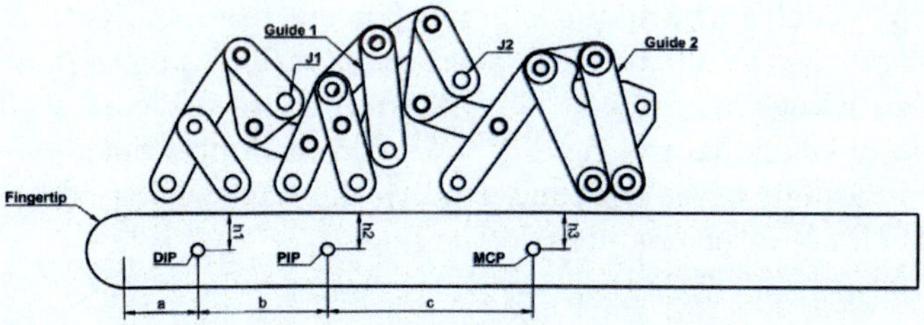

Fig. 2. Guidance joints are added to the redundant linkage design to prevent slipping between the exoskeleton and the hand. The linkage dimensions are based on the parameters a, b, c, h_1, h_2, h_3 derived from the 3D scan.

2.3 Mechanical Linkage Design

The mechanism is designed using the extracted parameters. A redundant linkage design is chosen due to the non-obstructive nature and the guidance added to each joint as illustrated in Fig. 2.

The redundant links are placed to connect each link of the finger. The distance between the joint axis and finger surface sets the height for the link bases by adding minimal room for the link corpus to rotate freely. Link pairs are placed in a way to not interfere with each other. The length of the links sets the range of motion for each joint, thus a minimum length is required to achieve set requirements. The design features additional link bases as this minimizes required link lengths and introduces room for additional components to be placed between each redundant link pair.

To transmit a rotation generated at the MCP joint to both Proximal Interphalangeal (PIP) and Distal Interphalangeal (DIP) joints, additional links are added to the design. For both stages of transmission, a pair of upper and lower links are introduced. The added links are attached to the existing redundant link pairs and to each other by the use of another component rotating around the bases J1 and J2. The lengths of the components are given by the set ROM of the joints. While a healthy DIP joint is capable of rotating 90°, the DIP ROM in the design is reduced to fit the design into the limited space and reduce link lengths. In case of a finger flexion or extension, the lower links create a rotation around J1 and J2, causing the upper links to push or pull on the redundant links, creating secondary rotational forces. The curvature of upper and lower links prevents a collision with other components during movement and a lower overall design. At this stage, the mechanism is capable of transmitting the force along the finger joints up to the distal finger. The RCM itself is achieved by a four-bar linkage driving the redundant joint link. The current design requires a rigid connection between finger links and link bases, commonly achieved by adjustable straps [11]. In reality, a perfectly rigid connection may not be always given due to e.g. a loose mounting of the device by the patient. To add additional guidance to the system similar to the RCM mechanism, additional guidance joints are introduced to the design. The added guides set the angle between redundant link pairs during movement and prohibit the mechanism from slipping in direction of the distal finger parts. As the links overlap at various points in the design, additional design planes are added. This allows links to drive adjacent to each other without interfering. To add rigidity to the design, outer links move in identical pairs. All link joint bases are connected to the finger using additional base components which are later mounted to the finger.

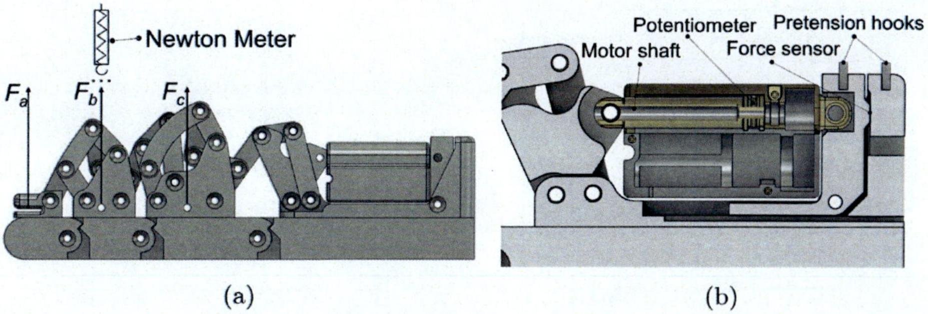

Fig. 3. Test setup. (a) Maximum force measurement at three axes for both flexion. For extension, the hand is flipped. (b) Cross section of the linear motor base with implemented force sensor and offset tension spring. The force sensor is measuring the internal link forces.

2.4 Actuation and Sensing

A motor with an internal position measurement provides a space-efficient solution. To cause the angular displacement, the linear motor (PQ12-P, *Actuonix*) with internal feedback to monitor its stroke length is chosen. To detect user intention, a force sensor is implemented. Due to the rigid finger design, any force applied by the patient on the mechanism is transferred directly to the motor. This enables the placement of a polymer think film force sensitive resister (FSR04CE, Ohmite) at the base of the motor as illustrated in Fig. 3(b). The motor is fixed to an axis that focuses the forces onto the sensor. To measure forces during extension and flexion, an offset is applied to the sensor using a tension spring.

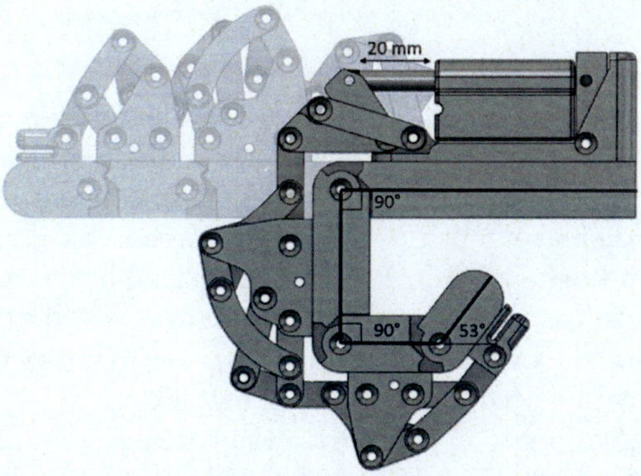

Fig. 4. Achieved ROM of the finger design with a fully extended linear motor.

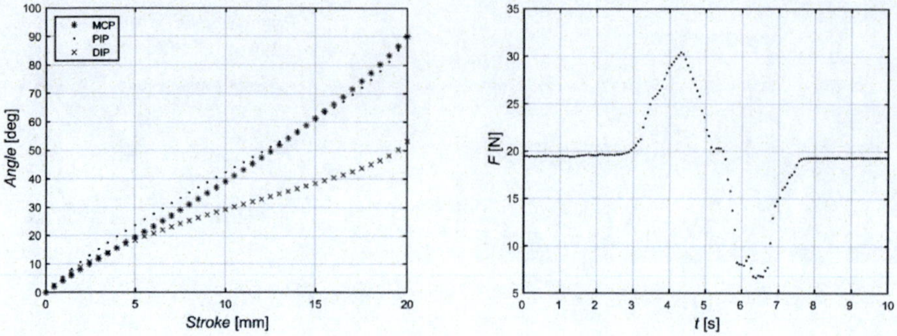

(a) (b)

Fig. 5. Angle and force measurements (a) Angular displacement of finger joints depending on stoke of the linear motor. (b) Force profile of one finger during both an external extension and flexion.

3 Evaluation

3.1 Test Setup

A 3D printed hand model based on the initial measurements is used to fix the designed mechanism. Forces are applied to the individual links of the index finger, perpendicular to the link axes, as seen in Fig. 3(a). An external force is applied until the design is no longer capable of moving on its own, thus marking the maximum force the mechanism can generate. Therefore, a spring-based newton meter is positioned inline with the indicated force axes (F_a, F_b, F_c).

3.2 Results

With a fully extended stroke of the linear motor at 20 mm, the mechanism is capable of closing the finger up to 90° at the MCP joint, 90° at the PIP joint and 53° in the DIP joint, as visualized in Fig. 4. As one motor actuates all three joints of one finger, the joint angles can be calculated using the known stroke length. The angular displacement in each finger joint is plotted over the whole travel of the motor and visualized in Fig. 5(a). External forces are applied to the finger to both simulate extension and flexion intention, and the measurements taken by the force sensor are shown in Fig. 5(b). Between seconds 6 to 10, an extension is applied, while seconds 11 to 15 show flexion.

The maximum link forces of the test setup are $F_a = 11\,\text{N}$, $F_b = 16\,\text{N}$, $F_c = 27\,\text{N}$ for extension and $F_a = 6\,\text{N}$, $F_b = 10\,\text{N}$, $F_c = 22\,\text{N}$ for flexion respectively. All five fingers with no motors attached measure a total weight of 198 g, the five motors together a total of 95 g. Both combined measure 284 g. The design is attached to a real finger using straps and does follow the finger during the flexible motion without adding disturbances. In Fig. 6 the complete assembly of the device in an exemplary use of grasping a spherical object.

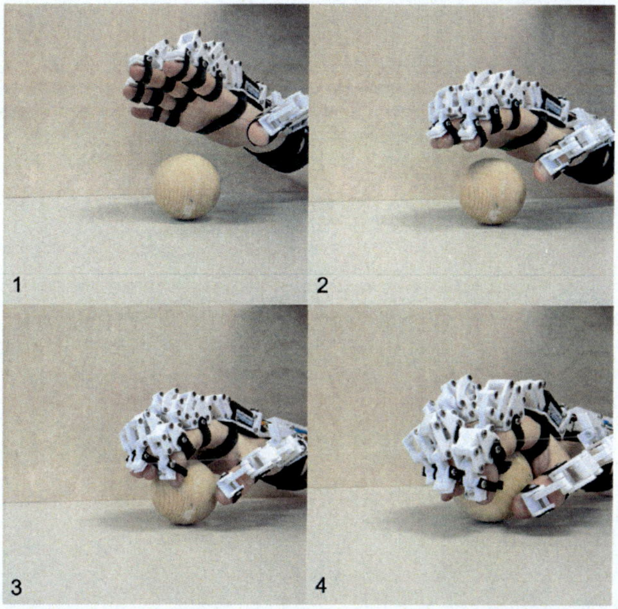

Fig. 6. The fully assembled exoskeleton worn by the hand it has been tailored to, while grasping a spherical object. Velcro straps are used to attach it to the hand.

4 Conclusion

In this paper, a compact and wearable hand exoskeleton is presented. The device is capable of performing extension as well as flexion movements for all finger joints. The design allows each finger and thumb to house a linear motor, creating five actively driven fingers that are controlled individually. With the achieved ROM, the exoskeleton can assist to grasp various objects of different shapes and sizes (e.g. pen, cup). The device was designed to fit a specific hand using a 3D hand model. Embedded force sensors for each finger enable a self-test procedure and the detection of user intention. Results show that the device is capable of applying sufficient forces on each link to enable basic operations such as holding various objects, yet further evaluation is required to test the performance during ADL. The device parts located on the hand weigh below the preferred weight limit of 300 g, with the option to place the rest of the required components on the arm. Due to the compact design, assembly of the finger is rather time intensive. Possible further improvements include a way to simplify the assembling process. While the results show that the developed design fulfils the main requirements, it was done for only this specific hand. Hence, it has to be explored how well the customization and manufacturing procedure works for other hands.

References

1. Lee, S.W., Landers, K.A., Park, H.S.: Development of a biomimetic hand exotendon device (BiomHED) for restoration of functional hand movement post-stroke. IEEE Trans. Neural Syst. Rehabil. Eng. **22**(4), 886–898 (2014)
2. Raghavan, P.: Upper Limb Motor Impairment After Stroke, pp. 599–610 (2015)
3. Dovat, L., et al.: HandCARE: a cable-actuated rehabilitation system to train hand function after stroke. IEEE Trans. Neural Syst. Rehabil. Eng. **16**(6), 582–591 (2008)
4. Ong, A.P.R., Bugtai, N.T.: A bio-inspired design of a hand robotic exoskeleton for rehabilitation. In: AIP Conference Proceedings, vol. 1933 (2018)
5. Troncossi, M., Mazzotti, C., Mozaffari Foumashi, M., Zannoli, D., Parenti-Castelli, V.: Design and manufacturing of a hand-and-wrist exoskeleton prototype for the rehabilitation of post-stroke patients. Quaderni del DIEM-Giornata Ettore Funaioli 1–10 (2012)
6. Polygerinos, P., Wang, Z., Galloway, K.C., Wood, R.J., Walsh, C.J.: Soft robotic glove for combined assistance and at-home rehabilitation. Robot. Auton. Syst. **73**, 135–143 (2015)
7. du Plessis, T., Djouani, K., Oosthuizen, C.: A review of active hand exoskeletons for rehabilitation and assistance. Robotics **10**(1), 40 (2021)
8. Boser, Q.A., Dawson, M.R., Schofield, J.S., Dziwenko, G.Y., Hebert, J.S.: Defining the design requirements for an assistive powered hand exoskeleton: a pilot explorative interview study and case series. Prosthet. Orthot. Int. (2020)
9. Chiri, A., Vitiello, N., Giovacchini, F., Roccella, S., Vecchi, F., Carrozza, M.C.: Mechatronic design and characterization of the index finger module of a hand exoskeleton for post-stroke rehabilitation. IEEE/ASME Trans. Mechatron. **17**(5), 884–894 (2011)
10. Tsai, Y.L., et al.: Usability assessment of a cable-driven exoskeletal robot for hand rehabilitation. Front. Neurorobot. **13**(February), 1–11 (2019)
11. Tong, K.Y., et al.: An intention driven hand functions task training robotic system. In: 2010 Annual International Conference of the IEEE Engineering in Medicine and Biology Society, EMBC 2010, pp. 3406–3409 (2010)
12. Otten, A., Voort, C., Stienen, A., Aarts, R., Van Asseldonk, E., Van Der Kooij, H.: LIMPACT: a hydraulically powered self-aligning upper limb exoskeleton. IEEE/ASME Trans. Mechatron. **20**(5), 2285–2298 (2015)
13. Gull, M.A., Bai, S., Bak, T.: A review on design of upper limb exoskeletons. Robotics **9**(1), 16 (2020)
14. Norkin, C., White, J.: Measurement of Joint Motion: A Guide To Goniometry. F. A. Davis Company (2016)
15. Wang, W.W., et al.: A joint localizer for finger length measurements. In: MeMeA 2013 - IEEE International Symposium on Medical Measurements and Applications, Proceedings, no. July 2014, pp. 111–115 (2013)
16. Fallis, A., Schlünke, M., Schulte, E., Schumacher, U. (ed.): Prometheus - LernAtlas der Anatomie Allgemeine Anatomie und Bewegungssystem, 2nd edn, vol. 53, no. 9. Georg Thieme Verlag, Stuttgart (2013)

Tree-Like Fractal Structures Modeling and Their Application in 3D Printed Bones

Anca Stanciu Birlescu(✉) and Nicolae Balc

Technical University of Cluj-Napoca, 400114 Cluj-Napoca, Romania
{Anca.Stanciu,Nicolae.Balc}@tcm.utcluj.ro

Abstract. Selective Laser Melting manufactured components can be modeled and built with internal structures (such as lattice), and these kinds of components have multiple applications in industry or biomechanics. The paper presents a mathematical model that generates tree-like fractal structures, that are intended as internal structures for Selective Laser Melting components. The mathematical model uses the language of homogeneous transformation matrices, and it is easily scalable (in terms of computing more complex tree-like fractals) due to its recursive nature. Numerical simulations are provided to show examples of fractals modeled with the proposed method. The use of fractals for internal structures is demonstrated on a CAD model of a femur bone.

Keywords: Additive Manufacturing · Fractals · Modeling · Biomechanics

1 Introduction

Additive Manufacturing (AM) represents a large engineering topic that develops rapidly worldwide. This kind of technology offers the possibility to create mechanical parts with complex geometries, and (equally important) manufacture components that use internal structures (e.g. lattice) [1, 2]. Furthermore, AM is still comparable with the classical manufacturing techniques, regarding quality, [3, 4], and offers a wide range of materials that can be used, from plastic to resins, to metals and ceramics and others [1, 3]. Selective Laser Melting (SLM) is a technology that uses metal powder as raw material to create final parts. The powder is evenly distributed on a building platform, then the lasers melts the material where necessary (as the CAD model) then another layer of power is applied, and the steps repeat until all necessary layers to build the part are completed [1]. This process is mostly used in industrial industries (aeronautics, automotive, military etc.) [4–6], but also in medicine, where implants can be easily adapted to the patients needs, here the process is more advantageous because of the shorter manufacturing time and lower material consumption [3, 7].

Fractals are complex mathematical structures that are found in nature. In additive manufacturing, fractals seem to have various applications such as: 1) describing imagines of surfaces of AM manufactured parts to study various properties [4, 8]; 2) developing new laser scan strategies [9]; manufacturing optimized components with tree like structure [10], sponge like structure [11], among others.

D. Tarnita et al. (Eds.): MESROB 2023, MMS 133, pp. 371–378, 2023.
https://doi.org/10.1007/978-3-031-32446-8_40

This article presents a mathematical model for tree-like fractal structures intended for the internal structures of metallic components obtained via SLM. The model uses the language of homogeneous transformation matrices and achieves a generalized description of each node (and branch) of the tree-like fractal structure. The fractals are then used for modeling a femur bone, to illustrate their application in creating nonhomogeneous components with application in biomechanics.

The paper is structured as follows: Sect. 2 presents the mathematical modeling of the tree-like fractal structures (on a plane). Section 3 presents numerical simulations of the mathematical model that generates fractals. Section 4 describes the application of fractals in medicine and in the end, Sect. 5 presents the conclusions.

2 Mathematical Modeling

Fractals are "self-similar scale invariant mathematical entities" and are based on an "iterative function system" [12] and have space filling properties [13]. In this paper tree-like fractals (Fig. 1) are studied, which are composed of branches, nodes (points of intersection of branches), and leaves (the final points of the fractal structure). It is important to note that the proposed tree-like fractal structure is a planar structure (even though the mathematical model is for the 3D Cartesian space).

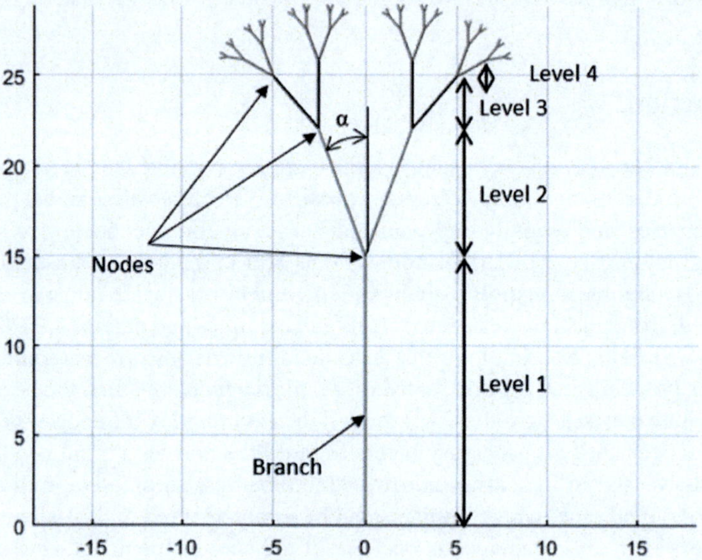

Fig. 1. A tree-like fractal.

For the mathematical modelling of the tree-like fractals the following equation is proposed using the language of homogeneous transformation matrices.

$$M_m = O_m \cdot R_0 \cdot T_1 \cdot R_1 \cdot \ldots \cdot T_{n-1} \cdot R_{n-1} \cdot T_n \tag{1}$$

where M_m represents the mth transformation matrix defining the mth fractal structure. O_m represents the mth origin of the mth fractal structure and has the form:

$$O_m = T_{org} \cdot R_Z \cdot R_Y \cdot R_X \tag{2}$$

with:

$$T_{org} = \begin{pmatrix} 1 & 0 & 0 & 0 \\ T_X & 1 & 0 & 0 \\ T_Y & 0 & 1 & 0 \\ T_Z & 0 & 0 & 1 \end{pmatrix}, R_Z = \begin{pmatrix} 1 & 0 & 0 & 0 \\ 0 & \cos(\alpha_0) & -\sin(\alpha_0) & 0 \\ 0 & \sin(\alpha_0) & cos(\alpha_0) & 0 \\ 0 & 0 & 0 & 1 \end{pmatrix}$$
$$R_Y = \begin{pmatrix} 1 & 0 & 0 & 0 \\ 0 & \cos(\beta_0) & 0 & \sin(\beta_0) \\ 0 & 0 & 1 & 0 \\ 0 & -\sin(\beta_0) & 0 & cos(\beta_0) \end{pmatrix}, R_X = \begin{pmatrix} 1 & 0 & 0 & 0 \\ 0 & 1 & 0 & 0 \\ 0 & 0 & \cos(\gamma_0) & -\sin(\gamma_0) \\ 0 & 0 & \sin(\gamma_0) & cos(\gamma_0) \end{pmatrix} \tag{3}$$

where T_X, T_Y, T_Z are Cartesian components of the origin of the fractal structure and α_0, β_0, γ_0, are the orientation angles of the fractal assuming *Z-Y-X* rotation sequence. Furthermore, the rotation matrices are assumed to be:

$$R_0 = I_4, R_i = \begin{pmatrix} 1 & 0 & 0 & 0 \\ 0 & \cos(\alpha_i) & -\sin(\alpha_i) & 0 \\ 0 & \sin(\alpha_i) & cos(\alpha_i) & 0 \\ 0 & 0 & 0 & 1 \end{pmatrix}, T_j = \begin{pmatrix} 1 & 0 & 0 & 0 \\ 0 & 1 & 0 & 0 \\ L_j & 0 & 1 & 0 \\ 0 & 0 & 0 & 1 \end{pmatrix} \tag{4}$$

where α_i represents the angle orientations for the fractal nodes and T_j describes the lengths of the fractal branches.

To determine the positions of each node and branch the following algorithm was used. First, the terms in Eq. (1) are grouped as following:

$$M_m = O_m \cdot \underline{R_0 \cdot T_1} \cdot \underline{\underline{R_1 \cdot T_2}} \cdot \ldots \tag{5}$$

By assigning:

$$\begin{gathered} node_0 : O_n \\ node_1 : node_0 \cdot R_0 \cdot T_1 \\ \vdots \\ node_n : node_{n-1} \cdot R_{n-1} \cdot T_n \end{gathered} \tag{6}$$

the transformation matrices of each node may be computed recursively from the nth node. To give an example for the transformation matrices computation let's consider a number of fractal nodes of $n = 4$. We start from:

$$\begin{aligned} node_4 &: node_3 \cdot R_3 \cdot T_4 \\ node_3 &: node_2 \cdot R_2 \cdot T_3 \\ node_2 &: node_1 \cdot R_1 \cdot T_2 \\ node_1 &: node_0 \cdot R_0 \cdot T_1 \\ node_0 &: O_n \end{aligned} \tag{7}$$

and we back-substitute each *node* after the numerical values for all angles (at nodes) and lengths (branches) were substituted in their respective transformation matrix.

Another important step in the computation algorithm is to determine the exact number of nodes and branches required for each level of the fractal. To compute this Table 1 is proposed, which generally describes the angle values for every tree-like fractal structure. Each row of the table describes the values of node angles required for a fractal node, or leaf. Leaves are in the right most column in the table (2^{n-1} column) and the root is in the 2^0 column. Furthermore, if the 2^{n-1} column is ignored (when the 2^{n-2} node is in discussion), row 1 and 2 in the table are the same, when the last two columns are ignored, row 1–4 are the same. We can deduce that with each column ignored (focusing form the leaves towards the root), each row becomes identical to the next 2^m rows (m = 0 at the leaves, m = 1 at the last node and so on). This pattern allows for the elimination of redundant computations. Table 1 offers a structured method for the numerical inputs (for the angle values) for the mathematical model described in Eqs. (1) and (7). The coordinates of each node of the fractal structure are extracted from $X = M_m[2]$, $Y = M_m$ [2,3], $Z = M_m$ [2,3], where M_m is the transformation matrix computed with Eqs. (1) and (7).

Table 1. Table of angle values.

	2^0	2^1	…	2^{n-3}	2^{n-2}	2^{n-1}
1	0	$-\alpha_1$	…	$-\alpha_{n-3}$	$-\alpha_{n-2}$	$-\alpha_{n-1}$
2	0	$-\alpha_1$	…	$-\alpha_{n-3}$	$-\alpha_{n-2}$	$+\alpha_{n-1}$
3	0	$-\alpha_1$	…	$-\alpha_{n-3}$	$+\alpha_{n-2}$	$-\alpha_{n-1}$
4	0	$-\alpha_1$	…	$-\alpha_{n-3}$	$+\alpha_{n-2}$	$+\alpha_{n-1}$
5	0	$-\alpha_1$	…	$+\alpha_{n-3}$	$-\alpha_{n-2}$	$-\alpha_{n-1}$
6	0	$-\alpha_1$	…	$+\alpha_{n-3}$	$-\alpha_{n-2}$	$+\alpha_{n-1}$
7	0	$-\alpha_1$	…	$+\alpha_{n-3}$	$+\alpha_{n-2}$	$-\alpha_{n-1}$
8	0	$-\alpha_1$	…	$+\alpha_{n-3}$	$+\alpha_{n-2}$	$+\alpha_{n-1}$
…	0	…	…	…	…	…
n	0	$+\alpha_1$	…	$+\alpha_{n-3}$	$+\alpha_{n-2}$	$+\alpha_{n-1}$

3 Numerical Simulations

As pointed out in Sect. 2, the mathematical model allows different parameters for the length of the branches and the angles between them. Therefore, different configurations of fractals can result. Note that if the angle between two branches is under 30° on all levels, a longer fractal can result, but if the angles is bigger than 30° more surface can be covered. Two examples are presented in Fig. 2a where the angle is 20° Fig. 2b, the angle is 45° on all fractal levels, the length of the first branch is 15 mm, with the rule that on each level, the length is halved. Figure 2c and 2d represent tree-like fractals, where the previous length rule applies, but on each level the angle between two branches differ. So, a fractal can be designed, to have higher height, but still cover more surface, if the angles in the first levels are small, but are getting bigger on the last levels.

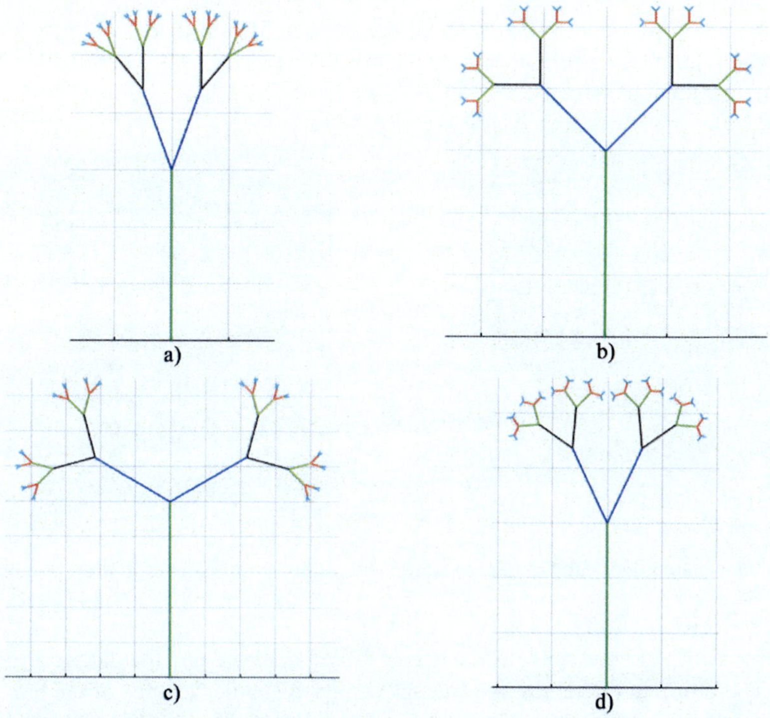

Fig. 2. Fractal configurations for different parameters: a) $l_1 = 15$ mm, $\alpha_1 = 20°$; b) $l_1 = 15$ mm, $\alpha_1 = 45°$; c) $l_1 = 10$ mm, $\alpha_1 = 60°$, $\alpha_2 = 45°$, $\alpha_3 = 30°$, $\alpha_4 = 30°$, $\alpha_5 = 15°$; d) $l_1 = 15$ mm, $\alpha_1 = 25°$, $\alpha_2 = 30°$, $\alpha_3 = 40°$, $\alpha_4 = 60°$, $\alpha_5 = 60°$.

Using the mathematical model, with different lengths and angles, allows to create different porosities or densities with the tree-like fractals, that can be used to create non-homogeneous mechanical parts (or even implants).

4 Application in Biomechanics

As mentioned before, SLM has a big influence not only in industry, but also in the medical area, where different implants or prosthesis can be designed and manufactured. It is showed that the homogenous structures, like lattice structure, that were included in the implants can have good results [14].

With the previous mathematical model, non-homogenous structures can be generated and with help of the Selective Laser Melting technology, these internal structures can be manufactured to be used in the medical field, using a variety of biocompatible materials.

To describe one possible application of the fractals, that can be generated by the mathematical model, the lower part of the femur bone (lateral condyle, medial condyle, and patellar surface) was filled with different configurations of tree-like fractals. A CAD representation of the femur bone and the tree like fractals, that creates different densities and porosities are presented in Fig. 3.

A main fractal was put in the center of the bone and from there, multiple smaller fractals were distributed, where necessary. Figure 3a shows the transparent hollow bone with the included net of fractals.

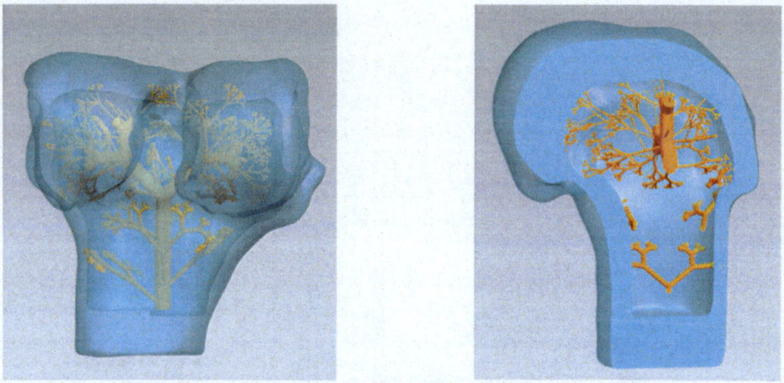

a) b)

Fig. 3. Femur bone filled with fractals: a) front view of the bone; b) net of fractals in section.

Some areas of the bone may need a denser filling, like the one that lattice structure can give. Therefore, in that areas, the fractals can have smaller lengths of the branches and can be more dens than in the base of the bone. Figure 3b shows a sections of the bone, where also the non-homogenous structure is represented, but also the different density levels in the areas of the bone.

In Table 2 some fractals parameters are defined including their origin, branches lengths and angles, and Fig. 4 highlights these tree-like fractals. For this example of application, the whole fractal net was designed manually, but for future work, with help of the mathematical model, the net will be generated automatically, only with the inputs of lengths, angles and strut diameters of the branches.

Table 2. Example of fractal parameters for 3D printed bone.

	O [mm]	V*	L_i [mm]	α_i [°]
1	X = 100.73, Y = −285.65, Z = −107.92	[0, −0.5, −0.87]	$L_1 = 12$	$\alpha_1 = 30$
2	X = 104.35, Y = −294.61, Z = −151.64	[−0.56, 0.82, 0.08]	$L_1 = 10$	$\alpha_1 = 30$
3	X = 129.95, Y = −301.95, Z = −141.14	[−0.91, −0.26, 0.33]	$L_1 = 7$	$\alpha_1 = 40$

*V is an orientation vector computed using Eq. (2)

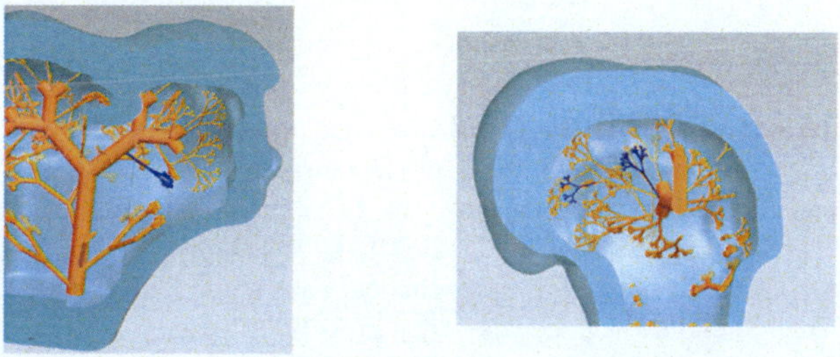

Fig. 4. Femur bone filled with fractals. The fractals modeled with the parameters from Table 2 are highlighted in blue.

5 Conclusions

The use of fractal geometry in additive manufacturing is not a novel approach, and multiple authors showed different applications for fractals. The paper focuses on developing a mathematical model for tree-like fractal structures, which are intended to build (non-homogeneous) metal components with internals structures using SLM technology. The mathematical model uses the language of homogeneous transformation matrices which makes it easy to compute numerically, and due to its recursive approach, it is easily scalable (to compute multiple levels of nodes) especially with vector programing paradigms such as Matlab.

As a first development stage in producing mechanical components with fractal internal structures (this approach was demonstrated in this paper on a femur bone), the model fully describes the proposed tree-like fractal structure in Cartesian coordinates, which can be used in automating the generation of internal structures to produce non-homogeneous components. Further work is intended for extending the model in 3 dimensions (as the tree-like fractals are plane structures at the moment), automatization of the fractal generation as internal structures of components, and most importantly testing the components in laboratory conditions (mostly mechanical tests) to determine various properties which in turn validates the use of tree-like fractals as internal structures for SLM manufactured components. Furthermore, a FEA comparison between fractals and lattice structures will be done to show differences in stiffness and strength, and also printing conditions and times will be analyzed.

Acknowledgement. This work was supported by the project POCU/380/6/13/123927–ANTRE-DOC, "Entrepreneurial competencies and excellence research in doctoral and postdoctoral studies programs", a project co-funded by the European Social Fund through the Human Capital Operationa. Furthermore, the infrastructure available from the European Development Fund and the Romanian Government through the Competitiveness Operational Programme 2014–2020, project ID P 34 466, MySMIS code 121349, contract no.5/05.06.2018 is highly acknowledged. The research was also supported by the DiCoMI Horizon 2020 project (778068—Directional Composites through Manufacturing Innovation).

References

1. Gebhardt, A., Kessler, J., Thurn, L.: 3D-Drucken: Grundlagen und Anwendungen des Additive Manufacturing. Carl Hanser Verlag GmbH Co KG, Germany (2016)
2. Alomar, Z., Concli, F.: A review of the selective laser melting lattice structures and their numerical models. Adv. Eng. Mater. **22**(12), 2000611 (2020)
3. Cosma, C., et al.: Theoretical analysis and practical case studies of powder-based additive manufacturing. Acta Technica Napocensis **61**(3), 369–378 (2018)
4. Girelli, L., et al.: Evaluation of the impact behavior of AlSi10Mg alloy produced using laser additive manufacturing. Mater. Sci. Eng. A **748**, 38–51 (2019)
5. Du, Y., et al.: Laser additive manufacturing of bio-inspired lattice structure: forming quality, microstructure and energy absorption behavior. Mater. Sci. Eng. A **773**, 138857 (2020)
6. Xiao, Z., et al.: Evaluation of topology-optimized lattice structures manufactured via selective laser melting. Mater. Des. **143**, 27–37 (2018)
7. Cosma, C., et al.: Physical-mechanical characteristics and microstructure of Ti6Al7Nb lattice structures manufactured by selective laser melting. Materials **13**(18), 4123 (2020)
8. Farhad, I., et al.: Fractal pattern recognition of image profiles for manufacturing process monitoring and control. In: Proceedings of the ASME 2018 13th International Manufacturing Science and Engineering Conference, MSEC 2018 (2018)
9. Catchpole-Smith, S., et al.: Fractal scan strategies for selective laser melting of 'unweldable' nickel superalloys. Addit. Manuf. **15**, 113–122 (2017)
10. Bai, P., et al.: Failure analysis of the tree column structures type AlSi10Mg alloy branches manufactured by selective laser melting. Materials **13**(18), 3969 (2020)
11. Zhao, M., et al.: Superelastic behaviors of additively manufactured porous NiTi shape memory alloys designed with Menger sponge-like fractal structures. Mater. Des. **200**, 109448 (2021)
12. Ullah, A., Omori, R., Nagara, Y., Kubo, A., Tamaki, J.: Toward error-free manufacturing of fractals. Procedia CIRP **12**, 43–48 (2013). https://doi.org/10.1016/j.procir.2013.09.00
13. Mazur, M., et al.: Additively manufactured, highly-uniform flow distributor for process intensification. Chem. Eng. Process. Process Intensification **143**, 107595 (2019)
14. Ilea, A., et al.: Osseointegration of titanium scaffolds manufactured by selective laser melting in rabbit femur defect model. J. Mater. Sci. Mater. Med. **30**, 26 (2019). https://doi.org/10.1007/s10856-019-6227-9

Basics of Hand Prosthesis Design

Isabela Todiriţe, Corina Radu Frenţ(✉), and Mihaiela Iliescu

Institute of Solid Mechanical, Romanian Academy, Bucharest, Romania
corinagabrielaradu@gmail.com

Abstract. The paper presents basic aspects and research results obtained by the authors, on the thematic of hand prosthesis. The objective is that of designing an innovative hand prosthesis. Some important aspects aspect considered in design are: relatively low cost, adequate and esthetic aspect, low weight. For these purposes, small, light mechanical parts were designed and most of them (gears, levers, shells) were made by 3D printing techniques (DLP) on high precision printer. Given the small mechanical components, there had to be chosen customized electronic components (micro-controllers, micro-motors, micro-sensors).

Keywords: hand prosthesis · kinematic analysis · 3D model · sensors · control

1 Introduction

Since ancient times, there have been methods of prosthetics for amputated limbs and other parts of human body. The oldest mention of a prosthesis is from the Rig Veda – an iron leg for a warrior.

Archaeological evidence of the existence of prostheses dates back to ancient Egypt and can be found in most past civilizations, from antiquity to the Middle Ages. Replacing fingers or limbs, over time, involved a variety of materials that have been used, like: wood, leather, metals. In many cases, these ancient prostheses were made with great attention to detail and with the clear aim of improving the lives of the beneficiaries, being very comfortable, easy to use and with acceptable appearance. They stand as the bases of contemporary prosthetics.

Prosthetic components include the socket, suspension and control system(s), joints, and appendage. There are many different options for prostheses, but all options aim to achieve a stable, comfortable and optimum function.

Hook-type hand prostheses are light, cheap devices with a very good grip capacity. They can be made of various metals: aluminum, stainless steel, titanium and chrome. These prostheses are only used to control body-powered devices.

The prehensile prosthesis represents the intermediate version between the hook and the artificial hand. They are part of the family of body-powered prostheses, just like hook prostheses. They are used for recreational and sports activities and from an aesthetic point of view they are not attractive.

Artificial hands have an aesthetic appearance, but a lower functionality compared to hook-and prehensile prostheses. These prostheses can be controlled by EMG signals,

D. Tarnita et al. (Eds.): MESROB 2023, MMS 133, pp. 379–385, 2023.
https://doi.org/10.1007/978-3-031-32446-8_41

indicating the user's intention. The artificial hand can be controlled through the neural interface and through targeted re-innervation of the muscles - TMR.

Unlike body-powered prostheses, electrically powered hand prostheses can to some extent imitate the gestures of the human hand through the bio-signals received by the electrodes. These electrodes can be placed on the surface of the skin, or surgically implanted, depending on the type and constructive model of the hand prosthesis.

The collection of the skin EMG signal is carried out with the help of sEMG sensors through the electrical signals generated by the healthy muscles of the arm and forearm. These signals are detected by sensors placed on the surface of the skin and are then transmitted to the microprocessor of the prosthesis, which interprets the signal and triggers the movements of the artificial hand.

The myoelectric prosthesis for the hand is composed of: electronic and mechanical components and components that ensure the aesthetic appearance. Electronic components include sensors, amplifiers, processors and batteries. The electrical signals generated by the user's healthy muscles are amplified to control the motors. The control unit is responsible for detecting electrical signals and decoding them into movements of the prosthesis [1].

Smart Bionic hand prosthesis is made of modern, waterproof and flexible materials, motion sensors, electric motors, control algorithms and a user interface that allows it to recognize and interpret the electromyography (EMG) signals generated by the healthy muscles from the user's arm. The fingers of this prosthetic hand are made in such a way as to reproduce the natural movement and a simple mechanism with 4 bars that moves 4 fingers is implemented. The four-bar link is the simplest closed movable link with only one degree of freedom. It has four components: crank, coupling, rocker and frame (see Fig. 1) [2].

In order to create a prosthetic hand that can replace the human one, Li Jiang in his work [3] defined the stages of a prosthetic hand design process.

The design process begins by defining the goals and requirements for the prosthetic hand (durability, weight, cost and system complexity).

The next stage is the one that defines the identification and evaluation of design concepts (sketches, 3D models of the prosthesis), then follows their testing through computer simulations.

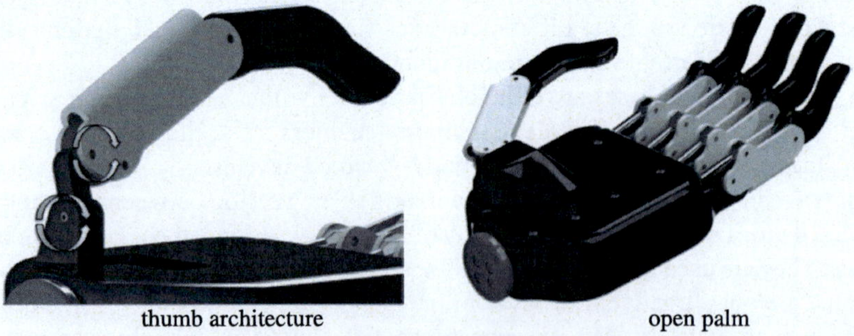

Fig. 1. Smart Bionic hand prosthesis [2].

Comfort and ergonomics of use, as well as durability and production costs are also taken into account. The quantified assessment of anthropomorphism refers to the assessment of the degree to which the prosthetic hand is perceived as human. This assessment can be done through questionnaires or psychological tests that measure the user's level of comfort and confidence in using the prosthetic hand.

The optimization and finalization stage of the prosthetic hand involves adjusting and improving the design and functionality to meet the user's requirements and needs.

Nowadays on the market there are several models of prosthetic hands, the manufacturing companies doing research studies in parallel to improve them.

2 Concept and Kinematics

Hand prostheses need to provide optimal function for general daily activities and for specific activities. The authors' concept and design for the hand prosthesis are innovative by some relevant aspects as follows:

- three rotations for each finger;
- independent motions for the fingers;
- solely electric drive;
- motions achieved by levers and gears (spur, worm) – no cables.
- command and control – by micro-motors, microcontroller and sensors' signals.
- sensors type: pressure, inclination, temperature, gyroscope and sEMG

The concept of prosthesis' finger is that of three phalanges, out of which the first one, P_1, (metacarpo-phalange) has two independent rotational motions. The other two phalanges (intermediate, P_2 and fingertip, P_3 phalanges) have dependent rotations, enabled by levers mechanism (see Fig. 2). The T notation is for the fingertip.

If there are cosidered the relative motions of the elements, the finger mehanism is made of lower pair joints, that are: H(0R1), A(1R2), B(1R4), C(3R4) and D(2R3), where the notation R stands for the rotational motion.

The mechanism has four mobile elements: 1(A, H), 2(A, D), 3(C, D) and 4(B, C).

Based on the above mentioned numbers of mobile elements and kinematic joints, it results the degree of mobility for the mechanism, $M = 2$.

Kinematic analysis of a mechanism consists in determimg the position, speed and acceleration parameters for each of its mobile elements.

For the studied mechanism this analysis was done aided by special procedures, named: A1R_G, A1RALFA_G and D1PVA_G [4, 5]. Position, speed and acceleration calculi were performed for 26 equidistant poition of element 1, considering the initial position: $\varphi_1 = \varphi_{10} = 3.2$ rad.

An example of the obtained results is shown in Fig. 3. It evidenced position and, consequently, trajectory for each of the finger mechanim's mobile elements.

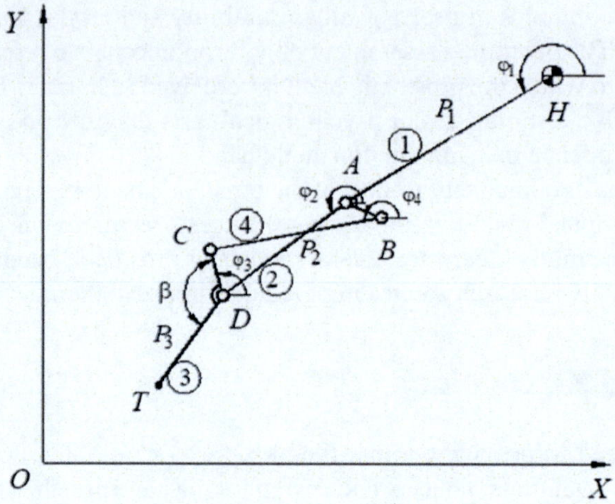

Fig. 2. Finger kinematic scheme.

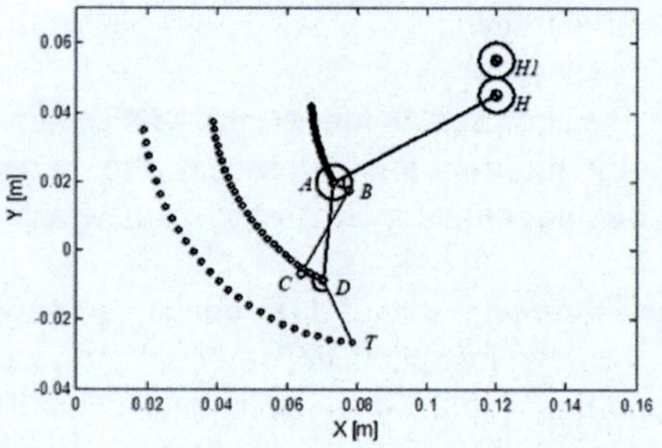

Fig. 3. Kinematic analysis result – mobile elements trajectories.

3 Design and Prototype

Designing the hand prosthesis has been a difficult process because of the conditions assumed, meaning:

- the prototype size and aspect to be similar to those of real hand;
- the mechanical parts have low dimensions (for example, module of 00.6 mm for gears) and high precision (for example, 0.005 and 0.01 mm tolerances);
- the mechatronic components with reduced dimensions and mass;
- low weight and friendly user interface; relatively affordable price.

Considering all the above mentioned and, not the least, the experience gained with various variants designed, the up to date design of the prosthesis is shown in Fig. 4.

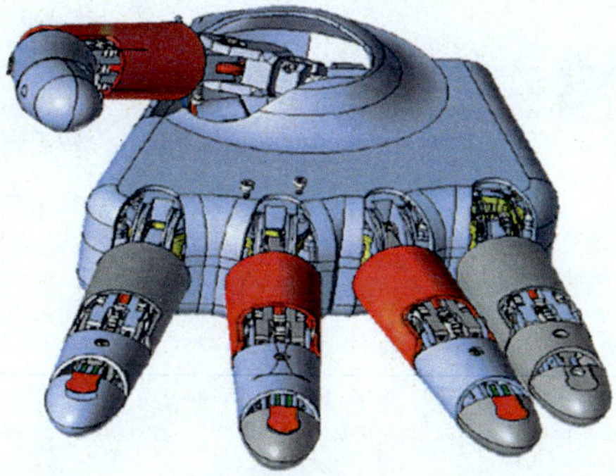

Fig. 4. Hand prosthesis design – 3D model.

The command and control system is made of subsystems, like: sensory subsystem (pressure, inclination, temperature, gyroscope, surface EMG); driving subsystem (15 micro-motors); control subsystem (microcomputer, micro-motor controllers, GPIO and power expanders) (see Fig. 5).

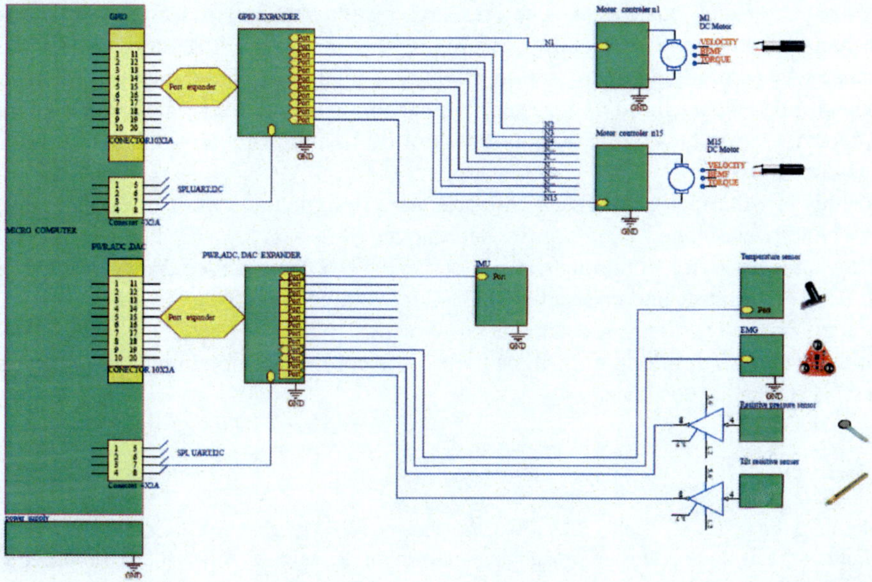

Fig. 5. Command and control scheme

Prototyping the hand prosthesis has been a challenge, as there were tested more rapid prototyping techniques: Fused Deposition Modeling (FDM) on Creality Ender 3-Pro; Scan, Spin and Selectively Photocure (3SP) Digital Light Processing (DLP) on Fig. 4 Standalone. Details on each of the applied printing techniques, as well as the appropriate selection for prototyping the hand prostheses mechanical components are presented in [6, 7]. Finally, up to date hand prosthesis prototype is shown in Fig. 6.

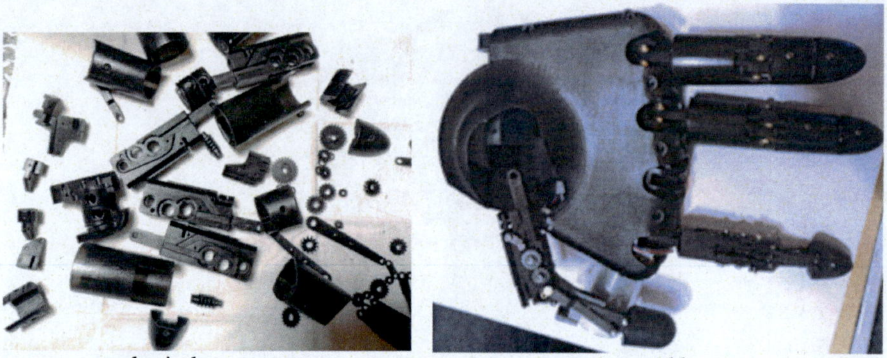

mechanical components assembly

Fig. 6. Hand prosthesis prototype

4 Conclusion

Prostheses for missing limbs have been used from ancient times, even there was only the aesthetic aspect or, both aesthetic and functional aspects envisaged.

The paper presents basic aspects and research results obtained in designing an innovative hand prosthesis. The specific features of this prosthesis, that could make the difference when comparing to the similar products available are: three rotations for each finger and independent motions for the fingers; motions achieved by levers and gears (spur, worm) – no cables; command and control by by micro-motors, microcontroller and sensors' signals.

For this prosthesis, light mechanical parts were designed and most of them (gears, levers, shells) were made by 3D printing techniques (DLP) on high precision printer.

Affordable costs for obtaining the prototype have been considered as a reachable target. Both 3D printing and conventional CNC machining were the techniques used for manufacturing the prosthesis mechanical components.

Further research development will be focused on completely obtaining the prototype and testing the hand prosthesis.

References

1. Bahrami Moqadam, S., Elahi, S.M., Mo, A., Zhang, W.: Hybrid control combined with a voluntary biosignal to control a prosthetic hand. Robot. Biomim. **5**, 4 (2018). https://doi.org/10.1186/s40638-018-0087-5
2. Badawy, A., Alfred, R.: Myoelectric prosthetic hand with a proprioceptive feedback system. J. King Saud Univ. Eng. Sci. **32**(6), 388–395 (2020). ISSN: 1018-3639. https://doi.org/10.1016/j.jksues.2019.05.002. https://www.sciencedirect.com/science/article/pii/S1018363918311681
3. Jiang, L., Liu, Y., Yang, D., Liu, H.: A synthetic framework for evaluating and designing an anthropomorphic prosthetic hand. J. Bionic Eng. **15**(1), 69–82 (2018). https://doi.org/10.1007/s42235-017-0005-5
4. Moise, V., Simionescu, I., Ene, M., Rotaru, A.: Analiza mecanismelor plane cu bare articulate. Aplicaţii în Matlab./Analysis of planar mechanism with links/Matlab application, Bucharest (2015)

5. Moise, V., Simionescu, I., Ene, M., Ungureanu, L.M., Rotaru, A.: Studiul şi animaţia mecanismelor aplicate. Aplicaţii în Matlab./The study and animation of applied mechanisms/Matlab application, Bucharest (2020)
6. Roşu, M.M., Radu (Frenţ), C., Iliescu, M.: Technical and economic analysis of manufacturing process for high precision customized part. In: Modern Technologies in Industrial Engineering, ModTech 2022, June 2022
7. Radu, C., Roşu, M.M., Matei, L., Ungureanu, L.M., Iliescu, M.: Concept, design, initial tests and prototype of customized upper limb prosthesis. Appl. Sci. **11**, 3077 (2021). https://doi.org/10.3390/app11073077

Rapid Prototyping Techniques for Innovative Hand Prosthesis

Emilia Furdu Lunguţ[1], Corina Radu Frenţ[2], Maria Magdalena Roşu[3], Luige Vlădăreanu[2], Mihaiela Iliescu[2], and Lucian Matei[4](✉)

[1] Titu Maiorescu University, CF2 Hospital, Mărăşti 63, Bucharest, Romania
[2] Institute of Solid Mechanics, Romanian Academy, Constantin Mille 15, 010141 Bucharest, Romania
[3] Faculty of Industrial Engineering and Robotics, University Politehnica of Bucharest, Bucharest, Romania
[4] Department of Automotive and Industrial Engineering, Faculty of Mechanics, University of Craiova, 107 Calea Bucuresti Street, Craiova, Romania
matei.lucian@ucv.ro, lucian.matei@edu.ucv.ro

Abstract. Missing limb is one of the challenges that life could give to any human being. There has always been high interest and, therefore, research on the way of trying to help and diminish this problem's influence on everyday life of the person involved. By prosthesis that would enable motions similar to that of a real human limb, every single day would be easier to take. The concept and design of innovative hand prosthesis, the rapid prototyping techniques considered for manufacturing, as well as finger's prototype are presented in this paper. The main conclusion is that these modern techniques are useful tools in any research but, there are still situations when conventional manufacturing techniques have to be considered.

Keywords: hand prosthesis · design · prototype · Digital Light Processing · Selective Laser Sintering

1 Introduction

Humans are so very complex beings, even when dealing with physical, psychological, feelings and, not the least, their social abilities. The human body is a complex whole made of systems (skeletal, muscular, nervous, etc. [1]) that work and interact so that to sustain life. There could be moments when something wrong happens and one of these systems gets damaged, more or less repairable. This is when attempt to get back to normal has to be done.

People with missing limb, caused by (car, work, war) accident and / or illness (diabetes) are to be met, unfortunately, more and more often. Doctors, engineers and many other specialized scientists have done thorough research to design and manufacture prostheses that could help these people have a, relatively, normal life.

D. Tarnita et al. (Eds.): MESROB 2023, MMS 133, pp. 386–393, 2023.
https://doi.org/10.1007/978-3-031-32446-8_42

A review on prosthetic hands is presented in [2] and one the significant conclusion is that even some of the human hand functions are simulated and achieved by modern bionic hand, still these (medical) devices can not completely replace the biological limb.

Still, the literature review proves deep research and encouraging results obtained in design, manufacture, test and validation for different type of hand prostheses.

One myoelectric prosthesis concept and prototype (see Fig. 1) are evidenced in [3]. In order to enable achievement of fingers' motion as close to that of real hand, the authors mention the proprioceptive feedback, based on the measured force on each finger. More of it, there are temperature sensors mounted on the hand system so that to avoid getting hot drink up to amputee's mouth.

Anthropomorphic prosthetic hand designed with five fingers driven by four independent actuators is described in [4]. There are used 2 sensors (sEMG) for capturing surface electromyography signal from the healthy limb. The control system is based on pat-tern recognition [5] and thus, eight hand gestures are recognizable and controlled in real time. Also, the hand prosthesis and grasp objects.

Innovative design of a mechanical finger used in hand prosthesis is mentioned in [6]. It is based on linkage-based mechanism [7, 8] but it has multiple groups of these mechanisms that do anthropomorphic motion-coupling and shape-adaptive grasping for objects with different shapes and sizes.

An important step in product development, once the concept and design are relatively set, is that of prototype/product manufacturing.

The modern trends in prototyping are that of 3D printing, with various techniques available, such as: Fused Deposition Modeling (FDM), PolyJet, Programmable PhotoPolymerization P3™ - by Stratysis [9]; MultiJet Modeling (MJM), Direct Metal Printing (DMP), Stereolithography (SLA) – by 3D Systems CADWORKS [10].

Review on 3D printing technologies for medical applications, pointing out their advantages over the conventional manufacturing technologies, is detailed in [11]. There are also mentioned the first application of 3D printing for bone rehabilitation and reconstruction [12]. An interesting aspect assessed is that of Intellectual property rights, as replicas of human parts prototypes could be reproduced much too easy.

Design of modular prosthetic hand, whose components are manufactured by additive manufacturing techniques, is presented in [13]. Kinematic analysis of the index finger mechanism, as well as the grasping tests proved correct motion of prosthesis fingers. As conclusion, a prosthetic hand prototyped by additive manufacturing technique was obtained, with low-costs.

All the above mentioned prove high interest on research and, consequently, results concerning missing limb prostheses - who would enable motions similar to that of a real human limb, would be light weight and, not the least, not too expensive. According to this idea, the present paper presents research results on: innovative concept of hand prosthesis; 3D printing techniques for the prototype components; geometric precision of the printed parts; conventional manufacturing as alternative for high precision parts and prototype of the prosthesis finger.

2 Materials and Methods

2.1 Upper Limb Motility

Medical aspects are important when designing limb prosthesis, due to the importance of knowing how the human body works as complex system. Once trying to get and adequate knowledge on its motility, the concept and design of prosthesis would follow up the natural information flux for ensuring the mobility similar to that of a real limb.

The motility of the upper limb is a complex function achieved by the interconnection of complex motor systems that are: pyramidal, extrapyramidal and peripheral.

Direct motor pathway transmits the voluntary motor impulse and consists of two neurons: the central and the peripheral ones.

Indirect motor pathway transmits automatic or semi-voluntary motor input and participates in the regulation of muscle tone. This pathway is called indirect because it relays in the brain before reaching the spinal cord and is made up of several types of central neurons and one peripheral neuron.

Motor unit is a functional unit made of motor neurons, an axon and the muscle fibers innervated by it. The motor neurons are located in the brain stem (motor nuclei of the cranial nerves) and in the spinal cord (anterior horn). In the anterior horn, the spinal reflex arcs close, a reflex being an involuntary response to a stimulus that depends on a reactive nervous circuit (see Fig. 1).

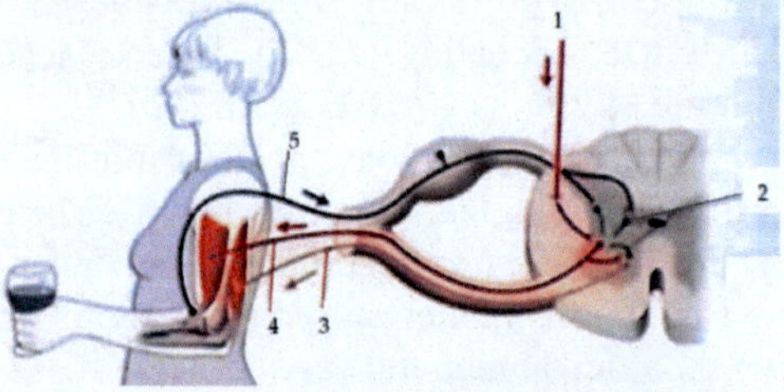

1. cortico-spinal tract
2. interneuron
3. antagonistic motor neurofiber
4. antagonistic motor neurofiber
5. sensitive neurofiber

Fig. 1. Cortical areas of motor pathways [14].

2.2 Upper Limb Concept and Design

The idea of an affordable, customized and, relatively, high functionality upper arm prosthesis has been raised as a way to help poor people get back to a, relatively, normal life. The designed prosthesis is aimed to have independent finger's motion, three rotations for the phalanges and one rotation for the whole finger, the motions are driven by independent micro motors and the signals generating action are given by sEMG sensors. Not the least, the prosthesis is low weight, easy to operate and, not the least, at affordable price.

The design of the upper limb prosthesis is evidenced in Fig. 2, so that it can be noticed details on the hand and finger components, with both mechanical parts (levers, worm – wheel gears, bearings) and electro-mechanical ones (micro-servomotors).

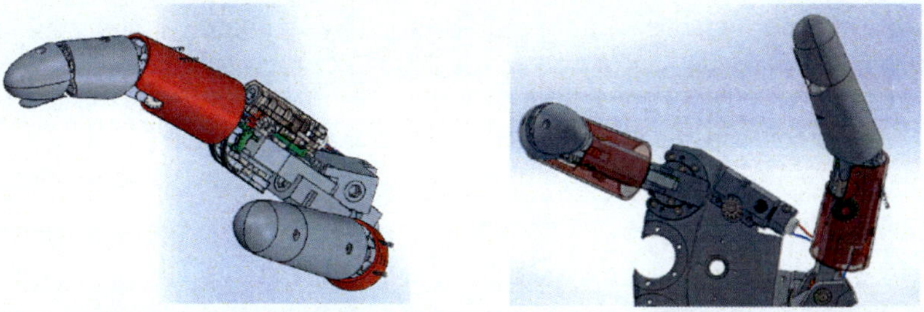

Fig. 2. Hand of the prosthesis – with thumb and index finger.

2.3 Prototyping the Components

Obtaining the prototype for the upper limb prosthesis stands as challenge, as the main issue is that of having a functional device, relatively fast and with affordable costs. The materials' aspect is also important, as the prosthesis is intended to be light and friendly user.

Considering all the above mentioned and, not the least, "screening" the available prototyping techniques (for the authors, at time being) two types of rapid prototyping techniques have been tested: Digital Light Processing (DLP) [15, 17] and Selective Laser Sintering (SLS) [16, 17].

The main problem that arises and determined different tests on 3D printing techniques, was that of geometric precision of the printed parts as, for example, the pitch for the worm should be of 0.5 mm and the module for the gear should be 0.6 mm. These are quite parts that need high geometric precision.

The *DLP printing technique* uses a projector with conventional light to cure the whole layer of the built surface in one flash. The resolution of the printed layer has been set to 0.01 mm, due to the precision required for the parts. A relevant image of how the parts are built inside the equipment chamber is presented in Fig. 3.

It was used "Fig. 4 Standalone" printer, from 3D Systems [18]. Detailed description of the printing process for hand prosthesis components is evidenced in [19].

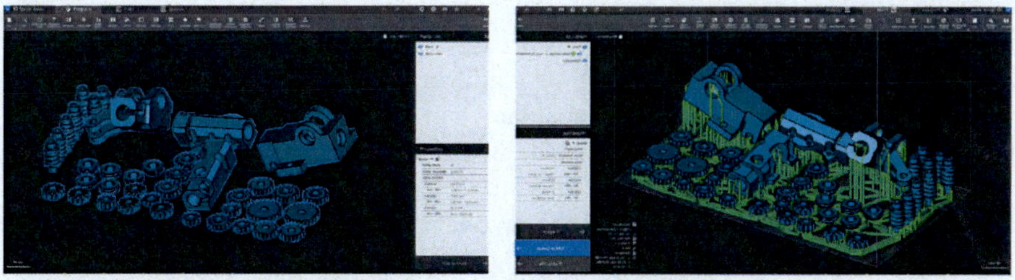

a. Preparing 3D model of the build table b. Finished processing of the build table

Fig. 3. Building process of the DLP printing (Fig. 4 printer)

The *SLS printing technique* uses a laser to accurately fuse the powder layer. The printer used is Fuse 1 [20], a key feature is that the non-sintered material (which acts as a support material during construction) can be reused by combining it with a minimum of 30% new material so that new parts can use up to 70% recycled powder. This printer uses the software platform Preform for the slicing process. All printed parts, after being imported into the software, can be adjusted on XYZ axes (see Fig. 4).

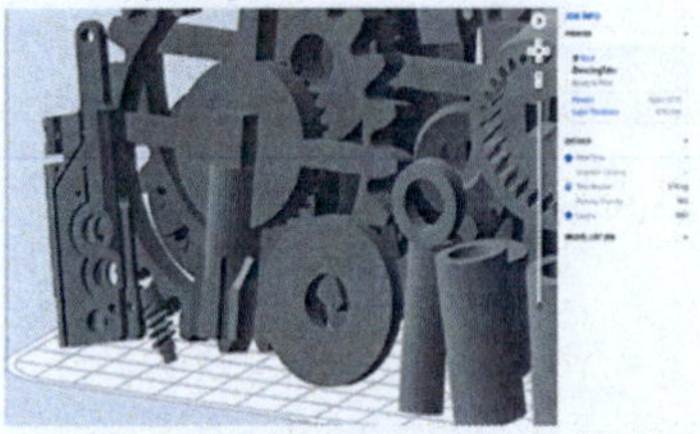

a. parts to be built into the building chamber

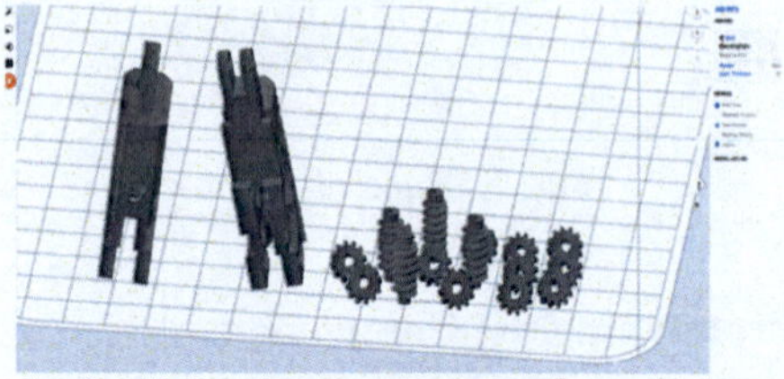

b. detail for the worm - wheel gear, phalanges

Fig. 4. Building parts by SLS printing - Preform orientation system (Fuse 1 printer)

For the printed parts the material used was Nylon12 and the refresh rate of the powder was set to 30% (30% new powder, 70% reclaimed powder).

3 Results

Most of the mechanical components for hand prosthesis prototype were manufactured by 3D printing, except from the bearings, screws, micro-motors.

The *SLS printing technique* (by Fuse 1 printer) resulted in parts that could be assembled into prototype's subassemblies. Still, there arises an important problem, that of high geometric precision that could not be achieved. For example, the gear could not be precisely printed, as its module value resulted different than 0.6 mm and, further, the associated wheel gear could not "work" for motion transmission.

This is why the *DLP printing* technique (by Fig. 4 printer) was further chosen and the resulted parts (right after the printing process is over) are shown in Fig. 5. After curing with UV light, the printed parts turned from "green parts" into final parts - ready to be assembled into hand prosthesis subsystems.

One important step further in having the whole prosthesis prototype ready, is that of assembling the parts. For checking the accuracy and the functioning, it was decided to assembly the index finger first and, after that the thumb. If all works right, then the rest of the three fingers would be assembled in a similar way.

Tests with the servo-motors, for the spur cylindrical gear were done (see Fig. 6).

One important aspect is that of mounting the rolling bears that ensure finger rotation around vertical (OZ) axis. For the index finger, the attempt to introduce 1 mm rollers into the pathway of the horseshoe part and, further, to generate the rotation failed. One careful check of this part evidenced materials deposition on the rolling pathway (see Fig. 7) and when randomly check dimension of the pathway width, it resulted values within the interval 0.92–0.102 mm. For the values lower than 0.99 mm, the rollers could not get into the pathway.

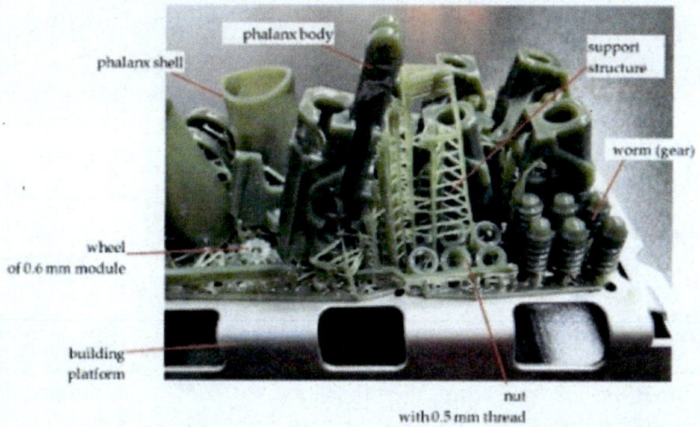

Fig. 5. Figure 4 built platform – with hand prosthesis parts

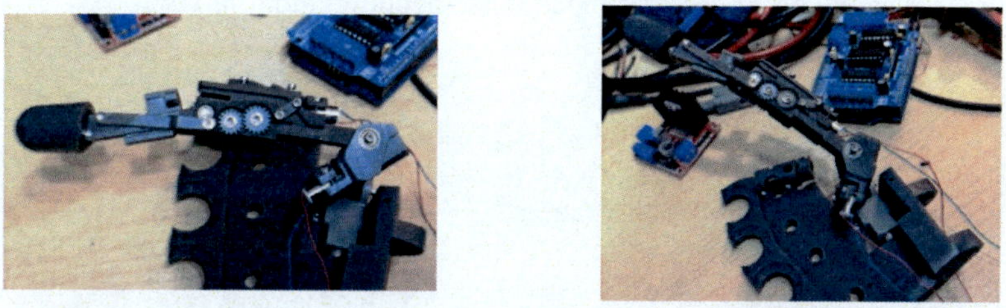

Fig. 6. Thumb prosthesis functional tests – tests for thumb motion

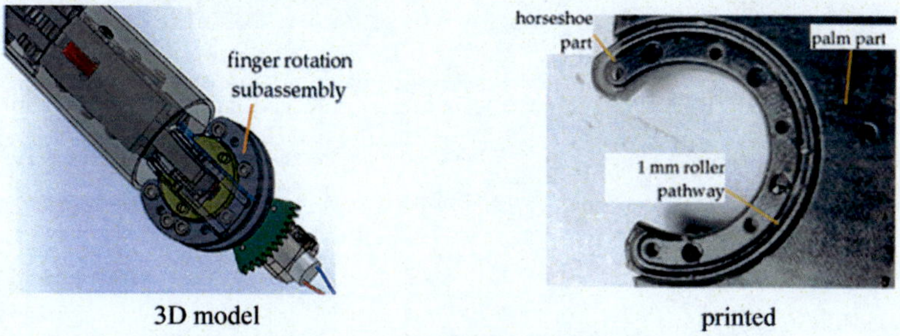

Fig. 7. Rotation subsystem for finger

4 Discussion

No matter how many attempts and careful check of the printing parameters, and materials, one problem could not be solved. This is that of accurate prototype for the bearing subsystem (with one hundred 1 mm roller balls and two horseshoe parts). This subsystem is component of the finger rotation subassembly (Fig. 7).

The solution, considering the available manufacturing systems and, not the least, the costs, was that of conventional manufacturing of the horseshoe parts and, therefore, choosing and adequate material for friction bearing, the copper-zinc alloy. The cutting (extractive) processing of these parts involved: turning, milling and drilling and customized devices for fixing the part while cutting (Fig. 8).

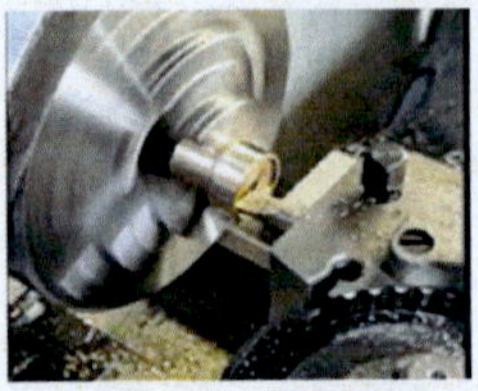
a. turning the horseshoe

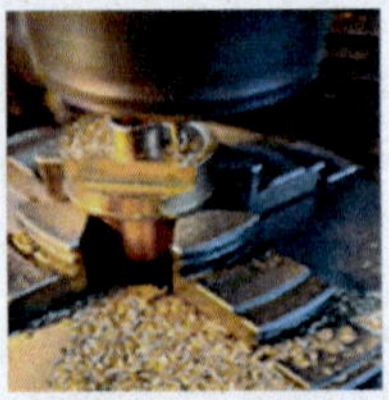
b. milling the horseshoe

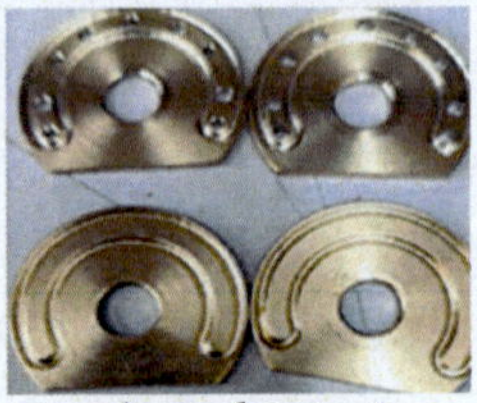
c. horseshoe parts

Fig. 8. Conventional manufacturing of the horseshoe parts

Finally, the assembled finger resulted and had accurate motions (Fig. 9).

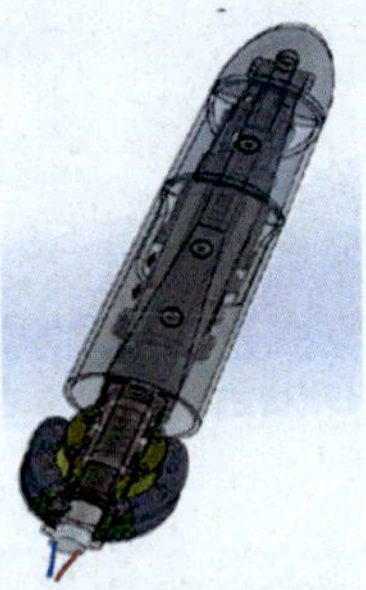
a. index finger 3D model

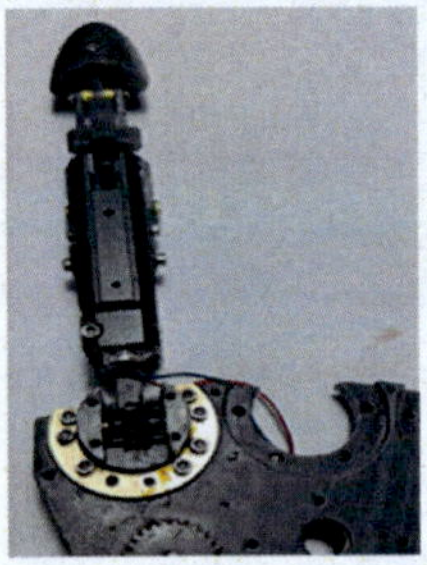
b. index finger prototype

Fig. 9. Hand prosthesis finger prototype.

5 Conclusions

This paper presents innovative concept and design for hand prosthesis and is focused on rapid prototyping techniques applied to manufacture its mechanical components. Based on the available 3D printing equipment and the up-to-date modern prototyping techniques (DLP, SLS) high precision parts were obtained.

The research results proved that, sometimes, the geometric precision generated by these techniques is not adequate for very small precise parts (tolerances lower than 0.01 mm and surface roughness less than 1.6 μm). So, conventional machining techniques had to be considered for finally obtaining prosthesis finger prototype.

Further research will be focused on: having the whole hand prosthesis prototype manufactured; tests of gripping, motions even with haptic feedback, validation and if possible, medical approval license.

References

1. Vasković, J.: Human body systems, 10 October 2022. https://www.kenhub.com/en/library/anatomy/human-body-systems. Accessed 10 Dec 2022
2. Clement, R.G., Bugler, K.E., Oliver, C.W.: Bionic prosthetic hands: a review of present technology and future aspirations. Surgeon **9**(6), 336–340 (2011). https://doi.org/10.1016/j.surge.2011.06.001
3. Badawy, A., Alfred, R.: Myoelectric prosthetic hand with a proprioceptive feedback system. J. King Saud Univ. Eng. Sci. **32**(6), 388–395 (2020). ISSN: 1018-3639. https://doi.org/10.1016/j.jksues.2019.05.002
4. Wang, N., Lao, K., Zhang, X.: Design and myoelectric control of an anthropomorphic prosthetic hand. J. Bionic Eng. **14**(1), 47–59 (2017). ISSN: 1672-6529. https://doi.org/10.1016/S1672-6529(16)60377-3
5. Scheme, E., Englehart, K.: Electromyogram pattern recognition for control of powered upper-limb prostheses: State of the art and challenges for clinical use. J. Rehabil. Res. Dev. **48**, 643–659 (2011)
6. Zhang, Y., Deng, H., Zhong, G.: Humanoid design of mechanical fingers using a motion coupling and shape-adaptive linkage mechanism. J. Bionic Eng. **15**(1), 94–105 (2018). https://doi.org/10.1007/s42235-017-0007-3
7. Bennett, D.A., Dalley, S.A., Truex, D., Goldfarb, M.: A multigrips hand prosthesis for providing precision and conformal grasps. IEEE-ASME Trans. Mechatron. **20**, 1697–1704 (2015)
8. Belter, J.T, Dollar, A.M., Leddy, M.: Multi-grasp prosthetic hand, US patent, 20170049583 (2017)
9. https://www.stratasys.com/en/guide-to-3d-printing/technologies-and-materials/p3-technology/. Accessed 7 Nov 2022
10. https://print3dcad.ro/tehnologii-print-3d/. Accessed 7 Nov 2022
11. Singh, P., Singh, G.: A review paper on 3D-printing technology and its application medical field. JETIR **5**(10) (2018)
12. Nyberg, E.L., et al.: 3D-printing technologies for craniofacial rehabilitation, reconstruction, and regeneration. Ann. Biomed. Eng. **45**(1), 45–57 (2017)
13. Soriano-Heras, E., Blaya-Haro, F., Molino, C., de Agustín del Burgo, J.M.: Rapid prototyping prosthetic hand acting by a low-cost shape-memory-alloy actuator. J. Artif. Organs **21**(2), 238–246 (2018). https://doi.org/10.1007/s10047-017-1014-1
14. Kamina, P.: Anatomie clinique. tome 5: neuroanatomie, 2e ed, ISBN: 13 978-2224033606
15. Cavallo, C.: All About Digital Light Processing 3D Printing. https://www.thomasnet.com/articles/custom-manufacturing-fabricating/digital-lightprocessing-dlp-3d-printing/. Accessed 7 Nov 2022
16. https://www.hannovermesse.de/apollo/hannover_messe_2022/obs/Binary/A1148232/2001507-SS-ENEU-0.pdf. Accessed 8 Nov 2022
17. https://print3dcad.ro/. Accessed 8 Nov 2022
18. https://www.3dsystems.com/3d-printers/figure-4-standalone. Accessed 10 June 2022
19. Radu, C., Roșu, M.M., Matei, L., Ungureanu, L.M., Iliescu, M.: Concept, design, initial tests and prototype of customized upper limb prosthesis. Appl. Sci. **11**(7), 3077 (2021). https://doi.org/10.3390/app11073077
20. https://cadworks.ro/fuse1-2/. Accessed 14 July 2022

Author Index

D. Tarnita et al. (Eds.): MESROB 2023, MMS 133, pp. 395–397, 2023.
https://doi.org/10.1007/978-3-031-32446-8